Lecture Notes
Clinical Biochemistry

Geoffrey Beckett

BSc PhD FRCPath
Consultant Clinical Scientist
Honorary Reader in Clinical Biochemistry
Department of Clinical Biochemistry
The Royal Infirmary of Edinburgh
Edinburgh

Simon Walker

MA MB BS DM FRCPath
Senior Lecturer in Clinical Biochemistry
Honorary Consultant Clinical Biochemist
Department of Clinical Biochemistry
The Royal Infirmary of Edinburgh
Edinburgh

Peter Rae

BA PhD MBChB FRCPE FRCPath
Consultant Clinical Biochemist
Honorary Senior Lecturer in Clinical Biochemistry
Department of Clinical Biochemistry
The Royal Infirmary of Edinburgh
Edinburgh

Peter Ashby

BA PhD FRCPath
Consultant Clinical Scientist
Honorary Senior Lecturer in Clinical Biochemistry
Department of Clinical Biochemistry
The Western General Hospital
Edinburgh

Eighth Edition

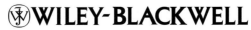
WILEY-BLACKWELL

A John Wiley & Sons, Ltd., Publication

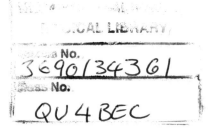
This edition first published 2010, © 2010 by Geoffrey Beckett, Simon Walker, Peter Rae, Peter Ashby
Previous editions 1975, 1980, 1984, 1988, 1993, 1998, 2005

Blackwell Publishing was acquired by John Wiley & Sons in February 2007. Blackwell's publishing programme has been merged with Wiley's global Scientific, Technical and Medical business to form Wiley-Blackwell.

Registered office: John Wiley & Sons Ltd, The Atrium, Southern Gate, Chichester, West Sussex PO19 8SQ, UK

Editorial offices: 9600 Garsington Road, Oxford OX4 2DQ, UK
                    The Atrium, Southern Gate, Chichester, West Sussex PO19 8SQ, UK
                    111 River Street, Hoboken, NJ 07030-5774, USA

For details of our global editorial offices, for customer services and for information about how to apply for permission to reuse the copyright material in this book please see our website at www.wiley.com/wiley-blackwell

Library of Congress Cataloging-in-Publication Data

Lecture notes. Clinical biochemistry. – 8th ed. / edited by Geoffrey
Beckett ... [et al.].
       p. ; cm.
  Includes bibliographical references and index.
  Includes bibliographical references and index.
  ISBN 978-1-4051-9305-4 (pbk. : alk. paper)
1. Clinical chemistry.   2. Clinical biochemistry.   I. Beckett, G. J.
  [DNLM: 1. Biochemistry.   2. Clinical Chemistry Tests.   3. Clinical Laboratory Techniques.   4. Pathology,
Clinical–methods.   QU 4 L4705 2010]
  RB40.L4 2010
  616.07′56–dc22

                              2009031374

A catalogue record for this book is available from the British Library.

Set in 8 on 12pt Stone Serif by Toppan Best-set Premedia Limited
Printed and bound in Malaysia by Vivar Prinitng Sdn Bhd

1   2010

Contents

Colour plate can be found facing p. 182

Preface

This is the eighth edition of the book first conceived by Professor Gordon Whitby, Dr Alistair Smith and Professor Iain Percy-Robb in 1975. As with the first edition, the book has been written primarily for medical students and junior doctors. The changes that have been introduced into the undergraduate medical teaching curriculum, including systems-based medicine, means that the book is now of relevance to each of the years of the course. In addition, we believe that the book is of value to specialist registrars, clinical scientists and biomedical scientists who are studying for higher qualifications to pursue a career in clinical biochemistry and metabolic medicine.

As with previous editions, the book has been modified in response to a number of suggestions made by a group of students commissioned by Wiley to review the previous edition. In response to their comments, Wiley have introduced a further colour into this edition and improved the format of the text and tables to make the content clearer. The order of the chapters has also been revised to allow all endocrine chapters to run consecutively. On our part, we have reviewed and updated all chapters to reflect current clinical practice and national guidelines, and we have included additional case studies since these have proved to be a very popular component of the book. It is interesting to note how lack of funding can prevent a useful test being introduced into clinical practice. In the 7th edition we were predicting that brain natriuretic peptide (BNP) measurements would play a pivotal role in the diagnosis of suspected heart failure in primary care. In the event, the introduction of BNP measurement into primary care in the UK has been slow due to lack of availability of adequate funding.

We have retained the objectives that have characterised the book throughout each of its previous editions. As a consequence, the reader should gain a knowledge and understanding of the value, limitations and interpretation of the many biochemical tests that are in common use in modern medicine. In addition we hope that this book will allow the reader to answer the questions first raised in Asher's Catechism published in the *British Medical Journal* in 1954 under the title 'Straight and Crooked Thinking in Medicine', namely:
Why do I request this test?
What will I look for in the result?
If I find what I am looking for, will it affect my diagnosis?
How will this investigation affect my management of the patient?

We would like to thank Dr Jean Kirk for her help with the paediatric biochemistry section; Dr Allan Deacon for his views regarding the investigation of porphyria; and Dr Gordon Brydon for helpful comments concerning tests of gastrointestinal function. We also wish to thank the staff at Wiley for their continued interest and support towards this title since its conception in 1975, and for this edition particularly Laura Murphy and Ben Townsend.

Geoff Beckett
Simon Walker
Peter Rae
Peter Ashby

List of abbreviations

ABP androgen-binding protein
A&E Accident and (&) Emergency
ACE angiotensin-converting enzyme
ACTH adrenocorticotrophic hormone
ADH antidiuretic hormone
AFP α-fetoprotein
AI angiotensin I
AII angiotensin II
AIP acute intermittent porphyria
ALA aminolaevulinic acid
ALP alkaline phosphatase
ALT alanine aminotransferase
AMP adenosine 5-monophosphate
ANP atrial natriuretic peptide
API α₁-protease inhibitor
AST aspartate aminotransferase
ATP adenosine triphosphate
ATPase adenosine triphosphatase
BChE butylcholinesterase
BMI body mass index
BMR basal metabolic rate
BNP B-type natriuretic peptide
CAH congenital adrenal hyperplasia
cAMP cyclic adenosine monophosphate
CBG cortisol-binding globulin
CCK-PZ cholecystokinin-pancreozymin
CDT carbohydrate-deficient transferrin
CEA carcinoembryoinic antigen
ChE cholinesterase
CK creatine kinase
CKD chronic kidney disease
CNS central nervous system
CoA coenzyme A
COC combined oral contraceptive
COHb carboxyhaemoglobin
CRH corticotrophin-releasing hormone
CRP C-reactive protein
CSF cerebrospinal fluid
CT computed tomography
DDAVP 1-deamino,8-D-arginine vasopressin

DHEA dehydroepiandrosterone
DHEAS dehydroepiandrosterone sulphate
DHCC dihydrocholecalciferol
DHT dihydrotestosterone
DIT di-iodotyrosine
DKA diabetic ketoacidosis
DPP-4 dipeptidyl peptidase-4
DVT deep venous thrombosis
ECF extracellular fluid
ECG electrocardiogram/electrocardiography
EDTA ethylenediamine tetraacetic acid
eGFR estimated glomerular filtration rate
ERCP endoscopic retrograde cholangiopancreatography
ESR erythrocyte sedimentation rate
FAD flavin–adenine dinucleotide
FAI free androgen index
FBHH familial benign hypocalciuric hypercalcaemia
FOB faecal occult blood
FSH follicle-stimulating hormone
FT3 free tri-iodothyronine
FT4 free thyroxine
GAD glutamic acid decarboxylase
Gal-1-PUT galactose-1-phosphate uridylyl-transferase
GC–MS gas chromatography–mass spectrometry
GFR glomerular filtration rate
GGT γ-glutamyltransferase
GH growth hormone
GHD growth hormone deficiency
GHRH growth hormone-releasing hormone
GI gastrointestinal
GIP glucose-dependent insulinotrophic peptide
GLP-1 glucagon-like polypeptide-1
GnRH gonadotrophin-releasing hormone
GP general practitioner
GSA glucocorticoid-suppressible hyperaldosteronism
GTT glucose tolerance test

Hb haemoglobin
HC hereditary coproporphyria
HCC hydroxycholecalciferol
hCG human chorionic gonadotrophin
HDL high-density lipoprotein
HDU high dependency unit
HGPRT hypoxanthine-guanine phosphoribosyltransferase
5-HIAA 5-hydroxyindoleacetic acid
HIV human immunodeficiency virus
HLA human leucocyte antigen
HMG-CoA β-hydroxy-β-methylglutaryl-coenzyme A
HNF hepatic nuclear factor
HPA hypothalamic–pituitary–adrenal
HPLC high-performance liquid chromatography
HRT hormone replacement therapy
hsCRP high sensitive C-reactive protein
5-HT 5-hydroxytryptamine
5-HTP 5-hydroxytryptophan
ICF intracellular fluid
ICU intensive care unit
IDL intermediate-density lipoprotein
IFCC International Federation for Clinical Chemistry
IFG impaired fasting glycaemia
Ig immunoglobulin
IGF insulin-like growth factor
IGFBP insulin-like growth factor-binding protein
IGT impaired glucose tolerance
IM intramuscular
INR international normalised ratio
IV intravenous
LCAT lecithin cholesterol acyltransferase
LDH lactate dehydrogenase
LDL low-density lipoprotein
LH luteinising hormone
LHRH luteinising hormone-releasing hormone
Lp (a) lipoprotein (a)
LSD lysergic acid diethylamide
MCAD medium chain acyl-CoA dehydrogenase
MCV mean cell volume
MDRD Modification of Diet in Renal Disease
MEGX monoethylglycinexylidide
MEN multiple endocrine neoplasia

MGUS monoclonal gammopathy of unknown significance
MIH Mullerian inhibitory hormone
MIT mono-iodotyrosine
MODY maturity onset diabetes of the young
MOM multiples of the median
MRI magnetic resonance imaging
MSAFP maternal serum α-fetoprotein
NAD nicotinamide–adenine dinucleotide
NADP NAD phosphate
NAFLD non-alcoholic fatty liver disase
NASH non-alcoholic steatohepatitis
NICE National Institute for Health and Clinical Excellence
NTD neural tube defect
NTI non-thyroidal illness
OGTT oral glucose tolerance test
PAPP-A pregnancy-associated plasma protein A
PBG porphobilinogen
PCOS polycystic ovarian syndrome
PCT porphyria cutanea tarda
PE pulmonary embolism
PEM protein-energy malnutrition
PKU phenylketonuria
POCT point of care testing
POP progestogen-only pill
PP pyridoxal phosphate
PRA plasma renin activity
PRPP 5-phosphoribosyl-1-pyrophosphate
PSA prostate-specific antigen
PT prothrombin time
PTC percutaneous transhepatic cholangiography
PTH parathyroid hormone
PTHrP PTH-related protein
RDA recommended dietary allowance
RF rheumatoid factor
ROC receiver operating characteristic
SAH subarachnoid haemorrhage
SD standard deviation
SHBG sex hormone-binding globulin
SI Système International
SIADH inappropriate secretion of ADH
SUR sulphonylurea receptor
T3 tri-iodothyronine
T4 thyroxine
TBG thyroxine-binding globulin

TDM therapeutic drug monitoring
TIBC total iron-binding capacity
TPMT thiopurine methyltransferase
TPN total parenteral nutrition
TPOAb thyroid peroxidase antibody
TPP thiamin pyrophosphate
TRAb thyrotrophin receptor antibody
TRH thyrotrophin-releasing hormone
TSH thyroid-stimulating hormone

TSI thyroid-stimulating immunoglobulin
tTG tissue transglutaminase
U&Es urea and electrolytes
UFC urinary free cortisol
VIP vasoactive intestinal peptide
VLDL very low density lipoprotein
VMA vanillylmandelic acid
VP variegate porphyria
WHO World Health Organization

Chapter 1

Requesting and interpreting tests

Introduction

Biochemical tests are crucial to many areas of modern medicine. Most biochemical tests are carried out on blood using plasma or serum, but urine, cerebrospinal fluid (CSF), faeces, kidney stones, pleural fluid, etc. are sometimes required. Plasma is obtained by taking whole blood into an anti-coagulant and represents the aqueous supernatant obtained when all the cellular elements have been separated by centrifugation. Serum is the corresponding aqueous phase when blood is allowed to clot. For many (but not all) biochemical tests on blood, it makes little difference whether plasma or serum is used and the terms are often used interchangeably.

There are many hundreds of tests available in clinical biochemistry that include many specialist tests. However, a core of common tests makes up the majority of test requesting in clinical biochemistry. These core tests will be offered by almost all clinical biochemistry laboratories and will be available 24 h daily for more urgent situations. It is also sometimes appropriate to bring tests together in profiles, especially where a group of tests can provide better understanding of a problem than a single test (e.g. the liver function test profile).

Lecture Notes: Clinical Biochemistry, 8e. By G. Beckett, S. Walker, P. Rae & P. Ashby. Published 2010 by Blackwell Publishing.

Many of the other more specialist tests are restricted to larger laboratories or, in some cases, to a very small number of centres offering a regional or national service.

In dealing with the large number of routine test requests, the modern clinical biochemistry laboratory depends heavily on automated instrumentation. This is most often linked to a laboratory computing system which assigns test requests to electronic patient files, maintains a cumulative patient record and regulates the printing of reports. Increasingly, test requests can be electronically booked at the ward, clinic or even general practitioner (GP) surgery via a terminal linked to the main laboratory computer. Equally, the test results can be displayed on computer screens at distant locations, even negating the need for issuing printed reports.

In this first chapter, we set out some of the principles of requesting tests and of the interpretation of results. The effects of analytical errors and of physiological factors, as well as of disease, on test results are stressed. Biochemical testing in differential diagnosis and in screening is discussed.

Collection of specimens

Test requests require unambiguous identification of the patient (patient's name, sex, date of birth and, increasingly, a unique patient identification number), together with the location, the name of the requesting doctor and the date and time of sampling. Each test request must specify which analyses are requested and provide details of the nature of the specimen itself and relevant clinical diagnostic information. Traditionally, this information is provided through the request form with appropriate parallel labelling of the specimen itself. Increasingly, this information is provided electronically so that only the sample itself need be sent to the laboratory with its own unique identifier (e.g. a bar code which links it to the electronic request).

Because of the large number of samples which are processed by most clinical biochemistry laboratories, every step needs to be taken to avoid errors. Regrettably, errors do rarely occur and can be divided according to the error source:

• Pre-analytical. For example, assigning a specimen to the wrong patient at the ward end or taking a sample at the wrong time (e.g. digoxin level is requested on a sample shortly after

digoxin has been administered (pp. 279)) or mislabelling of an aliquot of serum taken at specimen reception. Most errors fall into this category (see Table 1.1).

• Analytical. For example, a small sample volume may lead to a pipetting error where insufficient sample is used for the assay. Again, developments in automated sample detection and pipetting mean these problems are very unusual.

• Post-analytical. These are increasingly rare because of electronic download of results from the analyser but might include transcription errors when entering results into the lab computer manually.

On the scale of the requesting of biochemical tests, errors are fortunately rare. However, occasional blunders do arise and, if very unexpected results are obtained, it is incumbent on the requesting doctor to contact the laboratory immediately to look into the possibility that a blunder may have occurred.

Table 1.1 Some more common causes of pre-analytical errors arising from use of the laboratory

Error	Consequence
Crossover of addressograph labels between patients	This can lead to two patients each with the other's set of results. Where the patient is assigned a completely wrong set of results, it is important to investigate the problem in case there is a second patient with a corresponding wrong set of results.
Timing error	There are many examples where timing is important but not considered. Sending in a blood sample too early after the administration of a drug can lead to misleadingly high values in therapeutic monitoring. Interpretation of some tests (e.g. cortisol) is critically dependent on the time of day when the blood was sampled.
Sample collection tube error	For some tests the nature of the collection tube is critical, which is why the Biochemistry Laboratory specifies this detail. For example, using a plasma tube with lithium–heparin as the anti-coagulant invalidates this sample tube for measurement of a therapeutic lithium level! Electrophoresis requires a serum sample; otherwise, the fibrinogen interferes with the detection of any monoclonal bands. Topping up a biochemistry tube with a haematology (potassium ethylenediamine tetraacetic acid (EDTA) sample) will lead to high potassium and low calcium values in the biochemistry sample.
Sample taken from close to the site of an intravenous (IV) infusion	The blood sample will be diluted so that all the tests will be correspondingly low with the exception of those tests which might be affected by the composition of the infusion fluid itself. For example, using normal saline as the infusing fluid would lead to a lowering of all test results, but with sodium and chloride results which are likely to be raised.

The use of clinical biochemistry tests

Biochemical tests are most often *discretionary*, meaning that the test is requested for defined diagnostic purposes, as distinct from screening, where a disease is sought without there being any specific indication of its presence in the individual. The justification for discretionary testing is well summarised by Asher (1954):

1 Why do I request this test?
2 What will I look for in the result?
3 If I find what I am looking for, will it affect my diagnosis?
4 How will this investigation affect my management of the patient?
5 Will this investigation ultimately benefit the patient?

The principal reasons for requesting biochemical tests are as follows (where the first two categories would be defined as discretionary):

• To assist in diagnosis. For example, the diagnosis of diabetes mellitus is crucially dependent on the measurement and interpretation of plasma [glucose]. Biochemical tests may also aid the differential diagnosis or indicate the severity of a disease (see also Table 1.2).

• In disease monitoring. A good example is the use of arterial blood gases to follow the progress of someone admitted with a severe pneumonia or creatinine in an individual with chronic renal failure (see also Table 1.2).

• In prognosis or disease risk assessment. Serum cholesterol (pp. 192) or high-sensitive C-reactive protein (hsCRP) (pp. 192) are used in the assessment of cardiovascular risk, for example.

• In screening for disease. An example here would be measurement of thyroid-stimulating hormone (TSH) to screen for neonatal hypothyroidism.

• Miscellaneous, for example for forensic purposes or ethically approved research.

Screening may take two forms:

• In well-population screening a spectrum of tests is carried out on individuals from an apparently healthy population in an attempt to detect pre-symptomatic or early disease. It is easy to miss significant abnormalities in the 'flood' of data coming

Table 1.2 Test selection for the purposes of discretionary testing

Category	Example
To confirm a diagnosis	Serum [free T4] and [thyroid-stimulating hormone, (TSH)] in suspected hyperthyroidism
To aid differential diagnosis	To distinguish between different forms of jaundice
To refine a diagnosis	Use of adrenocorticotrophic hormone (ACTH) to localise Cushing's syndrome
To assess the severity of disease	Serum [creatinine] or [urea] in renal disease
To monitor progress	Plasma [glucose] and serum [K⁺] to follow treatment of patients with diabetic ketoacidosis (DKA)
To detect complications or side effects	Alanine aminotransferase (ALT) measurements in patients treated with hepatotoxic drugs
To monitor therapy	Serum drug concentrations in patients treated with anti-epileptic drugs

Table 1.3 Requirements for well-population screening

The disease is common or life-threatening
The tests are sensitive and specific
The tests are readily applied and acceptable to the population to be screened
Clinical, laboratory and other facilities are available for follow-up
Economics of screening have been clarified and the implications accepted

from the laboratory, even when the abnormalities are 'flagged' in some way. Most of the abnormalities detected will be of little or no significance, yet may need additional time-consuming and often expensive tests to clarify their importance (or lack of it). For these and other reasons, the value of well-population screening has been called into question and certainly should only be initiated under certain specific circumstances which are listed in Table 1.3.

Table 1.4 Examples of tests used in case-finding programmes

Programmes to detect diseases in	Chemical investigations
Neonates	
PKU	Serum [phenylalanine]
Hypothyroidism	Serum [TSH] and/or [thyroxine]
Adolescents and young adults	
Substance abuse	Drug screen
Pregnancy	
Diabetes mellitus in the mother	Plasma and urine [glucose]
Open neural tube defect (NTD) in the foetus	Maternal serum [α-fetoprotein]
Industry	
Industrial exposure to lead	Blood [lead]
Industrial exposure to pesticides	Serum cholinesterase activity
Elderly	
Malnutrition	Serum vitamin D levels
Thyroid dysfunction	Serum [TSH] and/or [thyroxine]

- In case-finding screening programmes appropriate tests are carried out on a population sample known to be at high risk of a particular disease. These are inherently more selective and yield a higher proportion of useful results (Table 1.4).

Point of care testing (POCT) (Table 1.5)

There are occasions when the urgency of the clinical situation requires that blood testing on patient samples is performed near the patient (point of care testing). Furthermore in the UK the government, in outlining the future of the National Health Service, has indicated a desire to move laboratory testing from the hospital laboratory into the community setting. High street pharmacies have taken up these opportunities and can, for example, provide cholesterol and glucose testing while you wait. In addition, there is an increasing number of urine test sticks that are sold for home use (e.g. pregnancy and ovulation testing by measuring human chorionic gonadotrophin (hCG) and luteinising hormone (LH), respectively).

POCT eliminates the need to send the specimen to the laboratory, and will usually allow a more rapid turnaround time. POCT is particularly suitable for use in intensive care units (ICUs), high-dependency units (HDUs), Accident and Emergency (A&E) departments and specialist clinics. Small dedicated analysers are often introduced into these centres.

Since decisions to initiate treatment are often made on the basis of POCT it is vital that confidence can be placed in the results obtained by such methods, such that the risk to the patient is minimised. It is thus essential that POCT is carried out by staff who are suitably trained and that the reliability of the tests is monitored on a regular basis using appropriate quality control measures.

If POCT is to be introduced into a ward or outpatient department it is essential that:
- The laboratory is consulted to advise on the choice of method, staff training and quality control issues.
- Only properly trained staff should be permitted to use the equipment.
- There are simple sets of written instructions, which must include simple quality control procedures and what to do when the instrument seems to be performing unreliably.
- Health and safety issues must be considered, e.g. risk of exposure to hepatitis or human immunodeficiency virus (HIV).
- Quality control is monitored on a regular basis, preferably by the main laboratory.
- Records are kept of patient results, quality control and the personnel that performed the test.

Advantages include:
- Rapid access to results on acutely ill patients.
- Closer (more frequent) monitoring, whether acutely ill (e.g. blood gases in ICU) or in the home (e.g. glucose meters).
- 24 h availability.

Disadvantages include:
- Typically more expensive than a main analytical laboratory test.

Table 1.5 Examples of POCT that are in common use

Common POCT in blood	Common POCT in urine
Blood gases	Glucose
Glucose	Ketones
Urea and creatinine	Red cells/haemoglobin
Na, K and Ca	Bilirubin
Bilirubin	Urobilinogen
Salicylate	pH
Paracetamol	Protein
Alcohol	hCG
Troponin	Drugs of abuse

- Requires wider staff training with less ability to regulate access by untrained individuals.
- Calibration and quality control requirements are potentially less robust.
- Results not often integrated into the full electronic patient record.

As outlined above, where it is appropriate to introduce POCT, it is critical that matters of training, analytical performance, quality control, and health and safety are properly addressed. 'Smart' systems are also available which only allow password access to trained individuals and can also prevent issue of results if calibration is unsatisfactory or quality control failure occurs. POCT instruments can also be networked and performance monitored from the central laboratory.

Interpretation of clinical biochemistry tests

Most reports issued by clinical biochemistry laboratories contain numerical measures of concentration or activity, expressed in the appropriate units. Typically, the result is interpreted in relation to a reference range (see p. 7) for the analyte in question.

The following questions should be considered when interpreting the results:

1 Is each result normal or abnormal? Reference ranges (often incorrectly called normal ranges) are needed in order to answer questions about quantitative data.

2 Does each result fit in with my previous assessment of this patient? If not, can I explain the discrepancy?

3 Has a significant change occurred in any of the results from those previously reported?

4 Do any of the results alter my diagnosis of this patient's illness or influence the way in which the illness should be managed?

5 If I cannot explain a result, what do I propose to do about it?

This section discusses the interpretation of laboratory results and the factors that may cause them to vary, under the following main headings:

1 *Analytical factors* These cause errors in measurement.

2 *Biological and pathological factors* Both these sets of factors affect the concentrations of analytes in blood, urine and other fluids sent for analysis.

Sources of variation in test results

Analytical sources of variation

Systematic and random variation

Analytical results are subject to error, no matter how good the laboratory and no matter how skilled the analyst. These errors may be due to lack of accuracy, that is, always tend to be either high or low, or may be due to random effects and lack precision, that is, may be unpredictably high or low.

Accuracy

An accurate method will, on average, yield results close to the true value of what is being measured. It has no systematic bias.

Precision

A precise method yields results that are close to one another (but not necessarily close to the true value) on repeated analysis. If multiple measurements are made on one specimen, the spread of results will be small for a precise method and large for an imprecise one.

The 'dartboard' analogy is often used to illustrate the different meanings of the terms accuracy and precision, and this is illustrated in Figure 1.1.

The standard deviation (SD) is the usual measure of scatter around a mean value. If the spread of results is wide, the SD is large, whereas if the spread is narrow, the SD is small. For data that have a Gaussian distribution, as is nearly always the

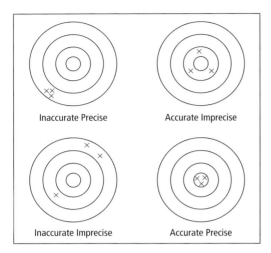

Figure 1.1 The 'dartboard' analogy can be used to illustrate accuracy and precision.

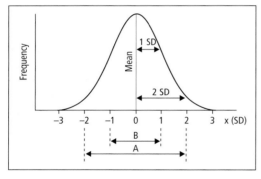

Figure 1.2 Diagram of a Gaussian (normal or symmetrical) distribution curve. The span (A) of the curve, the distance between the mean ± 2 SD, includes about 95% of the 'population'. The narrower span (B), the distance between the mean ± 1 SD, includes about 67% of the 'population'.

case for analytical errors, the shape of the curve (Figure 1.2) is completely defined by the mean and the SD, and these characteristics are such that:

- About 67% of results lie in the range mean ± 1 SD.
- About 95% of results lie in the range mean ± 2 SD.
- Over 99% of results lie in the range mean ± 3 SD.

Blunders

These are grossly inaccurate results that bear no constant or predictable relationship to the true value. They arise, for instance, from mislabelling of specimens at the time of collection, or transcription errors when preparing or issuing reports (see Table 1.1).

Serial results in the same patient

Doctors often have to interpret two or more sets of results for the same analysis or group of analyses performed on different occasions on the same patient. An important question is whether an analytical change is due mainly to laboratory imprecision or a to true change in the patients's clinical condition. Without elaborating on the statistical aspects of this, the following rule may be applied: if the results for analyses performed on specimens collected on different occasions, but under otherwise identical conditions, differ by more than 2.8 times the analytical SD then there is a chance of over 95% that a genuine change in concentration of the substance has occurred.

Biological causes of variation

As well as analytical variation, test results also show biological variation in both health and disease. Key questions are:

- How do results vary in health?
- How do results vary in disease?

How do results vary in health?

The concentrations of all analytes in blood vary with time due to diverse physiological factors *within* the individual. There are also differences *between* individuals.

Within-individual variation

The following may be important causes of within-individual variation:

1 *Diet* Variations in diet can affect the results of many tests, including serum [triglyceride], the response to glucose tolerance tests and urinary calcium excretion.

2 *Time of day* Several plasma constituents show diurnal variation (variation with the time of day), or a sleep/wake cycle. Examples include iron, adrenocorticotrophic hormone (ACTH) and cortisol concentrations.

3 *Posture* Proteins and all protein-bound constituents of plasma show significant differences in concentration between blood collected from upright individuals and blood from recumbent individuals. Examples include serum calcium, cholesterol, cortisol and total thyroxine concentrations.

4 *Muscular exercise* Recent exercise, especially if vigorous or unaccustomed, may increase serum creatine kinase (CK) activity and blood [lactate], and lower blood [pyruvate].

5 *Menstrual cycle* Several substances show variation with the phase of the cycle. Examples include serum [iron], and the serum concentrations of the pituitary gonadotrophins, ovarian steroids and their metabolites, as well as the amounts of these hormones and their metabolites excreted in the urine.

6 *Drugs* These can have marked effects on chemical results. Attention should be drawn particularly to the many effects of oestrogen-containing oral contraceptives on serum constituents (p. 166).

Even after allowing for known physiological factors that may affect plasma constituents and for analytical imprecision, there is still considerable residual individual variation (Table 1.6). The magnitude of this variation depends on the analyte, but it may be large and must be taken into account when interpreting successive values from a patient.

Between-individual variation

Differences between individuals can affect the concentrations of analytes in the blood. The following are the main examples:

Table 1.6 Residual individual variation of some serum constituents (expressed as the approximated day-to-day, within-individual coefficient of variation)

Serum constituent	CV (%)	Serum constituent	CV (%)
Sodium	1	ALT activity	25
Calcium	1–2	AST activity	25
Potassium	5	Iron	25
Urea	10		

CV = coefficient of variation.

1 *Age* Examples include serum [phosphate] and alkaline phosphatase (ALP) activity, and serum and urinary concentrations of the gonadotrophins and sex hormones.

2 *Sex* Examples include serum creatinine, iron, urate and urea concentrations and γ-glutamyltransferase (GGT) activity, and serum and urinary concentrations of the sex hormones.

3 *Race* Racial differences have been described for serum [cholesterol] and [protein]. It may be difficult to distinguish racial from environmental factors, such as diet.

Reference ranges

When looking at results, we need to compare each result with a set of results from a particular defined (or reference) population. This reference range is determined, in practice, by measuring a set of reference values from a sample of that population, usually of healthy individuals. The nature of the reference population should be given whenever reference ranges are quoted, although a healthy population is usually assumed. Even age-matched and sex-matched reference ranges are often difficult to obtain, since fairly large numbers of individuals are needed. In practice, blood donors are very often selected as the most readily available reference population.

Distribution of results in a reference population

When results of analyses for a reference population are analysed, they are invariably found to cluster around a central value, with a distribution that may be symmetrical (often Gaussian, Figure 1.3a) or asymmetrical (often log-Gaussian, Figure 1.3b). However, reference ranges can be calculated from these data without making any assumptions about the distribution of the data, using non-parametric methods.

Because of geographical, racial and other biological sources of variation between individuals, as well as differences in analytical methods, each laboratory should ideally define and publish its own reference ranges. Conventionally, these include the central 95% of the results obtained for each analysis from the reference population. This 95%

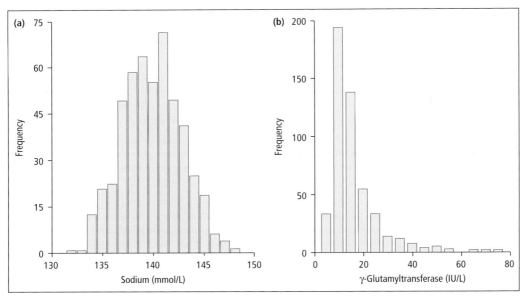

Figure 1.3 Histograms showing the relative frequency with which results with the values indicated were obtained when serum [Na⁺] and γ-glutamyltransferase (GGT) activities were measured in a reference population of healthy adult women. (a) The sodium data are symmetrically distributed about the mean whereas (b) the GGT data show a log-Gaussian distribution.

figure is arbitrary, selected in order to minimise the overlap between results from diseased populations and from healthy individuals.

Analytical factors can affect the reference ranges for individual laboratories. If an *inaccurate* method is used, the reference range will reflect the method bias. If an *imprecise* method is used, the reference range will be widened, that is, the observed span of results (reflected in the SD) will be greater. In statistical terms, the observed variance (i.e. the square of the SD) of the population results will equal the sum of the true or biological variance of the population plus the analytical variance of the method.

How do results vary in disease?

Biochemical test results do not exist in isolation, since, by the time tests are requested, the doctor will often have made a provisional diagnosis and a list of differential diagnoses based on each patient's symptoms and signs.

For example, in a patient with severe abdominal pain, tenderness and rigidity, there may be several differential diagnoses to consider – including, for example, acute pancreatitis, perforated peptic ulcer and acute cholecystitis. In all three conditions, the serum amylase activity may be raised, that is, above the upper reference value for healthy adults. So healthy adult reference ranges (in this instance) are irrelevant, since healthy adults do not have abdominal pain, tenderness and rigidity! Instead, we need to know how the serum amylase activity might vary in the clinically likely differential diagnoses. It would be useful to know, for instance, whether very high serum amylase activities are associated with one of these diagnostic possibilities, but not with the other two.

To summarise, to interpret results on patients adequately, we need to know:
• the reference range for healthy individuals of the appropriate age range and of the same sex;
• the values to be expected for patients with the disease, or diseases, under consideration;

- the prevalence of the disease, or diseases, in the population to which the patient belongs.

The assessment of diagnostic tests

In evaluating and interpreting a test, it is necessary to know how it behaves in health and disease. Central to understanding here are the terms sensitivity and specificity.

- Test sensitivity refers to how effective the test is in detecting individuals who have the disease in question. It is expressed as the percentage of true positives in all the individuals who have disease (all the individuals with disease will encompass the true positives (TP) and false negatives (FN)). So:

$$\text{Sensitivity} = TP/(TP + FN) \times 100\%$$

- Test specificity is a measure of how good the test is at providing a negative result in the absence of disease. It is expressed as the percentage of true negatives in all those without the disease (all the individuals without disease will encompass the true negatives (TN) and the false positives (FP)). So:

$$\text{Specificity} = TN/(TN + FP) \times 100\%$$

The ideal test is 100% sensitive (positive in all patients with the disease) and 100% specific (negative in all patients without the disease), shown diagrammatically in Figure 1.4a. This ideal is rarely achieved; there is usually overlap between the healthy and diseased populations (Figure 1.4b). In practice, we have to decide where to draw dividing lines that most effectively separate 'healthy' from 'diseased' groups, or disease A from disease B. We can illustrate this by means of the following hypothetical example.

The effectiveness of a test can also be defined in terms of the predictive value of a positive result and the predictive value of a negative result. The positive predictive value is:

$$TP/(TP + FP) \times 100\%$$

A test with a high positive predictive value will, by definition, have few false positives. This would be important in a situation where a high number of false positives would otherwise lead to extensive and costly further investigation.

The negative predictive value is defined as follows:

$$TN/(TN + FN) \times 100\%$$

A test with a high negative predictive value would, by definition, have few false negatives. This would be particularly important, for example, in a test which was used for a screening programme where it is essential not to miss a case of the disease in question.

In defining the presence or absence of a disease, a cut-off may be assigned to a test. Consider the situation where a high value for a particular test equates with the presence of a particular disease. A value above the cut-off would then define the presence of the disease and a value below the cut-off, the absence of disease. A cut-off which is set at a

Figure 1.4 Diagrammatic representations of the distributions of results obtained with a test (a) that completely separates healthy people from people with a disease without any overlap between the distribution curves (i.e. an ideal test with 100% sensitivity and 100% specificity), and a test (b) that is less sensitive and less specific, in which there is an area of overlap between the distribution curves for healthy people and people with disease.

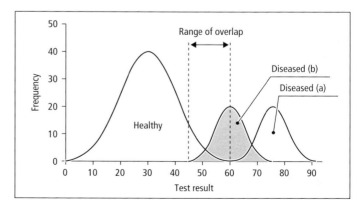

higher level will increase the test specificity at the expense of test sensitivity (more false negatives), whilst a cut-off set at a lower value will increase test sensitivity at the expenses of test specificity (more false positives).

In evaluating tests for decision making, it is clearly important to decide on the relative importance of sensitivity versus specificity in the context for which a test is used. To that end, it is helpful to be able to make comparisons of different tests with respect to sensitivity and specificity. This is often best carried out by plotting the test sensitivity against specificity and constructing a so-called receiver operating characteristic (ROC) curve. These curves will highlight which test is best suited to which requirement and will also help to define which cut-off to select in order to balance specificity versus sensitivity. This is illustrated in Figure 1.5.

Screening for rare diseases

For diseases that are rare, tests of extremely high sensitivity and specificity are required. To illustrate this, consider an inherited metabolic disorder with an incidence of 1:5000; this is similar to that of some of the more common, treatable, inherited metabolic diseases such as phenylketonuria (PKU) or congenital hypothyroidism. Assume that we have a test with a good performance, that is, a sensitivity and specificity of 99.5% (Table 1.7).

Table 1.7 shows that for every neonate affected by the disorder who has a positive test result, there will be about 25 (4999/199) neonates who also have a positive test but who do not have the disease. Two important points emerge:
1 Tests with very high sensitivity and with very low false-positive rates are required when screening for rare disorders.
2 A heavy investigative load will result from the screening programme, since all the false positives will have to be followed up to determine whether or not they indicate the presence of disease.

The traditional 95% reference range (see above) is not relevant to screening for rare conditions, since the rate of false positives would be far too

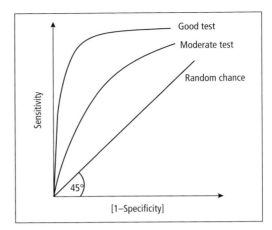

Figure 1.5 Schematic representation of a receiver operating characteristic (ROC) plot. A random test produces a straight line set at 45° to the axes. A discriminatory, good test produces a graph with a steep slope from the origin, displaying high sensitivity at high specificity. Less discriminatory tests produce curves at intermediate positions, as shown.
(Adapted with the authors' permission from: Roulston, J.E. and Leonard, R.F.C. 'Serological tumour markers: an Introduction' Publ. Churchill Livingstone 1993)

Table 1.7 A hypothetical set of results of a screening test for a relatively common inherited metabolic disorder in neonates

Diagnostic category	Positive results	Negative results	Total
Disease present	199	1	200
Disease absent	4999	994801	999800
Total	5198	994802	1000000
Predictive value	3.8%	100%	

Assumptions: sensitivity of the test 99.5%, false-positive rate 0.5% (specificity 99.5%), prevalence of the disorder, 1:5000; 1000000 neonates screened.
Note that the prevalence of PKA and of hypothyroidism in the UK is about 1:5000 live births, and that about 800000 neonates in the UK are screened annually.

high. The cut-off value has to be altered to decrease the false-positive rate, at the probable expense of missing some patients who have the condition for which screening is being carried out.

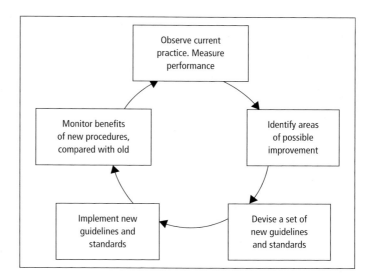

Figure 1.6 The audit cycle.

Audit in clinical biochemistry

Audit is the process whereby the procedures involved in patient care are monitored in order to give high priority to the delivery of an efficient and cost-effective service. The measure of health outcome is benefit to the patient.

The value of audit can most readily be seen in those specialties concerned directly with patient care, but the principles are applicable to all clinical and investigational specialties (e.g. radiology), as well as laboratory-based specialties such as clinical biochemistry. For example, the monitoring of laboratory performance may identify that reports are arriving too late and too often at the wrong location. This would precipitate a review of the form printing and delivery process, implementation of a change in the arrangements and a re-monitoring of the delivery process to ensure that the original problem had been overcome.

The audit process

There is an essential sequence to auditing activities (Figure 1.6):

1 Identify an area of concern or interest, particularly if it is felt that there is room for improvement in the service, or if the same quality of service can be provided more economically.
2 Review and analyse the present procedures.
3 Identify specific aspects that might be capable of improvement.
4 Identify alternative procedures or standards that might lead to improvement.
5 Take the practical steps necessary to implement any changes proposed.
6 Compare the performance after the changes with those before them.
7 It must be emphasised that the final stage of analysis of the effects of any change is an integral part of the audit process; it is essential to know whether the measures taken have improved the service or made it more cost-effective. Sometimes, changes have no effect, or even adverse effects.

Reference

Asher, R. (1954) Straight and crooked thinking in medicine. *British Medical Journal*, **2**, 460–2.

Keypoints

- As a rule, only those tests that may contribute to diagnosis and management of patients should be requested.
- Population screening is indicated where reliable tests are able to detect important and treatable disease; case-finding screening is valuable in groups at high risk of a specific disorder.
- There is an overlap between test results obtained in health and those obtained in disease or (where the test is being used for screening) results from affected individuals.
- Effective tests reduce this overlap to a minimum, but there will always be a trade-off between maximising the sensitivity of a test, that is, detecting as many affected individuals as possible, and maximising its specificity, that is, minimising the number of non-affected individuals classified as abnormal by the test.
- Strategies to maximise a test's value depend both on the test itself and on the prevalence of the disease in the population being studied.

Case 1.1

A new test is marketed which claims to diagnose heart failure. The test has a specificity of 70% and a sensitivity of 95% at the manufacturer's recommended cut-off for diagnosis. The Admissions Unit decides to use the test as part of an admission profile on breathless patients admitted for further assessment over the age of 65 years in order to exclude heart failure. Assuming a prevalence of 20% for heart failure in this population, calculate how many false negatives would be recorded after the first 1000 patients meeting the testing criteria had passed through the unit. Given that other tests can be used to establish a diagnosis of heart failure, do you think that the cut-off selected is sensible? (prevalence figures are for illustrative purposes only).

Comment: This is best examined by constructing a table as follows:

	Positive results	Negative results	Totals
Heart failure present	190 TP	10 FN	200
Heart failure absent	240 FP	560 TN	800
Total	430	570	1000

   Because the test has a relatively high sensitivity, the table shows that it identifies the majority of patients with heart failure which is what is required in a test to rule out heart failure. Because the test lacks specificity, it can also be seen from the table that it identifies a considerable number of patients with positive results who do not have heart failure. In fact, the test is positive on more occasions in patients who do not have heart failure than in those with heart failure. Because other tests are available to the clinician, the false-positive patients can be separated from the true-positive patients on the basis of these further investigations. The 560 patients where the result is a true negative would then not need to go through more expensive further investigations. In this example, the test has been valuable in ruling out patients who would not require further investigation but ruling in those who would benefit. Clearly, it is not a perfect test but would potentially prevent costly further investigations in a significant number of patients and, provided that the test itself is not too expensive, ultimately be worthy of consideration in terms of health economics.

Case 1.2

A 72-year-old man is admitted vaguely unwell with some nausea and associated vomiting, though not severe. He appears rather pale and wasted with a low blood pressure. He is on treatment with digoxin for his atrial fibrillation and the suspicion arises that his symptoms may arise from digoxin toxicity. This would also help explain the raised potassium result for which there is no other clear cause. The most recent digoxin dose had been taken just before his admission to the hospital. The house officer telephones to request an additional digoxin measurement on the admission sample and this is reported back as raised. On this basis, the digoxin is withheld and his condition monitored. Little improvement is noted and the nausea becomes worse, accompanied by a worsening of his atrial fibrillation. Further advice is sought.

Comment on this case with particular reference to the raised digoxin and the worsening of his atrial fibrillation.

Comment: The timing of a blood test is crucial to the interpretation of a number of drugs whose concentration in blood is monitored for therapeutic purposes. This is most certainly the case with digoxin where the blood sample should *not* be taken within 6 h of the most recent digoxin dose. The House Officer has requested digoxin as an additional test on the patient's admission sample, without reference to the exact time when the patient took his dose of digoxin prior to admission. In fact, the time elapsed between taking the drug and the blood sample was about 1 h. The raised digoxin concentration is uninterpretable and it may well be that the patient has digoxin levels within the therapeutic range or even on the low side. This turned out to be the case, explaining the worsening in his condition when the drug was inappropriately withheld.

An isolated raised potassium result can be a very important finding which reflects underlying pathology such as renal disease, DKA, etc. Although there was no immediate explanation for this man's raised potassium, it became evident what the problem was when the full blood count report was received. This showed a very high lymphocyte count consistent with chronic lymphocytic leukaemia. In this condition, the white cells are fragile and can lyse on blood sampling. With the high white cell count, it is then possible to measure a spuriously high potassium level in the corresponding biochemistry sample.

Case 1.3

The following results were obtained on a 54-year-old woman after surgery for ovarian cancer. Can you account for the abnormalities found?

Serum	Result	Reference range
Urea	2.0	2.5–6.6 mmol/L
Sodium	147	135–145 mmol/L
Potassium	2.0	3.6–5.0 mmol/L
Total CO$_2$	10.0	22–30 mmol/L
Bilirubin	7.0	3–16 µmol/L
ALT	11.0	10–50 U/L
ALP	35.0	40–125 U/L
Total protein	42.0	60–80 g/L
Calcium	1.6	2.1–2.6 mmol/L

Comments: Many of these results are abnormal and, with the exception of the sodium result, are abnormally low. In a post-operative patient, a set of results like this should immediately raise the suspicion that the blood sample was taken close to the site of an IV infusion. The fluid infused would dilute the blood at the site of sampling, leading to a consequent lowering of the concentration of all the analytes measured. If the IV infusion was normal saline, this would then account for the fact that only the sodium value is high while all the other values are low. When the Duty Biochemist contacted the House Officer on the ward, he did admit that he had had difficulty taking a blood sample from the patient and did recollect that he sampled from close to the site of the IV infusion. A repeat blood sample was requested from a site away from the infusion and confirmed the original error since all the results were within the reference range, apart from the sodium which was slightly low at 132 mmol/L.

Case 1.4

The following set of results was obtained on a young man admitted with a fractured femur after a motorcycle accident. He appeared stable and had no previous past medical history of note. The houseman was at a loss to explain the results but remembered that he had topped up the sample shortfall in the Biochemistry tube from the haematology full blood count tube. Can you account for the results?

Serum	Result	Reference range
Urea	6.4	2.5–6.6 mmol/L
Sodium	138	135–145 mmol/L
Potassium	16.1	3.6–5.0 mmol/L
Total CO_2	32	22–30 mmol/L
Bilirubin	14	3–16 μmol/L
ALT	40	10–50 U/L
ALP	38	40–125 U/L
Total protein	75	60–80 g/L
Calcium	0.6	2.1–2.6 mmol/L
Albumin	32	35–50 g/L

Comments: This particular case illustrates the importance of using the correct blood sample tube. In transferring some of the blood from the Haematology tube to the Biochemistry tube, the doctor had not appreciated that the anti-coagulant in the Haematology (pink) tube was potassium EDTA. This explains the high potassium and the low calcium since the EDTA chelates the calcium. leading to a low result on analysis.

Chapter 2

Disturbances of water, sodium and potassium balance

Fluid loss, retention or redistribution are common clinical problems in many areas of clinical practice. The management of these conditions is often urgent, and requires a rapid assessment of the history and examination, and of biochemical and other investigations.

In this chapter we consider:
- The distribution of water, Na^+ and K^+ in the different fluid compartments of the body, and their control by hormonal and other factors.
- Clinical effects and management of different types of loss, retention or redistribution of fluid.
- Causes and investigation of hypernatraemia and hyponatraemia.
- Causes and investigation of hyperkalaemia and hypokalaemia.
- Fluid and electrolyte problems in surgical patients, and the metabolic response to trauma.

Water and sodium balance

Both the internal and external balance of any substance must be considered. The internal balance is the distribution between different body compartments, while the external balance matches input with output. The movements of Na^+ and water that occur all the time between plasma and glomerular

Lecture Notes: Clinical Biochemistry, 8e. By G. Beckett, S. Walker, P. Rae & P. Ashby. Published 2010 by Blackwell Publishing.

filtrate, or between plasma and gastrointestinal (GI) secretions, provide the potential for large losses, with consequent serious and rapid alterations in internal balance. For example, about 25 000 mmol of Na^+ are filtered at the glomerulus over 24 h, normally with subsequent reabsorption of more than 99%. Likewise, 1000 of mmol Na^+ enter the GI tract in various secretions each day, but less than 0.5% (5 mmol) is normally lost in the faeces.

Internal distribution of water and sodium

In a 70 kg adult, the total body water is about 42 L comprising about 28 L of intracellular fluid (ICF) and 14 L of extracellular fluid (ECF) water. The ECF water is distributed as 3 L of plasma water and 11 L of interstitial water. The total body Na^+ is about 4200 mmol and is mainly extracellular – about 50% is in the ECF, 40% in bone and 10% in the ICF.

Two important factors influence the distribution of fluid between the ICF and the intravascular and extravascular compartments of the ECF:

1 *Osmolality* This affects the movement of water across cell membranes.

2 *Colloid osmotic pressure* Together with hydrodynamic factors, this affects the movement of water and low molecular mass solutes (predominantly NaCl) between the intravascular and extravascular compartments.

Osmolality, osmolarity and tonicity

The *osmolality* is the number of solute particles per unit weight of water, irrespective of the size or nature of the particles. Therefore, a given weight of low molecular weight solutes contributes much more to the osmolality than the same weight of high molecular weight solutes. The units are mmol/kg of water. This determines the osmotic pressure exerted by a solution across a membrane. Most laboratories can measure plasma osmolality, but it is also possible to calculate the approximate osmolality of plasma using a number of formulae of varying complexity. The following formula has the benefit of being easy to calculate and performs as well as more complex versions (all concentrations must be in mmol/L):

Calculated osmolality
$$= 2[Na^+] + 2[K^+] + [glucose] + [urea]$$

This formula includes all the low molecular weight solutes contributing to plasma osmolality. Values for Na^+ and K^+ are doubled so as to allow for their associated anions, such as chloride. The formula is approximate and is not a complete substitute for direct measurement. Calculated osmolality is usually close to measured osmolality, but they may differ considerably for two different types of reason. First, there may be large amounts of unmeasured low molecular mass solutes (e.g. ethanol) present in plasma. These will contribute to the measured osmolality, but will obviously not be taken into account in the osmolality calculated from this formula. This will cause an 'osmole gap', with measured osmolality being greater than calculated osmolality. The other cause of a discrepancy is when there is a gross increase in plasma protein or lipid concentration, both of which decrease the plasma water per unit volume. This affects some methods of measurement of [Na^+], giving an artefactually low result ('pseudohyponatraemia', see p. 23). This will result in an erroneously low calculated osmolality.

The osmolality of urine is usually measured directly, but is also linearly related to its specific gravity (which can be measured using urine dipsticks), unless there are significant amounts of glucose, protein or X-ray contrast media present.

The *osmolarity* is the number of particles of solute per litre of solution. Its units are mmol/L. Its measurement or calculation has been largely replaced by osmolality.

Tonicity is a term often confused with osmolality. However, it should only be used in relation to the osmotic pressure due to those solutes (e.g. Na^+) that exert their effects across cell membranes, thereby causing movement of water into or out of the cells. Substances that can readily diffuse into cells down their concentration gradients (e.g. urea, alcohol) contribute to plasma osmolality but not to plasma tonicity, since after equilibration their concentration will be equal on both sides of the cell membrane. Tonicity is not readily measurable.

The tonicity of ICF and ECF equilibrate with one another by movement of water across cell membranes. An increase in ECF tonicity causes a reduction in ICF volume as water moves from the ICF to the ECF to equalise the tonicity of the two compartments, whereas a decrease in ECF tonicity causes an increase in ICF volume as water moves from the ECF to the ICF.

Colloid osmotic pressure (oncotic pressure)

The osmotic pressure exerted by plasma proteins across cell membranes is negligible compared with the osmotic pressure of a solution containing NaCl and other small molecules, since they are present in much lower molar concentrations. In contrast, small molecules diffuse freely across the capillary wall, and so are not osmotically active at this site, but plasma proteins do not readily do so. This means that plasma [protein] and hydrodynamic factors together determine the distribution of water and solutes across the capillary wall, and hence between the intravascular and interstitial compartments (Figure 2.1).

Regulation of external water balance

Typical daily intakes and outputs of water are given in Table 2.1. Water intake is largely a consequence

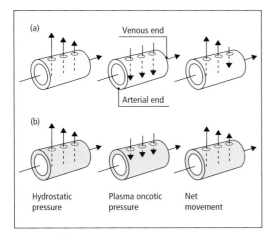

Figure 2.1 Movements of water and low molecular mass solutes across the capillary wall when the plasma [protein] is (a) normal and (b) low. The effects shown are: hydrostatic pressure, which drives water and low molecular mass solutes *outwards* and decreases along the length of the capillary; and plasma oncotic pressure, which attracts water and low molecular mass solutes *inwards* and is constant along the length of the capillary. The net movement of water and low molecular mass solutes across the capillary wall is governed by the net effect of hydrostatic and plasma oncotic pressures.

Table 2.1 Average daily water intake and output of a normal adult in the UK

Intake of water	mL	Output of water	mL
Water drunk	1500	Urine volume	1500
Water in food	750	Water content of faeces	50
Water from metabolism of food	250	Losses in expired air and insensible perspiration	950
Total	2500	Total	2500

of social habit and is very variable, but is also controlled by the sensation of thirst. Its output is controlled by the action of vasopressin, also known as antidiuretic hormone (ADH). In states of pure water deficiency, plasma tonicity increases, causing a sensation of thirst and stimulating vasopressin secretion, both mediated by hypothalamic osmoreceptors. Vasopressin then promotes water reab-

sorption in the distal nephron, with consequent production of small volumes of concentrated urine. Conversely, a large intake of water causes a fall in tonicity, suppresses thirst and reduces vasopressin secretion, leading to a diuresis, producing large volumes of dilute urine.

Secretion of vasopressin is normally controlled by small changes in ECF tonicity, but it is also under tonic inhibitory control from baroreceptors in the left atrium and great vessels on the left side of the heart. Where haemodynamic factors (e.g. excessive blood loss, heart failure) reduce the stretch on these receptors, often without an accompanying change in ECF tonicity, a reduction in tonic inhibitory control stimulates vasopressin secretion. The resulting water retention causes hyponatraemia and is relatively ineffective in expanding the intravascular compartment, since water diffuses freely throughout all compartments (Figure 2.2).

Regulation of external sodium balance

Dietary intakes of Na$^+$ (and Cl$^-$) are very variable worldwide. A typical 'Western' diet provides 100–200 mmol of both Na$^+$ and Cl$^-$ daily, but the total body Na$^+$ can be maintained even if intake is less than 5 mmol or greater than 750 mmol daily. Urinary losses of Na$^+$ normally closely match intake. There is normally little loss of these ions through the skin or in the faeces, but in disease the GI tract can become a major source of Na$^+$ loss.

The amount of Na$^+$ excreted in the urine controls the ECF volume since, when osmoregulation is normal, the amount of extracellular water is controlled to maintain a constant concentration of extracellular Na$^+$. A number of mechanisms are important regulators of Na$^+$ excretion:

• *The renin–angiotensin–aldosterone system* Renin is secreted in response to a fall in renal afferent arteriolar pressure or to a reduction in supply of Na$^+$ to the distal tubule. It converts angiotensinogen in plasma to angiotensin I (AI), which in turn is converted to angiotensin II (AII) by angiotensin-converting enzyme (ACE). Both AII and its metabolic product angiotensin III (AIII) are pharmacologi-

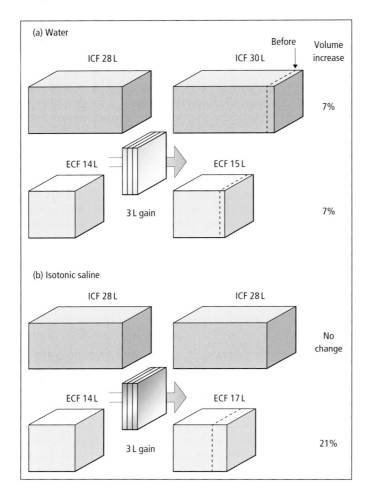

(a) Water

Before   Volume
increase

ICF 28 L   ICF 30 L

7%

ECF 14 L   ECF 15 L

3 L gain   7%

(b) Isotonic saline

ICF 28 L   ICF 28 L

No
change

ECF 14 L   ECF 17 L

3 L gain   21%

Figure 2.2 Different effects on the body's fluid compartments of fluid gains of 3 L of (a) water and (b) isotonic saline. The volumes shown relate to a 70 kg adult.

cally active, and stimulate the release of aldosterone from the adrenal cortex. Aldosterone acts on the distal tubule to promote Na^+ reabsorption in exchange for urinary loss of H^+ or K^+. Since Na^+ cannot enter cells freely, its retention (with iso-osmotically associated water) contributes solely to ECF volume expansion, unlike pure water retention (Figures 2.2 and 2.3). Although the renin–angiotensin–aldosterone system causes relatively slow responses to Na^+ deprivation or Na^+ loading, evidence suggests that this is the main regulatory mechanism for Na^+ excretion.

• *The glomerular filtration rate (GFR)* The rate of Na^+ excretion is often related to the GFR. When the GFR falls acutely, less Na^+ is filtered and excreted, and vice versa. However, this only becomes a limiting factor in Na^+ excretion at very low levels of GFR.

• *Atrial natriuretic peptide (ANP)* This peptide secreted by cardiocytes of the right atrium of the heart promotes Na^+ excretion by the kidney, apparently by causing a marked increase in GFR. The importance of the ANP regulatory mechanism is not yet clear, but it probably only plays a minor role. Other structurally similar peptides have been identified, including brain or B-type natriuretic peptide (BNP), secreted by the cardiac ventricles and with similar properties to ANP. BNP is increas-

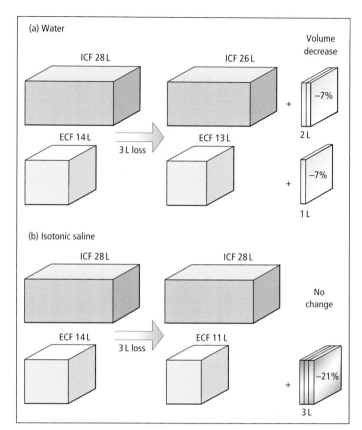

Figure 2.3 Different effects on the body's fluid compartments of fluid losses of 3 L of (a) water and (b) isotonic saline. The volumes shown relate to a 70 kg adult.

ingly being used in the assessment of patients suspected of having cardiac failure (see p. 182).

Disorders of water and sodium homeostasis

It is important to remember that the concentration of any substance is a consequence of the amount both of the solute (here Na^+) and of the solvent (here water). The concentration of the solute may change because of changes in either the amount of solute, the amount of solvent, or both. Although the physiological control mechanisms for water and for Na^+ are distinct, they need to be considered together when seeking an understanding of a patient's Na^+ and water balance, and of the plasma $[Na^+]$.

Whereas losses or gains of pure water are distributed across all fluid compartments, losses or gains of Na^+ and water, as isotonic fluid, are borne by the much smaller ECF compartment (Figures 2.2 and 2.3). Thus, it is usually more urgent to replace losses of isotonic fluid than losses of water. For the same reason, circulatory overload is more likely with excessive administration of isotonic Na^+-containing solutions than with isotonic dextrose (the dextrose is metabolised, leaving water behind).

Plasma $[Na^+]$ cannot be used as a simple measure of body Na^+ status since it is very often abnormal as a result of losses or gains of water rather than of Na^+. The plasma $[Na^+]$ must be interpreted in relation to the patient's history and the findings on clinical examination, and if necessary backed up by other investigations.

Table 2.2 Causes of depletion of and excess water

Categories	Examples
Depletion of water	
Inadequate intake	Infants, patients in coma or who are very sick, or have symptoms such as nausea or dysphagia
Abnormal losses via	
Lungs	Inadequate humidification in mechanical ventilation
Skin	Fevers and in hot climates
Renal tract	Diabetes insipidus, lithium therapy
Excess water	
Excessive intake	
Oral	Psychogenic polydipsia
Parenteral	Hypotonic infusions after operations
Renal retention	Excess vasopressin (SIADH, Table 2.5), hypoadrenalism, hypothyroidism

Table 2.3 Causes of depletion of and excess sodium

Categories	Examples
Depletion of sodium	
Inadequate oral intake	Rare, by itself
Abnormal losses via	
Skin	Excessive sweating, dermatitis, burns
GI tract	Vomiting, aspiration, diarrhoea, fistula, paralytic ileus, blood loss
Renal tract	Diuretic therapy, osmotic diuresis, renal tubular disease, mineralocorticoid deficiency
Excess of sodium	
Excessive intake	
Oral	Sea water (drowning), salt tablets, hypertonic NaCl administration (this is rare)
Parenteral	Post-operatively, infusion of hypertonic NaCl
Renal retention	Acute and chronic renal failure, primary and secondary hyperaldosteronism, Cushing's syndrome

The main causes of depletion and excess of water are summarised in Table 2.2, and of Na$^+$ in Table 2.3. Although some of these conditions may be associated with abnormal plasma [Na$^+$], it must be emphasised that this is not necessarily always the case. For example, patients with acute losses of isotonic fluid (e.g. plasma, ECF, blood) may be severely and dangerously hypovolaemic and Na$^+$ depleted, and very possibly in shock, but their plasma [Na$^+$] may nevertheless be normal or even raised.

Hyponatraemia

Hyponatraemia is the most common clinical biochemical abnormality. Most patients with hyponatraemia also have a low plasma osmolality. Unless an unusual cause of hyponatraemia is suspected (see 'Other causes of hyponatraemia', p. 23), measurement of plasma osmolality contributes little or no extra information.

Patients with hyponatraemia can be divided into three categories, on the basis of the ECF volume being low, normal or increased. These categories in turn reflect a total body Na$^+$ that is low, normal or increased, respectively. The value of this classification is two-fold. First, the clinical history and examination often indicate the ECF volume and therefore the total body Na$^+$ status. Secondly, treatment often depends on the total body Na$^+$ status rather than the [Na$^+$]. One possible way of narrowing the differential diagnosis of a patient with hyponatraemia, based on this subdivision, is shown in Figure 2.4.

Hyponatraemia with low ECF volume

The patient has lost Na$^+$ and water in one or more body fluids (e.g. GI tract secretions, urine, inflammatory exudate) or may have been treated with a diuretic (Table 2.4). The low ECF volume leads to tachycardia, orthostatic hypotension,

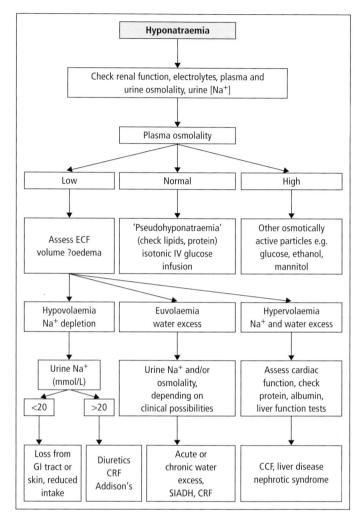

Figure 2.4 Schematic diagram to assist in the diagnosis of some of the more common causes of hyponatraemia. In practice more than one cause may be present, and the findings may be influenced by the recent clinical history and oral or IV fluid intake. (CCF = congestive cardiac failure; CRF = chronic renal failure; GI = gastrointestinal; SIADH, syndrome of inappropriate secretion of antidiuretic hormone.)

reduced skin turgor and oliguria. The hypovolaemia causes secondary aldosteronism with a low urinary [Na⁺] (usually <20 mmol/L), unless diuretic treatment is the cause when urinary [Na⁺] remains high. The hypovolaemia also provides a 'volume stimulus' to vasopressin secretion, resulting in oliguria and a concentrated urine. The consequent water retention can further contribute to the hyponatraemia.

Treatment requires administration of isotonic saline.

Hyponatraemia with normal ECF volume

The hyponatraemia results from excessive water retention, due to inability to excrete a water load. This may develop acutely, or it may be chronic (Table 2.4).

● *Acute water retention* Plasma [vasopressin] is acutely increased after trauma or major surgery, as part of the metabolic response to trauma, and during delivery and postpartum. Administration of excessive amounts of water (e.g. as 5% dex-

Table 2.4 Causes of hyponatraemia

ECF volume	Categories	Examples
Decreased total body Na$^+$ (loss of Na$^+$ > H$_2$O)		
Extrarenal losses of Na$^+$ (urine [Na$^+$] <20 mmol/L)	GI tract	Vomiting, diarrhoea
	Skin	Burns, severe dermatitis
	'Internal'	Paralytic ileus, peritoneal fluid
Renal losses of Na$^+$ (urine [Na$^+$] > 20 mmol/L)	Diuretics	
	Kidneys	Diuretic phase of renal tubular necrosis
	Adrenals	Mineralocorticoid deficiency
Normal or near-normal total body Na$^+$	Acute conditions	Parenteral administration of water, after surgery or trauma, or during or after delivery
	Chronic conditions	
	Anti-diuretic drugs	Opiates, chlorpropamide
	Kidneys	Chronic renal failure
	Adrenals	Glucocorticoid deficiency
	Vasopressin excess	SIADH (Table 2.5)
	Osmoregulator	Low setting in carcinomatosis
Increased total body Na$^+$	Acute conditions	Acute renal failure
	Chronic conditions	Oedematous states (p. 23)

trose) in these circumstances may exacerbate the hyponatraemia and cause acute water intoxication.

• *Chronic water retention* Perhaps the most widely known chronic 'cause' of this form of hyponatraemia is the syndrome of inappropriate secretion of ADH (SIADH) (Table 2.5). Whether this concept is of value in understanding its aetiology, or valid in terms of altered physiology, is uncertain. As the name implies, ADH (or rather vasopressin) is being secreted in the absence of an 'appropriate' physiological stimulus, of either fluid depletion or hypernatraemia. As water is retained, the potential for expansion of the ECF volume is limited by a reduction in renin and an increase in sodium excretion. A new steady state is achieved, with essentially normal, or only mildly increased, ECF volume. If the causative disorder (Table 2.5) is transient, plasma [Na$^+$] returns to normal when the primary disorder (e.g. pneumonia) is treated. However, in patients with cancer, the hyponatraemia is presumably due to production of vasopressin or a

Table 2.5 SIADH

Characteristics of the syndrome	Causes (and examples)
Low plasma [Na$^+$] and osmolality	Malignant disease of the bronchus, prostate, pancreas, etc.
Inappropriately high urine osmolality	Chest diseases, e.g. pneumonia, bronchitis, tuberculosis
Excessive renal excretion of Na$^+$	Central nervous system (CNS) diseases, including brain trauma, tumours, meningitis
No evidence of volume depletion	
No evidence of oedema	Drug treatment, e.g. carbamazepine, chlorpropamide, opiates
Normal renal and adrenal function	Miscellaneous conditions, including porphyria, psychosis, postoperative states

related substance by the tumour, and is usually persistent. If symptoms are mild, they may be treated by severe fluid restriction (i.e. ≤500 mL/ day), but if this is ineffective, treatment with a drug that antagonises the renal effects of vasopressin (e.g. demeclocycline) may be tried.

Other causes of chronic retention of water include:

• *Chronic renal disease* Damaged kidneys may be unable to concentrate or to dilute urine normally, tending to produce a urine of osmolality about that of plasma. Thus, the ability to excrete a water load is severely impaired, and excess water intake (oral or IV) readily produces a dilutional hyponatraemia. These patients may also be overloaded with Na^+.

• *Glucocorticoid deficiency* Whether due to anterior pituitary disease or abrupt withdrawal of long-term glucocorticoid therapy, this may lead to inability to excrete a water load, and to hyponatraemia.

• *Resetting of the osmostat* Some patients with malnutrition, carcinomatosis and tuberculosis seem to have their osmostat reset at a low level, with plasma $[Na^+]$ of 125–130 mmol/L. The cause is uncertain.

Hyponatraemia with increased ECF volume

Significant increases in total body Na^+ give rise to clinically detectable oedema (Table 2.4). Generalised oedema is usually associated with secondary aldosteronism, caused by a reduction in renal blood flow, which stimulates renin production. Patients fall into at least three categories:

• *Renal failure* Excess water intake in a poorly controlled patient with acute or chronic renal disease can lead to hyponatraemia with oedema.

• *Congestive cardiac failure* In cardiac failure there is reduced renal perfusion and an 'apparent' volume deficit, and also increased venous pressure, with altered fluid distribution between the intravascular and interstitial compartments (Figure 2.1). These lead to secondary aldosteronism and increased vasopressin secretion, causing Na^+ overload and hyponatraemia.

• *Hypoproteinaemic states* Low plasma [protein], especially low [albumin], leads to excessive losses of water and low molecular mass solutes from the intravascular to the interstitial compartments (Figure 2.1). Hence interstitial oedema is accompanied by reduced intravascular volume, with consequent secondary aldosteronism and stimulation of vasopressin release.

'Sick cell syndrome'

Some ill patients may have a hyponatraemia that is very resistant to treatment, and has no immediately obvious cause. The effective arterial plasma volume may be contracted, with a consequent secondary hyperaldosteronism and Na^+ retention. The total ECF volume may in contrast be increased, possibly because of stress-induced vasopressin secretion, or other causes of SIADH. These, however, may not be the whole explanation for the observed pathophysiology, since plasma [aldosterone] and [vasopressin] are not always raised. The hyponatraemia may be due, at least in part, to the 'sick cell syndrome', in which there is an inability to maintain an Na^+ gradient across the cell membrane, because of an increase in permeability, with or without impaired Na^+ pump activity.

Other causes of hyponatraemia

In all the examples of hyponatraemia discussed above, the low plasma $[Na^+]$ occurs in association with reduced plasma osmolality. Where this is not the case, the following possibilities should be considered:

• *Artefact* 'Hyponatraemia' is often caused by collection of a blood specimen from a vein close to a site at which fluid (typically 5% dextrose) is being administered intravenously.

• *Pseudohyponatraemia* This is an artefactual result due to a reduction in plasma water caused by marked hyperlipidaemia or hyperproteinaemia (e.g. multiple myeloma). Normally, lipids and proteins make up a relatively small proportion, by volume, of plasma. Na^+ and other electrolytes are dissolved in the plasma water, and do not enter the lipid or protein fraction of the plasma. This means that methods which measure $[Na^+]$ in the plasma water give similar results to those which measure [Na$^+$] in total plasma. Most commonly used methods for measuring [Na$^+$] measure the amount of Na$^+$ in a given volume of plasma. These methods include flame photometry, and ion-selective electrode methods in which the plasma is diluted before measurement. If the lipid or protein fraction is markedly increased, even if the [Na$^+$] in plasma water is normal, the amount of Na$^+$ in a given volume of plasma will be lower than normal, since there will be less water present than normal. The diagnosis can be confirmed by measuring plasma [Na$^+$] in undiluted plasma using a direct ion-selective electrode, which measures the [Na$^+$] in the plasma water (strictly speaking, the Na$^+$ activity), or by measuring plasma osmolality. In the absence of another cause of true hyponatraemia, the results of these measurements will be normal.

• *Hyperosmolar hyponatraemia* This may be due to hyperglycaemia, administration of mannitol or occasionally other causes. The hyponatraemia mainly reflects the shift of water out of the cells into the ECF in response to osmotic effects, other than those due to Na$^+$, across cell membranes. Treatment should be directed to the cause of the hyperosmolality rather than to the hyponatraemia.

Hypernatraemia

This is the most common cause of increased tonicity of body fluids. It is nearly always due to water deficit rather than Na$^+$ excess. The ICF volume is decreased due to movement of water out of cells.

Hypernatraemia with decreased body sodium

This is the most common group (Table 2.6). It is usually due to extrarenal loss of hypotonic fluid. The nature and effects of the disturbance of fluid balance can be thought of as comprising the consequences of the combination of two components:

• Loss of isotonic fluid, which causes reduction in ECF volume, with hypotension, shock and oliguria. The physiological response is high urine osmolality and low urine [Na$^+$] of less than 20 mmol/L.

• Loss of water, which causes volume reduction of both ICF and ECF and consequent hypernatraemia.

Urinary loss of hypotonic fluid sometimes occurs due to renal disease or to osmotic diuresis; in these patients, urine [Na$^+$] is likely to be greater than 20 mmol/L. The most common cause of hypernatraemia associated with an osmotic diuresis is hyperglycaemia.

Treatment should initially aim to replace the deficit of isotonic fluid by infusing isotonic saline or, if the deficit is large, hypotonic saline.

Hypernatraemia with normal body sodium

These patients (Table 2.6) have a pure water deficit, as may occur when insensible water losses are very high and insufficient water is drunk as replacement (e.g. in hot climates, in unconscious patients or in patients with a high fever). The urine has a

Table 2.6 Causes of hypernatraemia

Body sodium	Categories	Examples
Decreased body Na$^+$ (loss of H$_2$O > Na$^+$)	Extrarenal	Sweating, diarrhoea
	Renal	Osmotic diuresis (e.g. diabetes mellitus)
Normal body Na$^+$ (loss of H$_2$O only)	Extrarenal	Fever, high-temperature climates
	Via kidneys	Diabetes insipidus, prolonged unconsciousness
Increased body Na$^+$ (retention of Na$^+$ > H$_2$O)	Steroid excess	Steroid treatment, Cushing's syndrome, Conn's syndrome
	Intake of Na$^+$	Self-induced or iatrogenic, oral or parenteral

high osmolality, and its Na$^+$ content depends on Na$^+$ intake.

Hypernatraemia with normal body Na$^+$ also occurs in diabetes insipidus (p. 58) due to excessive renal water loss. This loss is normally replaced by drinking. However, dehydration may develop if the patient is unable to drink, as may occur in very young children or in unconscious patients. The urine has a low osmolality and its Na$^+$ content depends on Na$^+$ intake.

Treatment should aim to rehydrate these patients fairly slowly, to avoid causing acute shifts of water into cells, especially those of the brain, which may have accommodated to the hyperosmolality by increasing its intracellular solute concentration. Water, administered orally, is the simplest treatment. IV therapy may be necessary, with 5% glucose or glucose–saline.

Hypernatraemia with increased body sodium

This is relatively uncommon (Table 2.6). Mild hypernatraemia may be caused by an excess of mineralocorticoids or glucocorticoids. More often, it occurs if excess Na$^+$ is administered therapeutically (e.g. NaHCO$_3$ during resuscitation). Treatment may be with diuretics or, rarely, by renal dialysis.

Other chemical investigations in fluid balance disorders

Several other chemical investigations, in addition to plasma [Na$^+$], may help when the history or clinical examination suggests that there is a disorder of fluid balance.

Blood specimens

Plasma urea and plasma creatinine Hypovolaemia is usually associated with a reduced GFR, and so with raised plasma [urea] and [creatinine]. Plasma [urea] may increase before plasma [creatinine] in the early stages of water and Na$^+$ depletion (p. 55).

Plasma chloride Alterations in plasma [Cl$^-$] parallel those in plasma [Na$^+$], except in the presence of

some acid–base disturbances (p. 44). Chloride measurements are rarely of value in assessing disturbances of fluid balance.

Plasma albumin This may help to assess acute changes in intravascular volume, and may be useful in following changes in patients with fluid balance disorders over time. Plasma [albumin] should be measured in patients with oedema, to find out whether hypoalbuminaemia is present as a contributory cause, and to determine its severity.

Plasma osmolality Plasma osmolality usually parallels plasma [Na$^+$] and can be estimated by calculation (p. 16), but may be of value when a defect in vasopressin action is suspected to be responsible for a fluid–electrolyte disorder. Plasma osmolality measurements are also of interest when it seems likely that the calculated osmolality and measured osmolality might differ significantly. This occurs when:

• There is marked hyperproteinaemia or hypertriglyceridaemia, causing a low plasma water concentration.

• Significant amounts of foreign low molecular mass materials (e.g. ethanol, ethylene glycol, glycine) which will not contribute to calculated osmolality are present in plasma.

In both these examples, the finding of a marked discrepancy between the measured osmolality and the calculated osmolarity may be of diagnostic value.

Urine specimens

Urine osmolality

Measurements of urine osmolality are of value in the investigation of:

• *Polyuria* A relatively concentrated urine suggests that polyuria is due to an osmotic diuretic (e.g. glucose), whereas a dilute urine suggests that there is primary polydipsia or diabetes insipidus (p. 57). Patients with chronic renal failure may also have polyuria, with a urine osmolality that is usually within 50 mmol/kg of the plasma value.

- *Oliguria* Where acute renal failure is suspected (p. 61).
- *SIADH* In patients with SIADH (p. 22), the urine osmolality is not maximally dilute, despite a dilutional hyponatraemia.

Urine sodium

This normally varies with Na$^+$ intake. Measurements of 24 h output, taken with the clinical findings, may be useful in the diagnosis of disturbances in Na$^+$ and water handling, and in planning fluid replacement.

Patients with low urine [Na$^+$] This is an appropriate response in patients who are volume depleted, with oliguria and normally functioning kidneys; urine [Na$^+$] is usually less than 10 mmol/L, and urine flow increases after volume repletion. Na$^+$ retention and low urine [Na$^+$] occur in the secondary hyperaldosteronism associated with congestive cardiac failure, liver disease and hypoproteinaemic states, and in Cushing's syndrome and Conn's syndrome.

Patients with natriuresis In hyponatraemic patients with evidence of ECF volume depletion, continuing natriuresis (i.e. urine [Na$^+$] > 20 mmol/L) suggests either:
- Volume depletion that is so severe as to have led to acute renal failure. The patient will be oliguric, with rising plasma [urea] and [creatinine]; diuresis fails to occur after volume repletion.
- In the absence of acute renal failure, this occurs with overzealous diuretic use, with salt-losing nephritis and with defects in the hypothalamic–pituitary–adrenal (HPA) axis, including Addison's disease.

Natriuresis may also occur in hyponatraemic states associated with SIADH or acute water intoxication and where ECF volume is normal or even increased.

Potassium balance

Potassium is the main intracellular cation. About 98% of total body K$^+$ is in cells, the balance (~50 mmol) being in the ECF. There is a large concentration gradient across cell membranes, the ICF [K$^+$] being about 150 mmol/L compared with about 4 mmol/L in ECF.

Internal distribution

This is determined by movements across the cell membrane. Factors causing K$^+$ to move out of cells include hypertonicity, acidosis, insulin lack and severe cell damage or cell death. Potassium moves into cells if there is alkalosis, or when insulin is given.

External balance

This is mainly determined, in the absence of GI disease, by intake of K$^+$ and by its renal excretion. A typical 'Western' diet contains 20–100 mmol of K$^+$ daily; this intake is normally closely matched by the urinary excretion. The control of renal K$^+$ excretion is not fully understood, but the following points have been established:
- Nearly all the K$^+$ filtered at the glomerulus is reabsorbed in the proximal tubule. Less than 10% reaches the distal tubule, where the main regulation of K$^+$ excretion occurs. Secretion of K$^+$ in response to alterations in dietary intake occurs in the distal tubule, the cortical collecting tubule and the collecting duct.
- The distal tubule is an important site of Na$^+$ reabsorption. When Na$^+$ is reabsorbed, the tubular lumen becomes electronegative in relation to the adjacent cell, and cations in the cell (e.g. K$^+$, H$^+$) move into the lumen to balance the charge. The rate of movement of K$^+$ into the lumen depends on there being sufficient delivery of Na$^+$ to the distal tubule, as well as on the rate of urine flow and on the concentration of K$^+$ in the tubular cell.
- The concentration of K$^+$ in the tubular cell depends largely on adenosine triphosphatase-dependent (ATPase-dependent) Na$^+$/K$^+$ exchange with peritubular fluid (i.e. the ECF). This is affected by mineralocorticoids, by acid–base changes and by ECF [K$^+$]. The tubular cell [K$^+$] tends to be increased by hyperkalaemia, by mineralocorticoid excess and by alkalosis, all of which tend to cause an increase in K$^+$ excretion.

Abnormalities of plasma potassium concentration

The reference range for plasma [K$^+$] is 3.3–4.7 mmol/L. The important, and often life-threatening, clinical manifestations of abnormalities of plasma [K$^+$] are those relating to disturbances of neuromuscular excitability and of cardiac conduction. Any patient with an abnormal plasma [K$^+$], who also shows signs of muscle weakness or of a cardiac arrhythmia, should have cardiac monitoring with electrocardiography (ECG). The abnormal plasma [K$^+$] should be corrected, with appropriate monitoring during treatment.

Hypokalaemia (Table 2.7) must not be equated with K$^+$ depletion, and hyperkalaemia (Table 2.8) must not be equated with K$^+$ excess. Although most patients with K$^+$ depletion have hypokalaemia, and most patients with K$^+$ excess may have hyper-kalaemia, acute changes in the distribution of K$^+$ in the body can offset any effects of depletion or excess. To generalise, acute changes in plasma [K$^+$] are usually caused by redistribution of K$^+$ across cell membranes, whereas chronic changes in plasma [K$^+$] are usually due to abnormal external K$^+$ balance.

Hypokalaemia

Altered internal distribution: shift of K$^+$ into cells

- *Acute shifts* of K$^+$ into the cell may occur in alkalosis, but the hypokalaemia may be more closely related to the increased renal excretion of K$^+$. Patients with respiratory alkalosis caused by voluntary hyperventilation rarely show hypokalaemia, but patients on prolonged assisted ventilation may have low plasma [K$^+$] if the alveolar P_{CO_2} is low for a relatively long period.
- *Insulin* in high dosage, given intravenously, promotes the uptake of K$^+$ by liver and muscle. Acute shifts of K$^+$ into cells may occur in diabetic ketoacidosis (DKA) shortly after starting treatment.
- *Adrenaline* and other β-adrenergic agonists stimulate the uptake of K$^+$ into cells. This may contribute to the hypokalaemia appearing in patients after myocardial infarction, since catecholamine levels are likely to be increased in these patients. Hypokalaemic effects of salbutamol (a synthetic β-adrenergic agonist) have also been described.
- *Cellular incorporation of K$^+$* may cause hypokalaemia in states where cell mass rapidly increases. Examples include the treatment of severe megaloblastic anaemia with vitamin B$_{12}$ or folate, and the parenteral re-feeding of wasted patients (especially if insulin is also administered). It also occurs when there are rapidly proliferating leukaemic cells.

Altered external balance: deficient intake of K$^+$

Prolonged deficient intake of K$^+$ can lead to a decrease in total body K$^+$, eventually manifested as hypokalaemia. This may occur in chronic and

Table 2.7 Causes of hypokalaemia

Cause	Categories	Examples
Artefact		Specimen collected from an infusion site or near to one
Redistribution of K$^+$ between ECF and ICF		Alkalosis, familial periodic paralysis (hypokalaemic form), treatment of hyperglycaemia with insulin
Abnormal external balance	Inadequate intake	Anorexia nervosa, alcoholism (both rare)
	Abnormal losses from the GI tract	Vomiting, nasogastric aspiration, diarrhoea, fistula, laxative abuse, villous adenoma of the colon
	Abnormal losses from the renal tract	Diuretics, osmotic diuresis, renal tubular acidosis, aldosteronism, Cushing's syndrome, Bartter's syndrome

severe malnutrition in the developing world, in the elderly on deficient diets, and in anorexia nervosa.

Altered external balance: excessive losses of K$^+$

- *Hyperaldosteronism*, both primary and secondary, and Cushing's syndrome (including that due to steroid administration) cause excessive renal K$^+$ loss due to increased K$^+$ transfer into the distal tubule in response to increased reabsorption of Na$^+$ from the tubular lumen. Mineralocorticoid excess also favours transfer of K$^+$ into the tubular cell from the interstitial fluid in exchange for Na$^+$. Urinary K$^+$ loss in hyperaldosteronism returns to normal if there is dietary Na$^+$ restriction, which limits distal tubular delivery of Na$^+$.
- *Diuretic therapy* increases renal K$^+$ excretion by causing increased delivery of Na$^+$ to the distal tubule and increased urine flow rate. Diuretics may also cause hypovolaemia, with consequent secondary hyperaldosteronism.
- *Acidosis and alkalosis* both affect renal K$^+$ excretion in ways that are not fully understood. Acute acidosis causes K$^+$ retention, and acute alkalosis causes increased K$^+$ excretion. However, chronic acidosis and chronic alkalosis both cause increased K$^+$ excretion.
- *GI fluid losses* often cause K$^+$ depletion. However, if gastric fluid is lost in large quantity, renal K$^+$ loss (due to the combined effects of the resultant secondary hyperaldosteronism and the metabolic alkalosis) is the main cause of the K$^+$ depletion, rather than the direct loss of K$^+$ in gastric juice. In diarrhoea or laxative abuse, the increased losses of K$^+$ in faeces may cause K$^+$ depletion.
- *Renal disease* does not usually cause excessive K$^+$ loss. However, a few tubular abnormalities are associated with K$^+$ depletion, in the absence of diuretic therapy:
  - *Renal tubular acidosis* The K$^+$ loss is caused both by the chronic acidosis and, in patients with proximal renal tubular acidosis (p. 59), by increased delivery of Na$^+$ to the distal tubule. In distal renal tubular acidosis, the inability to excrete H$^+$ may cause a compensatory transfer of K$^+$ to the tubular fluid.
  - *Bartter's syndrome* The syndrome consists of persistent hypokalaemia with secondary hyperaldosteronism in association with a metabolic alkalosis; patients are normotensive. There is increased delivery of Na$^+$ to the distal tubule, caused by an abnormality of chloride reabsorption in the loop of Henle.

Table 2.8 Causes of hyperkalaemia

Cause	Categories	Examples
Artefact		Trauma during blood collection, delay in separating plasma/serum, freezing blood
Redistribution of K$^+$ between ECF and ICF		Acidosis, hypertonicity, tissue and tumour necrosis (e.g. burns, leukaemia), haemolytic disorders, hyperkalaemic familial periodic paralysis, insulin deficiency
Abnormal external balance	Increased intake	Excessive oral intake of K$^+$ (rare by itself)
	Decreased renal output*	
	Renal causes	**1** Renal failure, oliguric (acute and chronic); inappropriate oral intake in chronic failure
		2 Failure of renal tubular response, due to systemic lupus erythematosus, K$^+$-sparing diuretics, chronic interstitial nephritis
	Adrenal causes	Addison's disease, selective hypoaldosteronism

* With or without inappropriate intake.

- *Excessive sweating* Sweat [K$^+$] is higher than ECF concentrations, so excessive sweat losses can result in potassium depletion and hypokalaemia.

Other causes of hypokalaemia

Artefact Collection of a blood sample from a vein near to a site of an IV infusion, where the fluid has a low [K$^+$].

Hyperkalaemia

Plasma [K$^+$] over 6.5 mmol/L requires urgent treatment. IV calcium gluconate has a rapid but short-lived effect in countering the neuromuscular effects of hyperkalaemia. Treatment with glucose and insulin causes K$^+$ to pass into the ICF. However, treatment with ion-exchange resins or renal dialysis may be needed.

Altered internal distribution of K$^+$

- *Acidosis* The effects of acidosis on internal K$^+$ balance are complicated. As a general rule, acidotic states are often accompanied by hyperkalaemia, as K$^+$ moves from the ICF into the ECF. Although this is the case for acute respiratory acidosis, and for both acute and chronic metabolic acidosis, it is more unusual to find hyperkalaemia in chronic respiratory acidosis. It is important to note that a high plasma [K$^+$] may be accompanied by a reduced total body K$^+$ as a result of excessive urinary K$^+$ losses in both chronic respiratory acidosis and metabolic acidosis.
- *Hypertonic states* In these, K$^+$ moves out of cells, possibly because of the increased intracellular [K$^+$] caused by the reduction in ICF volume.
- *Uncontrolled diabetes mellitus* The lack of insulin prevents K$^+$ from entering cells. This results in hyperkalaemia, despite the K$^+$ loss caused by the osmotic diuresis.
- *Cellular necrosis* This may lead to excessive release of K$^+$ and may result in hyperkalaemia. Extensive cell damage may be a feature of rhabdomyolysis (e.g. crush injury), haemolysis, burns or tumour necrosis (e.g. in the treatment of leukaemias).

- *Digoxin poisoning* causes hyperkalaemia by inhibiting the Na$^+$/K$^+$ ATPase pump. Therapeutic doses do not have this effect.

Altered external balance: increased intake of K$^+$

Increased K$^+$ intake only rarely causes accumulation of K$^+$ in the body, since the normal kidney can excrete a large K$^+$ load. However, if there is renal impairment, K$^+$ may accumulate if salt substitutes are administered, or excessive amounts of some fruit drinks are drunk or if excessive potassium replacement therapy accompanies diuretic administration.

Altered external balance: decreased excretion of K$^+$

- *Intrinsic renal disease* This is an important cause of hyperkalaemia. It may occur in acute renal failure and in the later stages of chronic renal failure. In patients with renal disease that largely affects the renal medulla, hyperkalaemia may occur earlier. This may be because increased K$^+$ secretion from the collecting duct, an important adaptive response in the damaged kidney, is lost earlier in patients with medullary disease.
- *Mineralocorticoid deficiency* This may occur in Addison's disease and in secondary adrenocortical hypofunction. In both, K$^+$ retention may occur. This is not an invariable feature, presumably because other mechanisms can facilitate K$^+$ excretion. Selective hypoaldosteronism, accompanied by normal glucocorticoid production, may occur in patients with diabetes mellitus in whom juxtaglomerular sclerosis probably interferes with renin production. ACE inhibitors, by reducing AII (and therefore aldosterone) levels, may lead to increased plasma [K$^+$], but severe problems are only likely to occur in the presence of renal failure.
- Patients treated with *K$^+$-sparing diuretics* (e.g. spironolactone, amiloride) may fail to respond to aldosterone. If the K$^+$ intake is high in these

patients, or if they have renal insufficiency or selective hypoaldosteronism, this can lead to dangerous hyperkalaemia.

Other causes of hyperkalaemia

• *Artefact* This is the most common cause of hyperkalaemia. When red cells, or occasionally white cells or platelets, are left in contact with plasma or serum for too long, K^+ leaks from the cells. In any blood specimen that does not have its plasma or serum separated from the cells within about 3 h, $[K^+]$ is likely to be spuriously high. Blood specimens collected into potassium EDTA, an anti-coagulant widely used for haematological specimens, have greatly increased plasma $[K^+]$. Sometimes, doctors decant part of a blood specimen initially collected by mistake into potassium EDTA into another container, and send this for biochemical analysis. A clue to the source of this artefact, which may increase plasma $[K^+]$ to 'lethal' levels (e.g. >8 mmol/L), is an accompanying very low plasma [calcium], due to chelation of Ca^{2+} with EDTA.

• *Pseudohyperkalaemia* Pseudohyperkalaemia can occur in acute and chronic myeloproliferative disorders, chronic lymphocytic leukaemia and severe thrombocytosis as a result of cell lysis during venepuncture, or if there is any delay in the separation of plasma following specimen collection, since there are large numbers of abnormally fragile white cells present.

Other investigations in disordered K^+ metabolism

• *Urine K^+* measurements may be of help in determining the source of K^+ depletion in patients with unexplained hypokalaemia, but are otherwise of little value. A 24-h urine collection should be made. If the patient is Na^+ depleted, this will induce aldosterone secretion, making the results difficult or impossible to interpret, so urine $[Na^+]$ should also be checked to ensure this is adequate.

• *Plasma total* $[CO_2]$ (p. 43) may prove helpful in the investigation of disorders of K^+ balance, since

metabolic acidosis and metabolic alkalosis are commonly associated with abnormalities of K^+ homeostasis. It is rarely necessary to assess acid–base status fully when investigating disturbances of K^+ metabolism; plasma [total CO_2] often suffices.

• Other investigations may be indicated by the history of the patient's illness and the findings on clinical examination. Hypomagnesaemia may be associated with hypokalaemia, so $[Mg^{2+}]$ should be checked in cases of prolonged or unexplained hypokalaemia.

Fluid and electrolyte balance in surgical patients

Accidental and operative trauma produce several metabolic effects. These include breakdown of protein, release of K^+ from cells and a consequent K^+ deficit due to urinary loss, temporary retention of water, use of glycogen reserves, gluconeogenesis, mobilisation of fat reserves and a tendency to ketosis that sometimes progresses to a metabolic acidosis. Hormonal responses include increased secretion of adrenal corticosteroids, with temporary abolition of negative feedback control and increased secretion of aldosterone and vasopressin.

These metabolic responses to trauma are physiological and appropriate. They are the reason why post-operative states are such frequent causes of temporary disturbances in electrolyte metabolism. Most patients after major surgery have a temporarily impaired ability to excrete a water load or a Na^+ load; they also have a plasma [urea] that is often raised due to tissue catabolism. Injudicious fluid therapy, especially in the first 48 h after operation, may 'correct' the chemical abnormalities, for example by lowering the plasma [urea], but only by causing retention of fluid and the possibility of acute water intoxication.

Patients who present for emergency surgery with disturbances of water and electrolyte metabolism already developed should have the severity of the disturbances assessed and corrective measures instituted pre-operatively. This usually

Table 2.9 Compostion of intravenous fluids

	Na+ (mmol/L)	K+ (mmol/L)	Cl- (mmol/L)	Osmolarity (mosm/L)
Plasma	136–145	3.5–5.0	98–105	280–300
0.9% ('normal') saline	154	0	154	308
5% dextrose	0	0	0	278
Dextrose 4%, saline 0.18%	30	0	30	283
Ringer's lactate	130	4	109	273
Hartmann's	131	5	111	275

involves clinical assessment and the measurement of plasma urea, creatinine, [Na+] and [K+] as an emergency (and see below). Ideally, fluid and electrolyte disturbances should be corrected before surgery.

Patients admitted for major elective surgery, who may be liable to develop disturbances of water and electrolyte balance post-operatively, require pre-operative determination of baseline values for plasma urea, creatinine, [Na+] and [K+].

Post-operatively, any tendency for patients to develop disturbances of water and electrolyte balance can be minimised by regular clinical assessment. In addition to plasma 'electrolytes', fluid balance charts and measurement of 24-h urinary losses of Na+ and K+, or losses from a fistula, can provide information of value in calculating the approximate volume and composition of fluid needed to replace continuing losses.

Intravenous fluid administration

Fluid administration, whether oral or intravenous, may be required for normal daily maintenance, the replacement of abnormal losses, or for resuscitation. Food and fluids should be provided orally or enterally when possible, and any intravenous infusion should not be continued longer than necessary. Decisions regarding prescription of fluids should take the stress responses described above into account as well as an assessment of any current excesses or deficits, normal maintenance requirements, and the volumes and compositions of any abnormal (e.g. intestinal) losses.

The most reliable assessment of patients' fluid status uses invasive cardiac monitoring, but this is unlikely to be practical except in the setting of intensive care. Under most circumstances fluid requirements are assessed and monitored by the usual clinical approaches of history, examination and laboratory measurements. Items of note in the history and examination are any abnormal losses or excesses, changes in weight, fluid balance charts, urine output, blood pressure, capillary refill, autonomic responses, skin turgor and dry mouth. Laboratory measurements include serum [Na+], [K+], [HCO₃⁻] and [Cl⁻] (the latter two on point of care blood gas machines) and urine [Na+] (and possibly urine [K+] and [urea]).

Normal daily maintenace requirements for an adult are 50–100 mmol of sodium, 40–80 mmol of potassium and 1.5–2.5 L of water. Historically these requirements have been met using a combination of 0.9% saline and 5% dextrose with added potassium as required (see Table 2.9). Current guidelines encourage the use of balanced salt solutions such as Hartmann's solutions or Ringer's lactate/acetate (see References), especially for the purposes of crystalloid fluid resuscitation or replacement of abnormal losses.

Further Reading

Intensive Care Society (2008) *British Consensus Guidelines on Intravenous Fluid Therapy for Adult Surgical Patients*. Intensive Care Society, London.

Keypoints

- Compared with the ECF compartment (volume ~14 L), the ICF is much larger (~28 L) and has a relatively low [Na⁺] and high [K⁺].
- Gains or losses of water are distributed through both the ECF and ICF. Intake and output are controlled by thirst and vasopressin, respectively.
- In general, the ECF volume parallels total body sodium, and is normally mainly controlled by aldosterone. Sodium retention will expand ECF volume, and vice versa.
- Acute losses of isotonic fluid cause hypovolaemia, with clinical symptoms of hypotension, etc., but not hyponatraemia, at least in the short term.
- Losses of hypotonic fluid, for example in sweat, or of water often result in hypernatraemia.
- Increased vasopressin secretion is part of the metabolic response to trauma or surgery. Care should be taken to avoid giving excess hypotonic fluids during or after surgery, since there is a risk of acute water intoxication.
- Changes in plasma [K⁺] usually result from acute movements across the cell membrane or, in the longer term, whole-body gains or losses.
- Hyperkalaemia, especially of acute onset, can cause potentially lethal neuromuscular abnormalities, and should be treated urgently with appropriate biochemical and ECG monitoring.

Case 2.1

A 45-year-old man was brought into the A&E department late at night in a comatose state. It was impossible to obtain a history from him, and clinical examination was difficult, but it was noted that he smelt strongly of alcohol. The following analyses were requested urgently.

Why is his measured osmolality so high?

Serum	Result	Reference range
Urea	4.7	2.5–6.6 mmol/L
Na⁺	137	132–144 mmol/L
K⁺	4.3	3.6–5.0 mmol/L
Total CO_2	20	24–30 mmol/L
Glucose	4.2	mmol/L
Osmolality	465	280–290 mmol/kg

Comments: The osmolality can be calculated as 291.5, using the formula on p. 16. The difference between this figure and the value for the directly measured osmolality (465 mmol/L) could be explained by the presence of another low molecular mass solute in plasma. From the patient's history, it seemed that ethanol might be contributing significantly to the plasma osmolality, and plasma [ethanol] was measured the following day, on the residue of the specimen collected at the time of emergency admission. The result was 170 mmol/L, very close to the difference between the measured and calculated osmolalities.

Case 2.2

A 76-year-old man was making reasonable post-operative progress following major abdominal surgery for a carcinoma of the colon. Two days after the operation he appeared well, and there were no signs of dehydration or oedema. The following results were obtained:

What is the most likely cause of this man's low plasma [Na⁺]?

Serum	Result	Reference range
Urea	4.3	2.5–6.6 mmol/L
Na⁺	128	132–144 mmol/L
K⁺	4.3	3.6–5.0 mmol/L
Total CO_2	25	24–30 mmol/L

Comments: Hyponatraemia is often seen in post-operative patients receiving IV fluids. At this time the ability to excrete water is reduced as part of the metabolic response to trauma. If excessive amounts of hypotonic fluids (usually 5% dextrose) are given, hyponatraemia will result. It may also be at least partly due to the 'sick cell syndrome'. There are usually no clinical features of water intoxication, and all that is required is review of the patient's fluid balance, and adjustment of the prescription for IV fluids. This man had received a total of 4.5 L of fluid since his operation, and his fluid balance chart showed that he had a positive balance of 2 L.

Case 2.3

A 63-year-old coal miner had had a persistent chest infection, with cough and sputum, for the previous 2 months. He was a smoker. Clinical examination revealed finger clubbing, crackles and wheezes throughout the chest, and a small pleural effusion. There were no signs of dehydration or oedema. Examination of blood and of a random urine specimen yielded the following results:

What is the most likely cause of this man's low plasma [Na^+] and osmolality?

Serum	Result	Reference range
Urea	2.3	2.5–6.6 mmol/L
Na^+	118	135–145 mmol/L
K^+	4.3	3.6–5.0 mmol/L
Total CO_2	26	22–30 mmol/L
Osmolality	260	280–296 mmol/L

Urine	Result	
Na^+	74	mmol/L
Osmolality	625	mmol/kg

Comments: This patient is not diluting his urine in response to low plasma osmolality and hyponatraemia: this suggests inappropriate ADH secretion. There tends to be a continuing natriuresis despite the hyponatraemia in these patients, as the retention of water leads to mild expansion of the ECF, and hence reduced aldosterone secretion. The presence of a dilutional hyponatraemia is also supported by the low plasma [urea]. Before diagnosing the syndrome of inappropriate ADH secretion (SIADH, p. 22), it is important to exclude adrenal, pituitary and renal disease. In this patient, possible explanations include the recurrent chest infections, and/or an underlying bronchogenic carcinoma, with ectopic secretion of ADH.

Case 2.4

A 71-year-old woman was found by a neighbour drowsy and unwell. She had had an upper respiratory tract infection several weeks previously, and had been very slow to recover from this. She had been increasingly thirsty over this period. The only past history was of diabetes mellitus, diagnosed about 5 years previously and controlled by diet. On examination, she was very dehydrated, but her breath did not smell of ketones. The following results were obtained:

Why is her sodium so high?

Serum	Result	Reference range
Urea	28.2	0.5–6.6 mmol/L
Na^+	156	135–145 mmol/L
K^+	4.4	3.6–5.0 mmol/L
Total CO_2	26	22–30 mmol/L
Glucose	38.2	mmol/L

Comments: She has hyperglycaemic, hyperosmolar, non-ketotic metabolic decompensation of her diabetes. The onset of this is usually slower than that of ketoacidosis and, possibly because vomiting is less likely, patients do not become acutely ill so rapidly. The prolonged osmotic diuresis due to the severe hyperglycaemia results in large losses of water, often in excess of the sodium loss, resulting in hypernatraemia. GFR is reduced, causing raised plasma [urea]. Treatment requires the replacement of the fluid and electrolyte losses, and the use of insulin to restore the glucose concentration to normal and prevent the continuing osmotic diuresis. (See also Chapter 12.)

Case 2.5

A young man was trapped underneath a car in a road traffic accident, and suffered multiple fractures. Despite adequate fluid intake over the next 36 h, he was noted to be oliguric. The following results were obtained:

Serum	Result	Reference range
Urea	22.1	2.5–6.6 mmol/L
Na$^+$	133	135–145 mmol/L
K$^+$	6.1	3.6–5.0 mmol/L
Creatinine	214	60–120 μmol/L

Why is the potassium high?

Comments: The crush injuries, with associated rhabdomyolysis, may have caused hyperkalaemia for at least two reasons: (1) release of K$^+$ from the damaged muscle and (2) acute renal failure caused by release of myoglobin, which is filtered at the glomerulus but precipitates in the distal nephron. This impairs the ability of the kidney to excrete K$^+$.

Case 2.6

A 64-year-old man was admitted on a Sunday for an elective operation on his nasal sinuses; his previous hospital notes were not available. He appeared to be fit for operation on clinical examination, and his pre-operative ECG was normal, but the following results were obtained on a blood specimen analysed as part of the routine pre-operative assessment:

How would you interpret the hyperkalaemia in relation to the findings on clinical examination and the normal ECG recording? Would your comments be influenced by the information that became available later that day, when the patient's medical records were received, that he had chronic lymphocytic leukaemia?

Serum	Result	Reference range
Urea	7.0	2.5–6.6 mmol/L
Na$^+$	135	135–145 mmol/L
K$^+$	8.8	3.6–5.0 mmol/L
Total CO$_2$	30	22–30 mmol/L

Comments: The ECG changes that are associated with hyperkalaemia are not correlated closely with the level of plasma [K$^+$], but it would be most unlikely for the ECG to be normal in a patient whose plasma [K$^+$] was 8.8 mmol/L. It is much more likely that the hyperkalaemia was an artefact caused by release of K$^+$ from blood cells (in this case from lymphocytes).

Chapter 3

Acid–base balance and oxygen transport

The hydrogen ion concentration of ECF is normally maintained within very close limits. To achieve this, each day the body must dispose of

1 About 20 000 mmol of CO_2 generated by tissue metabolism. CO_2 itself is not an acid, but combines with water to form the weak acid, carbonic acid.

2 About 40–80 mmol of non-volatile acids, mainly sulphur-containing organic acids, which are excreted by the kidneys.

This chapter deals with the clinical disturbances that may arise in respiratory disorders, when gaseous exchange in the lung of O_2 or CO_2 or both is impaired, and in metabolic disorders when there is either an excessive production, or loss, of non-volatile acid or an abnormality of excretion.

Transport of carbon dioxide

The CO_2 produced in tissue cells diffuses freely down a concentration gradient across the cell membrane into the ECF and red cells. This gradient is maintained because red blood cell metabolism is anaerobic, so that no CO_2 is produced there, and the concentration remains low. The following reactions then occur:

Lecture Notes: Clinical Biochemistry, 8e. By G. Beckett, S. Walker, P. Rae & P. Ashby. Published 2010 by Blackwell Publishing.

$$CO_2 + H_2O \leftrightarrow H_2CO_3 \qquad (3.1)$$

$$H_2CO_3 \leftrightarrow H^+ + HCO_3^- \qquad (3.2)$$

Reaction 3.1, the hydration of CO_2 to form carbonic acid (H_2CO_3), is slow, except in the presence of the catalyst carbonate dehydratase (also known as carbonic anhydrase). This limits its site in the blood mainly to erythrocytes, where carbonate dehydratase is located. Reaction 3.2, the ionisation of carbonic acid, then occurs rapidly and spontaneously. The H^+ ions are mainly buffered inside the red cell by haemoglobin (Hb). Hb is a more effective buffer when deoxygenated, so its buffering capacity increases as it passes through the capillary beds and gives up oxygen to the tissues. Bicarbonate ions, meanwhile, pass from the erythrocytes down their concentration gradient into plasma, in exchange for chloride ions to maintain electrical neutrality.

In the lungs, the P_{CO_2} in the alveoli is maintained at a low level by ventilation. The P_{CO_2} in the blood of the pulmonary capillaries is therefore higher than the P_{CO_2} in the alveoli, so the P_{CO_2} gradient is reversed. CO_2 diffuses into the alveoli down its concentration gradient, and is excreted by the lungs. The above reaction sequence shifts to the left, carbonate dehydratase again catalysing reaction 3.1, but this time in the reverse direction.

Renal mechanisms for HCO_3^- reabsorption and H^+ excretion

Glomerular filtrate contains the same concentration of HCO_3^- as plasma. At normal HCO_3^-, renal tubular mechanisms are responsible for reabsorbing virtually all this HCO_3^-. If this failed to occur, large amounts of HCO_3^- would be lost in the urine, resulting in an acidosis and reduction in the body's buffering capacity. In addition, the renal tubules are responsible for excreting 40–80 mmol of acid per day under normal circumstances. This will increase when there is an acidosis.

The mechanism of reabsorption of HCO_3^- is shown in Figure 3.1. HCO_3^- is not able to cross the luminal membrane of the renal tubular cells. H^+ is pumped from the tubular cell into the lumen, in exchange for Na^+. The H^+ combines with HCO_3^- to form H_2CO_3 in the lumen. This dissociates to give water and CO_2, which readily diffuses into the cell. In the cell, CO_2 recombines with water under the influence of carbonate dehydratase to give H_2CO_3. This dissociates to H^+ and HCO_3^-. The HCO_3^- then passes across the basal membrane of the cell into the interstitial fluid. This mechanism results in the reabsorption of filtered HCO_3^-, but no net excretion of H^+.

The net excretion of H^+ relies on the same renal tubular cell reactions as HCO_3^- reabsorption, but occurs after luminal HCO_3^- has been reabsorbed, and depends on the presence of other suitable buffers in the urine (Figure 3.2). The main urinary buffer is phosphate, most of which is present as HPO_4^{2-}, which can combine with H^+ to form

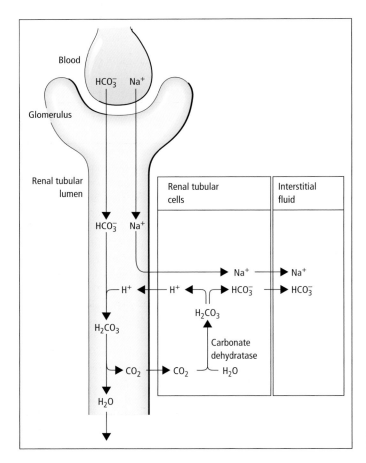

Figure 3.1 Reabsorption of bicarbonate in the renal tubule.

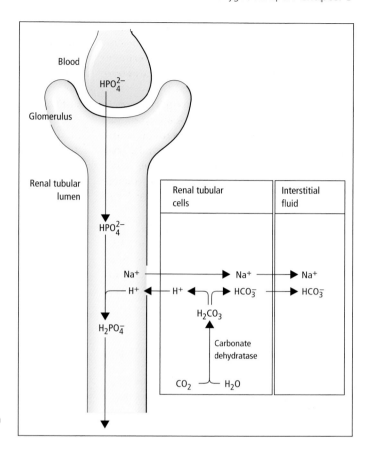

Figure 3.2 Renal hydrogen ion excretion.

$H_2PO_4^-$. Ammonia can also act as a urinary buffer, and is formed by the deamination of glutamine in renal tubular cells under the influence of the enzyme glutaminase. Ammonia readily diffuses across the cell membrane into the tubular lumen, where it combines with H^+ to form NH_4^+. This does not pass across cell membranes, so passive reabsorption is prevented. Glutaminase is induced in chronic acidoses, stimulating increased ammonia production and therefore increased H^+ excretion in the form of NH_4^+ ions.

Buffering of hydrogen ions

The lungs and the kidneys together maintain the overall acid–base balance. However, the ECF needs to be protected against rapid changes in [H^+]. This is achieved by various buffer systems. A buffer system consists of a weak (incompletely dissociated) acid in equilibrium with its conjugate base and H^+. The capacity of a buffer for H^+ is related to its concentration and the position of its equilibrium, being most effective at the [H^+] at which the acid and conjugate base are present in equal concentrations. Thus, Hb and plasma proteins act as efficient buffers in blood, since they are abundant, and at a physiological [H^+] of approximately 40 nmol/L have side groups that exist in an appropriate equilibrium. At this [H^+], the bicarbonate buffer system has an equilibrium that is far removed from the ideal, with HCO_3^- being about 20 times greater than [H_2CO_3]. However, the effectiveness of the bicarbonate system is greatly enhanced *in vivo* by the fact that H_2CO_3 is readily produced or disposed of by interconversion with CO_2. Furthermore, physiological control mechanisms act on this buffer system to maintain both P_{CO_2} and $[HCO_3^-]$ within limits, and hence to control $[H^+]$.

Any physiological buffer system could be used to investigate and define acid–base status, but the H_2CO_3/HCO_3^- buffer system is the most appropriate for this purpose, due to its physiological importance.

The Henderson equation simply applies the law of mass action to this buffer system, to give

$$[H^+] = K \times [H_2CO_3]/[HCO_3^-] \qquad (3.3)$$

The $[H_2CO_3]$ term can be replaced by SP_{CO_2}, where S is the solubility coefficient of CO_2, since H_2CO_3 is in equilibrium with dissolved CO_2. Substituting numerical values, at 37 °C, this equation becomes

$$[H^+] = 180 \times [P_{CO_2}]/[HCO_3^-] \qquad (3.4)$$

(where $[H^+]$ is measured in nmol/L, P_{CO_2} in kilopascals (kPa) and HCO_3^- in mmol/L).

The changes discussed above are caused by changes in the equilibria of chemical reactions, and must be distinguished from the acid–base changes that occur as a result of respiratory or renal physiological mechanisms operating to return plasma $[H^+]$ towards normal. For example, if there is a rise in P_{CO_2}, this will be reflected immediately by a rise in both plasma $[H^+]$ and $[HCO_3^-]$ due to a shift to the right in reactions 3.1 and 3.2 above. The concentrations of H^+ and HCO_3^- are very different, $[H^+]$ being measured in nanomoles per litre while HCO_3^- is measured in in millimoles per litre. The same rise in each may therefore result in a substantial relative increase in $[H^+]$, but a relatively imperceptible increase in HCO_3^-. Only after several hours would the effect of physiological renal compensatory changes become evident.

Investigating acid–base balance

The acid–base status of a patient can be fully characterised by measuring $[H^+]$ and P_{CO_2} in arterial or arterialised capillary blood specimens; HCO_3^- is then obtained by calculation (reaction 3.4).

Although standard bicarbonate, and base excess or deficit are still sometimes reported, these derived values are not necessary for the understanding of acid–base disturbances.

Collection and transport of specimens

Arterial blood specimens are the most appropriate for assessing acid–base status. However, unless an arterial cannula is *in situ*, these specimens may be difficult to obtain for repeated assessment of patients whose clinical condition is changing rapidly. Arterialised capillary blood specimens are also widely used, especially in infants and children. It is essential for the capillary blood to flow freely, and collection of satisfactory samples may be impossible if there is peripheral vasoconstriction or the blood flow is sluggish.

Patients must be relaxed, and their breathing pattern should have settled after any temporary disturbance (e.g. due to insertion of an arterial cannula) before specimens are collected. Some patients may hyperventilate temporarily because they are apprehensive.

Blood is collected in syringes or capillary tubes that contain sufficient heparin to act as an anticoagulant; excess heparin, which is acidic, must be avoided. If ionised Ca^{2+} is to be measured on the same specimen, as is possible with some instruments, calcium-balanced heparin must be used. Specimens must be free of air bubbles, since these will equilibrate with the sample causing a rise in P_{O_2} and a fall in P_{CO_2}.

Acid–base measurements should be performed immediately after the sample has been obtained, or the specimen should be chilled until analysis. Otherwise, glycolysis (with the production of lactic acid) occurs, and the acid–base composition of the blood alters rapidly. Specimens chilled in iced water can have their analysis delayed for as long as 4 h. However, the clinical reasons that gave rise to the need for full acid–base studies usually demand more rapid answers.

Temperature effects

Acid–base measurements are nearly always made at 37 °C, but some patients may have body temperatures that are higher or lower than 37 °C. Equations are available to relate [H⁺], P_{CO_2} and P_{O_2} determined at 37 °C, to 'equivalent' values that correspond to the patient's body temperature. However, reference ranges for acid–base data have only been established by most laboratories for measurements made at 37 °C. Analytical results adjusted to values that would have been obtained at the patient's temperature, according to these equations, may therefore be difficult to interpret. If treatment aimed at reducing an acid–base disturbance (e.g. $NaHCO_3$ infusion) is given to a severely hypothermic patient, the effects of the treatment should be monitored frequently by repeating the acid–base measurements (at 37 °C).

Disturbances of acid–base status

Acid–base disorders fall into two main categories, respiratory and metabolic.
- *Respiratory disorders* A primary defect in ventilation affects the P_{CO_2}.
- *Metabolic disorders* The primary defect may be the production of non-volatile acids, or ingestion of substances that give rise to them, in excess of the kidney's ability to excrete these substances. Alternatively, the primary defect may be the loss of H⁺ from the body, or it may be the loss or retention of HCO_3^-.

Acid–base status can be understood and described on the basis of the relationships represented by reactions 3.1 and 3.2, and consideration of the Henderson equation. The following discussion is restricted mainly to consideration of simple acid–base disturbances, in which there is a single primary disturbance, normally accompanied by compensatory physiological changes that usually tend to correct plasma [H⁺] towards normal. We shall not consider mixed disturbances, where two or more primary simple disturbances are present, in any detail. Sets of illustrative acid–base results for patients with the four categories of simple disorders of acid–base status are given in Table 3.1.

Respiratory acidosis

This is caused by CO_2 retention due to hypoventilation (Table 3.2). It may accompany intrinsic lung disease, or defects in the control of ventilation, or diseases affecting the nerve supply or muscles of the chest wall or diaphragm, or disorders affecting the ribcage.

In acute respiratory acidosis, a rise in P_{CO_2} causes the equilibria in reactions 3.1 and 3.2 to shift to the right, as a result of which plasma [H⁺] and [HCO_3^-] both increase (although, as explained above, because of the large difference in their basal concentrations, the change in [HCO_3^-] will be relatively small or imperceptible). Equilibration of H⁺ with body buffer systems limits the potential rise in [H⁺], and a new steady state is achieved within a few minutes.

Unless the cause of the acute episode of acidosis is resolved, or is treated quickly and successfully, renal compensation causes HCO_3^- retention and H⁺ excretion, thereby returning plasma [H⁺] towards normal while HCO_3^- increases. These compensatory changes can occur over a period of hours to days, by which time a new steady state is achieved and the daily renal H⁺ excretion and HCO_3^- reten-

Table 3.1 Illustrative data for patients with simple disturbances of acid–base balance

	[H⁺] (nmol/L)	P_{CO_2} (kPa)	Plasma [HCO₃] (mmol/L)	Plasma [total CO₂] (mmol/L)
Reference ranges	36–44	4.4–6.1	21.0–27.5	24–30
Respiratory acidosis	58	9.3	29	32
Respiratory alkalosis	29	3.2	20	22
Metabolic acidosis	72	3.2	8	11
Metabolic alkalosis	28	6.0	39	43

Table 3.2 Respiratory acidosis

Mechanism	Examples of causes
Alveolar P_{CO_2} increased due to defect in respiratory function	Pulmonary disease – chronic bronchitis, severe asthma, pulmonary oedema, fibrosis Mechanical disorders – thoracic trauma, pneumothorax, myopathies
Alveolar P_{CO_2} increased due to defect in respiratory control mechanisms	CNS disease – stroke, trauma CNS depression – anaesthetics, opiates, severe hypoxia Neurological disease – motor neuron disease, spinal cord lesions, poliomyelitis

Table 3.3 Respiratory alkalosis

Mechanism	Examples of causes
Alveolar P_{CO_2} lowered due to hyperventilation	Voluntary hyperventilation, mechanical ventilation Reflex hyperventilation – chest wall disease, decreased pulmonary compliance Stimulation of respiratory centre – pain, fever, salicylate overdose, hepatic encephalopathy, hypoxia

Table 3.4 Metabolic acidosis

Mechanism	Examples of causes
Increased H+ production in excess of body's excretory capacity	Ketoacidosis – diabetic, alcoholic Lactic acidosis – hypoxic, shock, drugs, inherited metabolic disease Poisoning – methanol, salicylate
Failure to excrete H+ at the normal rate	Acute and chronic renal failure Distal renal tubular acidosis
Loss of HCO_3	Loss from the GI tract – severe diarrhoea, pancreatic fistula Loss in the urine – ureteroenterostomy, proximal renal tubular acidosis, carbonate dehydratase inhibitors (acetazolamide)

excretion and reduce H+ excretion. Plasma [H+] returns towards normal, whereas plasma HCO_3^- falls further. A new steady state will be achieved in hours to days if the respiratory disorder persists. It is unusual for chronic respiratory alkalosis to be severe, and plasma HCO_3^- rarely falls below 12 mmol/L.

Metabolic acidosis

Increased production or decreased excretion of H+ leads to accumulation of H+ within the ECF (Table 3.4). The extra H+ ions combine with HCO_3^- to form H_2CO_3, disturbing the equilibrium in reaction 3.2, with a shift to the left. However, since there is no ventilatory abnormality, any increase in plasma $[H_2CO_3]$ is only transient, as the related slight increase in dissolved CO_2 is immediately excreted by the lungs. The net effect is that a new equilibrium rapidly establishes itself in which the product, $[H^+] \times [HCO_3^-]$, remains unchanged, since $[H_2CO_3]$ is unchanged. In consequence, the rise in plasma [H+] is limited, but at the expense of a fall

tion return to normal. The patient then has the pattern of acid–base abnormalities of chronic respiratory acidosis.

Respiratory alkalosis

This is due to hyperventilation (Table 3.3). The reduced P_{CO_2} that results causes the equilibrium positions of reactions 3.1 and 3.2 to move to the left. As a result, plasma [H+] and HCO_3^- both fall, although the relative change in HCO_3^- is small.

If conditions giving rise to a low P_{CO_2} persist for more than a few hours, the kidneys increase HCO_3^-

in [HCO$_3^-$], which has been consumed in this process and may be very low. Its availability for further buffering becomes progressively more limited. Less often, metabolic acidosis arises from loss of HCO$_3^-$ from the renal system or GI tract. Typically in these conditions, HCO$_3^-$ does not fall to such a great extent, rarely being less than 15 mmol/L.

The rise in ECF [H$^+$] stimulates the respiratory centre, causing compensatory hyperventilation. As a result, due to the fall in P_{CO_2}, plasma [H$^+$] returns towards normal, while plasma [HCO$_3^-$] falls even further. It is quite common for patients with metabolic acidosis to have very low plasma [HCO$_3^-$], often below 10 mmol/L. Plasma [H$^+$] will not, however, become completely normal through this mechanism, since it is the low [H$^+$] that drives the compensatory hyperventilation – as the [H$^+$] falls, the hyperventilation becomes correspondingly reduced. In addition, if renal function is normal, H$^+$ will be excreted by the kidney.

Metabolic alkalosis

This is most often due to prolonged vomiting, but may be due to other causes (Table 3.5). The loss of H$^+$ upsets the equilibrium in reaction 3.2,

Table 3.5 Metabolic alkalosis

Mechanism	Examples of causes
Saline-responsive	H$^+$ loss from GI tract – vomiting, nasogastric drainage
	H$^+$ loss in urine – thiazide diuretics (especially in cardiac failure), nephrotic syndrome
	Alkali administration – sodium bicarbonate
Saline-unresponsive	Associated with hypertension – primary and secondary aldosteronism, Cushing's syndrome
	Not associated with hypertension – severe K$^+$ depletion, Bartter's syndrome

causing it to shift to the right as H$_2$CO$_3$ dissociates to form H$^+$ (which is being lost) and HCO$_3^-$. However, because there is no primary disturbance of ventilation, plasma HCO$_3^-$ remains constant, with the net effect that plasma [H$^+$] falls and [HCO$_3^-$] rises. Respiratory compensation (i.e. hypoventilation) for the alkalosis is usually minimal, since any resulting rise in P_{CO_2} or fall in P_{O_2} will be a potent stimulator of ventilation. HCO$_3^-$ is freely filtered at the glomerulus, and is therefore available for excretion in the urine, which would rapidly tend to restore the acid–base status towards normal. The continuing presence of an alkalosis means there is inappropriate reabsorption of filtered HCO$_3^-$ from the distal nephron. This can be due to ECF volume depletion, potassium deficiency or mineralocorticoid excess.

Interpretation of results of acid–base assessment

Results of acid–base measurements must be considered in the light of clinical findings, and the results of other chemical tests (e.g. plasma creatinine, urea, Na$^+$ and K$^+$); other types of investigation (e.g. radiological) may also be important.

Interpretation of acid–base results is based on the equilibria represented by reactions 3.1 and 3.2 and the related Henderson equation. After reviewing the clinical findings, acid–base results can be considered in the following order:
- Plasma [H$^+$]. Reference range 36–44 nmol/L.
- Plasma P_{CO_2}. Reference range 4.5–6.1 kPa.
- Plasma [HCO$_3^-$]. Reference range 21.0–27.5 mmol/L.

This procedure immediately identifies those patients in whom there is an uncompensated acidosis or alkalosis, and is the starting point for their further classification, as considered below.

Alternatively, the results can be plotted on a diagram of [H$^+$] against P_{CO_2} (Figure 3.3). In this diagram, simple acid–base disturbances represent bands of results, as shown. Results falling between the bands due to metabolic acidosis and respiratory alkalosis, or between those due to respiratory acidosis and metabolic alkalosis need careful con-

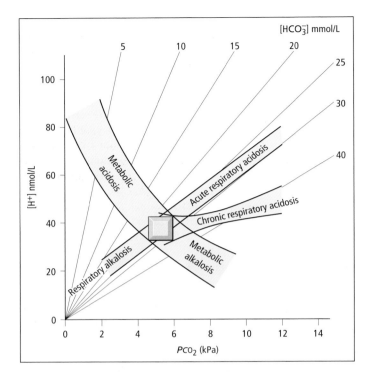

Figure 3.3 On this plot of [H⁺] against P_{CO_2}, lines of equal $[HCO_3^-]$ radiate from the origin, increasing in value towards the bottom right corner. The bands of values marked show the expected results in patients with simple acid–base disorders.

sideration. These may represent either a combination of two acid–base disorders, or compensation for a single disorder.

Plasma [H⁺] is increased

The patient has an acidosis. The P_{CO_2} result is considered next, as follows:

- P_{CO_2} is decreased. The patient has a *metabolic acidosis*. The reduced P_{CO_2} is due to hyperventilation, the physiological compensatory response (e.g. overbreathing in patients with diabetic ketoacidosis). Plasma $[HCO_3^-]$ is reduced in these patients, sometimes to below 10 mmol/L.

- P_{CO_2} is normal. The patient has an *uncompensated metabolic acidosis*. Plasma $[HCO_3^-]$ will be decreased. However, the normal compensatory response should lower the P_{CO_2} in patients with a simple metabolic acidosis (see above), so there is a co-existing respiratory pathology causing CO_2 retention – in other words, there is a simultaneous respiratory acidosis. This combination of results is seen, for example, in patients with combined respiratory and circulatory failure, such as occurs during a cardiac arrest.

- P_{CO_2} is increased. The patient has a *respiratory acidosis*. The pattern of results will depend on whether the respiratory acidosis is acute or chronic:

  - *Acute* The patient will have a high plasma [H⁺] and a high P_{CO_2}, with a slightly raised plasma $[HCO_3^-]$, since the renal response has not yet had time to develop.

  - *Chronic* The patient will have a normal or slightly raised plasma [H⁺], a high P_{CO_2} and a markedly raised plasma $[HCO_3^-]$, due to renal retention of HCO_3^-.

Plasma [H⁺] is decreased

The patient has an alkalosis. The P_{CO_2} result should be assessed next:

- P_{CO_2} is decreased. The patient has a *respiratory alkalosis*. If this is a simple disturbance, plasma $[HCO_3^-]$ will be decreased (not below ~12 mmol/L).

- P_{CO_2} is normal. The patient has an *uncompensated metabolic alkalosis*, and the plasma [HCO_3^-] will be increased.
- P_{CO_2} is increased. The patient may have a metabolic alkalosis with some respiratory compensation. However, it is unlikely that this patient has a simple acid–base disturbance since significant hypoventilation is not often a marked feature of the compensatory response to a metabolic alkalosis. A more common explanation for a low plasma [H^+] and an increased P_{CO_2} is that the patient has a mixed acid–base disturbance, consisting of a metabolic alkalosis and a respiratory acidosis. Plasma [HCO_3^-] will also be increased.

Plasma [H^+] is normal

The patient either has no acid–base disturbance, or no net acid–base disturbance, as a result of one of the mechanisms described below. Considering the P_{CO_2} result next:

- P_{CO_2} is decreased. The patient most probably has a mixed acid–base disturbance consisting of a respiratory alkalosis and a metabolic acidosis. Both these types of acid–base disturbance cause a decreased plasma [HCO_3^-], and the distinction can usually be made on clinical grounds. A fully compensated respiratory alkalosis is another possibility.
- P_{CO_2} is normal. There is no significant acid–base disturbance. Since both plasma [H^+] and P_{CO_2} are normal, plasma [HCO_3^-] must be normal; see reaction 3.4.
- P_{CO_2} is increased. The patient either has a fully compensated respiratory acidosis, or there is a mixed acid–base disturbance consisting of a respiratory acidosis and a metabolic alkalosis. Both these possibilities give rise to increased plasma [HCO_3^-], to over 30 mmol/L. They can usually be distinguished on clinical grounds.

Mixed acid–base disturbances

It may not always be possible to differentiate some mixed acid–base disturbances from simple ones by the scheme described above. For instance, some patients with chronic renal failure (which causes a primary metabolic acidosis) may also have chronic obstructive airways disease (which causes a primary respiratory acidosis). Plasma [H^+] will be increased in these patients, but the results for plasma P_{CO_2} and [HCO_3^-] cannot be predicted. The history and clinical findings must be taken into account.

Plotting the results on a diagram of [H^+] against P_{CO_2} (Figure 3.3) may help. Results falling between the bands of respiratory and metabolic acidoses are due to a combination of these two conditions. Similarly, results between the bands due to respiratory and metabolic alkaloses are due to a combination of these.

Other investigations in acid–base assessment

The full characterisation of acid–base status requires arterial or arterialised capillary blood samples, since venous blood P_{CO_2} (even if 'arterialised') bears no constant relationship to alveolar P_{CO_2}. However, other investigations can provide some useful information.

Total CO_2 (reference range 24–30 mmol/L)

This test, performed on venous plasma or serum, includes contributions from HCO_3^-, H_2CO_3, dissolved CO_2 and carbamino compounds. However, about 95% of 'total CO_2' is contributed by HCO_3^-. Total CO_2 measurements have the advantages of ease of sample collection and suitability for measurement in large numbers, but they cannot define a patient's acid–base status, since plasma [H^+] and P_{CO_2} are both unknown. For example, an increased plasma [total CO_2] may be due to either a respiratory acidosis or a metabolic alkalosis. However, when interpreted in the light of clinical findings, plasma [total CO_2] can often give an adequate assessment of whether an acid–base disturbance is present and, if one is present, provide an indication of its severity. This is particularly true when there is a metabolic disturbance.

Anion gap (reference range 10–20 mmol/L)

The anion gap (or *ion difference*) is obtained from plasma electrolyte results, as follows:

$$AG = ([Na^+] + [K^+]) - ([Cl^-] + [total\ CO_2])$$

The difference between the cations and the anions represents the unmeasured anions or anion gap and includes proteins, phosphate, sulphate and lactate ions. The anion gap may be increased because of an increase in unmeasured anions. This may be of help in narrowing the differential diagnosis in a patient with metabolic acidosis (Table 3.6). In the presence of metabolic acidosis, a raised anion gap points to the cause being excessive production of hydrogen ions or failure to excrete them. As the acid accumulates in the ECF (e.g. in DKA), the HCO_3^- is titrated and replaced with unmeasured anions (e.g. acetoacetate) and the anion gap increases. In contrast, if the cause is a loss of HCO_3^- (e.g. renal tubular acidosis), there is a compensatory increase in Cl^- and the anion gap remains unchanged (Table 3.4, and see below).

Plasma chloride (reference range 95–107 mmol/L)

The causes of metabolic acidosis are sometimes divided into those with an increased anion gap

Table 3.6 Causes of an increased anion gap

Mechanism	Examples of causes
Plasma [unmeasured anions] increased with or without changes in [Na$^+$] and [Cl$^-$]	Metabolic acidosis – uraemic acidosis, lactic acidosis, DKA, salicylate overdose, methanol ingestion
Increase in plasma [Na$^+$]	Treatment with sodium salts, e.g. salts of some high-dose antibiotics such as carbenicillin; this increases plasma [unmeasured anions]
Artefact	Improper handling of specimens after collection, causing loss of CO_2

(Table 3.6) and those with a normal anion gap. In the latter group, the fall in plasma [total CO_2], which accompanies the metabolic acidosis, is associated with an approximately equal rise in plasma [Cl$^-$]. Patients with metabolic acidosis and a normal anion gap are sometimes described as having hyperchloraemic acidosis.

Increased plasma [Cl$^-$], out of proportion to any accompanying increase in plasma [Na$^+$], may occur in patients with chronic renal failure, ureteric transplants into the colon, renal tubular acidosis, or in patients treated with carbonate dehydratase inhibitors. Increased plasma [Cl$^-$] may also occur in patients who develop respiratory alkalosis as a result of prolonged assisted ventilation. A iatrogenic cause of increased plasma [Cl$^-$] is the IV administration of excessive amounts of isotonic or 'physiological' saline, which contains 155 mmol/L NaCl.

Patients who lose large volumes of gastric secretion (e.g. due to pyloric stenosis) often show a disproportionately marked fall in plasma [Cl$^-$] compared with any hyponatraemia that may develop. They develop metabolic alkalosis, and are often dehydrated.

Treatment of acid–base disturbances

A thorough clinical assessment is the basis on which the results of acid–base analyses are interpreted, and treatment initiated. Having defined the nature of an acid–base disturbance, treatment should aim to correct the primary disorder and to assist the physiological compensatory mechanisms. In some cases, more active intervention may be necessary (e.g. treatment with NaHCO$_3$). It is often possible to correct an acid–base disturbance by treatment aimed only at the causative condition (e.g. DKA is usually corrected without the administration of NaHCO$_3$). Where active treatment of the acid–base disturbance is necessary, this is usually needed for metabolic disturbances.

In metabolic acidosis, treatment with HCO$_3^-$ is usually not indicated unless [H$^+$] is very high (e.g. >90 nmol/L), except for patients with proximal renal tubular acidosis, who lose HCO_3^- because of the primary defect.

In metabolic alkalosis, many patients inappropriately retain HCO_3^- because of volume depletion, potassium depletion or mineralocorticoid excess, perpetuating the alkalosis. These patients respond to the administration of isotonic saline. Non-responders include patients with mineralocorticoid excess, either due to primary adrenal hyperfunction or due to those causes of secondary adrenal hyperfunction that are not due to hypovolaemia and ECF depletion. These include renal artery stenosis, magnesium deficiency and Bartter's syndrome. Treatment of these is directed at the primary disorder.

Oxygen transport

Oxygen delivery to tissues depends on the combination of their blood supply and the arterial O_2 content. In turn the O_2 content depends on the concentration of Hb and its saturation. Tissue hypoxia can therefore be caused not just by hypoxaemia, but also by impaired perfusion (e.g. because of reduced cardiac output or vasoconstriction), anaemia and the presence of abnormal Hb species. The full characterisation of the oxygen composition of a blood sample requires measurement of P_{O_2}, Hb concentration and percentage oxygen saturation. Hb measurements are widely available, and P_{O_2} is one of the measurements automatically performed by most blood gas analysers as part of the full acid–base assessment of patients. Hb saturation is measured using an oximeter within the laboratory, or using a pulse oximeter at the bedside. This comprises a probe which is attached to the patient's finger or earlobe.

Measurements of P_{O_2} in arterial blood (reference range 12–15 kPa) are important, and are often valuable in assessing the efficiency of oxygen therapy, when high P_{O_2} values may be found. Above a P_{O_2} of 10.5 kPa, however, Hb is almost fully saturated with O_2 (Figure 3.4), and further increases in P_{O_2} do not result in greater O_2 carriage. Conversely, as P_{O_2} drops, initially there is little reduction in O_2 carriage on Hb, but when it falls

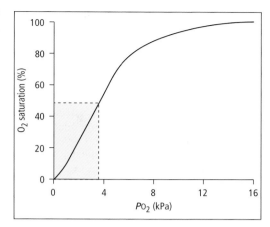

Figure 3.4 The oxygen dissociation curve of Hb. It is important to note that, above a P_{O_2} of approximately 9 kPa, Hb is over 95% saturated with O_2. Also shown in the figure is the value of the P_{O_2}, 3.8 kPa, that corresponds to 50% saturation with O_2; this value is called the P_{50} value.

below about 8 kPa, saturation starts to fall rapidly. In addition, results of P_{O_2} measurements may be misleading in conditions where the oxygen-carrying capacity of blood is grossly impaired, as in severe anaemia, carbon monoxide poisoning and when abnormal Hb derivatives (e.g. methaemoglobin) are present. Measurement of both the blood [Hb] and the percentage oxygen saturation are required in addition to P_{O_2} under these circumstances.

Indications for full blood acid–base and oxygen measurements

The main indications for full acid–base assessment, coupled with P_{O_2} or oxygen saturation measurements, are in the investigation and management of patients with pulmonary disorders, severely ill patients in ICUs and patients in the operative and peri-operative periods of major surgery who may often be on assisted ventilation. Other important applications include the investigation and management of patients with vascular abnormalities involving the shunting of blood.

Full acid–base assessment is less essential in patients with metabolic acidosis or alkalosis, for whom measurements of plasma [total CO_2] on venous blood may give sufficient information.

Respiratory insufficiency

This term is applied to two types of disorder in which lung function is impaired sufficiently to cause the P_{O_2} to become abnormally low, usually less than 8.0 kPa.

Type I: low P_{O_2} with normal or low P_{CO_2}

Hypoxia without hypercapnia occurs in patients in whom there is a preponderance of alveoli that are adequately perfused with blood, but inadequately ventilated. It occurs, for example, in emphysema, pulmonary oedema and asthma. Type II respiratory insufficiency can also occur in some of these conditions, if they are sufficiently severe.

In type I respiratory insufficiency, there is, in effect, a partial right-to-left shunt, bringing unoxygenated blood to the left side of the heart. Increased ventilation of the adequately perfused and ventilated alveoli is able to compensate for the tendency for the P_{CO_2} to rise. It cannot, however, restore the P_{O_2} to normal, since the blood perfusing the normal alveoli conveys Hb that is already nearly saturated with O_2.

Type II: low P_{O_2} with high P_{CO_2}

This combination means that there is hypoventilation. The cause may be central in origin, or due to airways obstruction, or it may be neuromuscular. There may be altered ventilation/perfusion relationships, with an excessive number of alveoli being inadequately perfused; this causes 'wasted' ventilation and an increase in 'dead space'.

Chronic obstructive airways disease is an important cause of type II respiratory insufficiency. It also occurs with mechanical defects in ventilation (e.g. chest injuries, myasthenia gravis). In severe asthma, if serial measurements show a rising P_{CO_2} and falling P_{O_2}, more intensive treatment is urgently needed.

Oxygen therapy

The most recent British guidelines for the administration of emergency oxygen emphasise that oxygen is a treatment for hypoxaemia, not breathlessness, since oxygen has not been shown to have any effect on the sensation of breathlessness in non-hypoxaemic patients. They stress the importance of oxygen saturation, measured by pulse oximetry, recommending that oxygen is administered to patients whose oxygen saturation falls below target ranges. These are 94–98% for most acutely ill patients, and 82–92% for patients at risk of hypercapnic respiratory failure. Oxygen therapy should be adjusted to achieve saturations within these target ranges, rather than using fixed doses. Most therapy will use nasal cannulae rather than masks.

Further Reading

British Thoracic Society Emergency Oxygen Guideline Group. (2008) Guidelines for emergency oxygen use in adult patients, *Thorax*, **63** (Suppl VI), vi1–vi68.

Keypoints

- Meaningful acid–base studies on blood usually require arterial specimens, and need to be analysed soon after collection.
- Respiratory acidosis is common in chronic obstructive airways disease. There is a raised P_{CO_2}, [H⁺] and [HCO_3^-]. Compensatory renal HCO_3^- retention tends to return [H⁺] towards normal.
- Respiratory alkalosis is usually transient and due to overbreathing, or occasionally artificial ventilation. P_{CO_2}, [HCO_3^-] and [H⁺] are reduced.
- Metabolic acidosis is due to acid overproduction, for example DKA, failure to excrete acid, for example renal disease, or loss of base. [H⁺] is increased and [HCO_3^-] is decreased, and there is often a compensatory reduction in P_{CO_2} due to overbreathing.
- Metabolic alkalosis is most often due to loss of gastric acid, for example in pyloric stenosis. [H⁺] is low and [HCO_3^-] is raised.
- Respiratory insufficiency is said to be present when P_{O_2} is below 8.0 kPa. In type I, the P_{CO_2} is normal or low whereas in type II it is raised.

Case 3.1

A 70-year-old man was admitted to a hospital as an emergency. He gave a history of dyspepsia and epigastric pain extending over many years. He had never sought medical attention for this. One week prior to admission, he had started to vomit, and had since vomited frequently, being unable to keep down any food. He was clinically dehydrated, and had marked epigastric tenderness, but no sign of abdominal rigidity. Analysis of an arterial blood specimen gave the following results:

Serum	Result	Reference range
Urea	17.3	2.5–6.6 mmol/L
Na$^+$	131	135–145 mmol/L
K$^+$	2.2	3.6–5.0 mmol/L
Creatinine	250	60–120 µmol/L

Blood gas analysis	Result	Reference range
H$^+$	26	37–45 nmol/L
P_{CO_2}	6.2	4.5–6.0 kPa
HCO$_3^-$	44	21–29 mmol/L
P_{O_2}	9.5	12–15 kPa

How would you describe this patient's acid–base status? What might have caused the various abnormalities revealed by these results? Why is the plasma [K$^+$] so low?

Comments: The patient had a metabolic alkalosis. This was caused by his persistent vomiting, the vomit being likely to consist almost entirely of gastric contents. In this age group, the cause could be carcinoma of the stomach or chronic peptic ulceration with associated scarring and fibrosis, leading to obstruction of gastric outflow.

Gastric juice [K$^+$] is about 10 mmol/L. Also, in the presence of an alkalosis, K$^+$ shifts from the ECF into cells. Furthermore, dehydration causes secondary hyperaldosteronism in order to maintain ECF volume, and Na$^+$ is avidly retained by the kidneys in exchange for H$^+$ and K$^+$. Patients such as this man, despite having an alkalosis and despite being hypokalaemic, often excrete an acid urine containing large amounts of K$^+$.

Case 3.2

The junior doctor first on call for the A&E department examined a 22-year-old man who was having an acute attack of asthma. The patient was very distressed, so the doctor treated him with a nebulised bronchodilator immediately and returned 10 min later to examine him, when he was more settled and was breathing air. He decided to check the patient's arterial blood gases, the results of which were

Blood gas analysis	Result	Reference range
H$^+$	44	37–45 nmol/L
P_{CO_2}	6.0	4.5–6.0 kPa
HCO$_3^-$	27.0	21–29 mmol/L
P_{O_2}	10.2	12–15 kPa

The doctor asked the A&E consultant whether he could send the patient home. Would you consider that these results suggested that it would be safe to do so?

(continued on p. 48)

Case 3.2 *(continued)*

Comments: It would not be safe to send this patient home. In a moderately severe asthmatic attack, the ventilatory drive from hypoxia and from mechanical receptors in the chest normally results in a P_{CO_2} at or below the lower end of the reference range. A P_{CO_2} greater than this is a serious prognostic sign, indicative either of extensive 'shunting' of blood through areas of the lung that are underventilated because of bronchoconstriction or plugging with mucus, or of the patient becoming increasingly tired. A rising P_{CO_2} in an asthmatic attack is an indication for ventilating these patients.

Case 3.3

A 75-year-old widow, a known heavy smoker and chronic bronchitic, and a patient in a long-stay hospital, became very breathless and wheezy. The senior nurse called the doctor who was on duty, but he was unable to come at once because he was treating another emergency. He asked the nurse to start the patient on 24% oxygen. One hour later, when the doctor arrived, he examined the patient and took an arterial specimen to determine her blood gases. The results were as follows:

Blood gas analysis	Result	Reference range
H^+	97	37–45 nmol/L
P_{CO_2}	21.8	4.5–6.0 kPa
HCO_3^-	42	21–29 mmol/L
P_{O_2}	22.5	12–15 kPa

How would you describe the patient's acid–base status? Do you think that she was breathing 24% oxygen?

Comments: This patient had a respiratory acidosis. Although she gave a long history of chest complaints, the history of her recent illness was short, and it was most unlikely that renal compensation could have accounted in that short time for the very high arterial plasma [HCO_3^-]. From the arterial P_{O_2} result, it was apparent that the patient was breathing a much higher concentration of O_2 than 24%. Atmospheric pressure is approximately 100 kPa, so the P_{O_2} of inspired air (in kilopascals) is numerically equal, approximately, to the percentage of O_2 inspired. Further, it is approximately true that:

$$\text{Inspired } P_{O_2} = \text{alveolar } P_{O_2} + \text{alveolar } P_{CO_2}$$

Since alveolar P_{CO_2} equals arterial P_{CO_2}, this equation can be rewritten as:

$$\text{Inspired } P_{O_2} = \text{alveolar } P_{O_2} + \text{alveolar } P_{CO_2}$$

Alveolar P_{O_2} *must* be greater than arterial P_{O_2}, so it was possible to conclude that the patient must have been breathing O_2 at a concentration of at least 40%. On checking, it was found that the wrong mask had been fitted, and that O_2 was being delivered at 60%.

It was concluded that the patient had an underlying chronic (compensated) respiratory acidosis with CO_2 retention (type II respiratory failure), and that the administration of oxygen at high concentration had removed the hypoxic drive to ventilation, thereby superimposing an acute respiratory acidosis on the underlying chronic acid–base disturbance.

Case 3.4

A young woman was admitted in a confused and restless condition. History taking was not easy, but it seemed that she had been becoming progressively unwell over the preceding week or two. Acid–base analysis was performed and results were as follows:

Blood gas analysis	Result	Reference range
H^+	78	37–45 nmol/L
P_{CO_2}	3.2	4.5–6.0 kPa
HCO_3^-	6	21–29 mmol/L
P_{O_2}	11.8	12–15 kPa

What is her acid–base disorder? What are the most likely causes, and what investigations could narrow this down?

Comments: She has a metabolic acidosis. Despite the long list of possible causes of metabolic acidosis, the most common causes are relatively few, and are DKA, renal failure, salicylate overdose and lactic acidosis. Usually these can be differentiated on the basis of the history; by measuring urea and electrolytes (U&Es) and glucose (and salicylate if indicated); and performing urinalysis (using a dipstick, and looking especially for ketones). Lactate can also be measured if required, but is often not necessary. This woman was a newly presenting type 1 diabetic.

Case 3.5

An elderly man was brought into the A&E department after collapsing in the street. He was deeply comatose and cyanosed, with unrecordable blood pressure. The results of acid–base analysis were as follows:

Blood gas analysis	Result	Reference range
H^+	124	37–45 nmol/L
P_{CO_2}	10.4	4.5–6.0 kPa
HCO_3^-	15.4	21–29 mmol/L
P_{O_2}	4.8	12–15 kPa

What is his acid–base status? What are the possible causes?

Comments: He has a combined metabolic and respiratory acidosis. The combination of the elevated H^+ and P_{CO_2} may initially suggest that he has respiratory acidosis, but the bicarbonate would not be reduced in a simple respiratory acidosis. This means that there is an additional component of metabolic acidosis present. Results of this sort are seen in patients with markedly impaired circulatory and respiratory function, such as that which occurs after a cardiac arrest. This man had a large abdominal aortic aneurysm that had ruptured.

Case 3.6

A 60-year-old man with insulin-treated type 2 diabetes experienced severe central chest pain, associated with nausea. He refused to let his wife call the doctor, but went to bed and, since he felt too ill to eat, he stopped taking his insulin. Two days later, he had another episode of chest pain and became breathless. His wife called an ambulance, and he was admitted. He was shocked, with central cyanosis, pulse 120/min, blood pressure 66/34, respiratory rate 30/min. An ECG demonstrated a large anterior myocardial infarct. The results of acid–base analyses were as follows:

Blood gas analyses	Results	Reference range
H^+	39	36–44 nmol/L
P_{CO_2}	2	4.4–6.1 kPa
HCO_3^-	9.4	21.0–27.5 mmol/L
P_{O_2} kPa	7	12–15 kPa

What is his acid–base status, and what may have caused it?

Comments: He has a combination of metabolic acidosis (causing elevated [H^+] and low P_{CO_2}) and respiratory alkalosis (causing low [H^+] and low P_{CO_2}). The combination explains the normal [H^+] with very low P_{CO_2}. The metabolic acidosis could be due to DKA (caused by inappropriately stopping insulin in the face of his severe illness) and/or to lactic acidosis (caused by impaired tissue perfusion because of his circulatory failure). The respiratory alkalosis is due to hyperventilation caused by pulmonary oedema and/or hypoxia and/or anxiety.

Chapter 4

Renal disease

The kidneys are paired retroperitoneal organs each comprising about 1 million nephrons, which act as independent functional units. They have multiple physiological functions, which can be broadly categorised as the excretion of waste products, the homeostatic regulation of the ECF volume and composition, and endocrine. In order to achieve these functions, they receive a rich blood supply, amounting to about 25% of the cardiac output.

The excretory and homeostatic functions are achieved through filtration at the glomerulus and tubular reabsorption. The glomeruli act as filters which are permeable to water and low molecular weight substances, but impermeable to macromolecules. This impermeability is determined by both size and charge, with proteins smaller than albumin (68 kDa) being filtered, and positively charged molecules being filtered more readily than those with a negative charge. The filtration rate is determined by the differences in hydrostatic and oncotic pressures between the glomerular capillaries and the lumen of the nephron, by the nature of the glomerular basement membrane and by the total glomerular area available for filtration. The total glomerular area available reflects the total number of functioning nephrons. The total volume of the glomerular filtrate amounts to about 170 L/day (12 times the typical ECF volume), and has a composition similar to plasma except that it is almost free of protein.

The renal tubules are presented with this volume of water, most of which needs to be reabsorbed, containing a complex mixture of ions and small molecules some of which have to be retained, some of them in a regulated manner; small amounts of small proteins which are reabsorbed and catabolised; and metabolic waste products such as urea, creatinine and sulphate ions, which are excreted. The proximal convoluted tubule is responsible for the obligatory reabsorption of much of the glomerular filtrate, with further reabsorption in the distal convoluted tubule being subject to homeostatic control mechanisms. In the proximal tubule, energy-dependent mechanisms reabsorb about 75% of the filtered Na^+ and all of the K^+, HCO_3^-, amino acids and glucose, with an iso-osmotic amount of water. In the ascending limb of the loop of Henle, Cl^- is pumped out into the interstitial fluid, generating the medullary hypertonicity on which the ability to excrete concentrated urine depends. This removal of Na^+ and Cl^- in the ascending limb results in the delivery to the distal convoluted tubule of hypotonic fluid containing only 10% of the filtered Na^+ and 20% of the filtered water. The further reabsorption of Na^+ in the distal convoluted tubule is under the control of aldosterone, and generates an electrochemical gradient which promotes the secretion of K^+ and H^+.

Lecture Notes: Clinical Biochemistry, 8e. By G. Beckett, S. Walker, P. Rae & P. Ashby. Published 2010 by Blackwell Publishing.

The collecting ducts receive the fluid from the distal convoluted tubules and pass through the hypertonic renal medulla. In the absence of vasopressin, the cells lining the ducts are impermeable to water, resulting in the excretion of dilute urine. Vasopressin stimulates the incorporation of aquaporins into the cell membranes. Water can then be passively reabsorbed under the influence of the osmotic gradient between the duct lumen and the interstitial fluid, and concentrated urine is excreted.

The endocrine functions of the kidney include the ability to synthesise hormones (e.g. renin, erythropoietin, calcitriol), to respond to them (e.g. aldosterone, parathyroid hormone (PTH)) and to inactivate or excrete them (e.g. insulin, glucagon). All of these functions may be affected by renal disease, with local or systemic consequences.

Many diseases affect renal function. In some, several functions are affected; in others, there is selective impairment of glomerular function or of one or more tubular functions. In this chapter, we discuss the use of chemical tests to investigate glomerular and tubular function. In general, chemical tests are mainly of value in detecting the presence of renal disease by its effects on renal function, and in assessing its progress. They are of less value in determining the causes of disease.

Tests of glomerular function

The GFR depends on the net pressure across the glomerular membrane, the physical nature of the membrane and its surface area, which in turn reflects the number of functioning glomeruli. All three factors may be modified by disease, but, in the absence of large changes in filtration pressure or in the structure of the glomerular membrane, the GFR provides a useful index of the numbers of functioning glomeruli. It gives an estimate of the degree of renal impairment by disease.

Accurate measurement of the GFR by clearance tests requires determination of the concentrations, in plasma and urine, of a substance that is filtered at the glomerulus, but which is neither reabsorbed nor secreted by the tubules; its concentration in plasma needs to remain constant throughout the period of urine collection. It is convenient if the substance is present endogenously, and important for it to be readily measured. Its clearance is given by

$$\text{Clearance} = U \cdot V / P$$

where U is the concentration in urine, V is the volume of urine produced per minute and P is the concentration in plasma. When performing this calculation manually, care should be taken to ensure consistency of units, especially for the plasma and urine concentrations.

Inulin (a complex plant carbohydrate) meets these criteria, apart from the fact that it is not an endogenous compound, but needs to be administered by IV infusion. This makes it completely impractical for routine clinical use, but it remains the original standard against which other measures of GFR are assessed.

Estimated GFR (eGFR) is now widely reported on laboratory report forms. This is a calculated estimate based on creatinine and a number of other variables. It gets around some of the problems associated with creatinine, described below, by incorporating age and sex in the calculation, but suffers from significant imprecision, and is not always applicable. It is further described on p. 56.

Measurement of creatinine clearance

Creatine is synthesised in the liver, kidneys and pancreas, and is transported to its sites of usage, principally muscle and brain. About 1–2% of the total muscle creatine pool is converted daily to creatinine through the spontaneous, non-enzymatic loss of water. Creatinine is an end-product of nitrogen metabolism, and as such undergoes no further metabolism, but is excreted in the urine. Creatinine production reflects the body's total muscle mass.

Creatinine meets some of the criteria mentioned above. Creatinine in the plasma is filtered freely at the glomerulus, but its concentration may not remain constant over the period of urine collection. A small amount of this filtered creatinine undergoes tubular reabsorption. A larger amount, up to 10% of urinary creatinine, is actively secreted into the urine by the tubules. Its measurement in plasma is subject to analytical overestimation. In practice, the effects of tubular secretion and analytical overestimation tend to cancel each other out at normal levels of GFR, and creatinine clearance is a fair approximation to the GFR. As the GFR falls, however, creatinine clearance progressively overestimates the true GFR.

Estimation of creatinine clearance

A number of formulae exist for predicting creatinine clearance (or GFR) from plasma [creatinine] and other readily available information, such as age, sex and weight. The best known of these is that of Cockcroft and Gault (1976):

Creatinine clearance =

$$\frac{(140 - age) \times wt \times (0.85 \text{ if patient is female})}{0.814 \times serum[creatinine]}$$

(creatinine clearance in ml/min, age in years, weight in kg, [creatinine] in µmol/L).

This equation has been shown to be as reliable an estimate of creatinine clearance as its actual measurement, since it avoids the inaccuracies inherent in timed urine collections. However, since it estimates creatinine clearance (not GFR), it suffers from the same overestimation of GFR as creatinine clearance when renal function declines. This calculation should not be used when serum [creatinine] is changing rapidly, when the diet is unusual (strict vegetarian diets, or creatine supplements), in extremes of muscle mass (malnutrition, muscle wasting, amputations) or in obesity.

The dosage of a number of potentially toxic chemotherapeutic agents is stratified by creatinine clearance calculated using the Cockcroft–Gault or a similar equation, so these calculations remain in use in pharmacy practice.

Plasma creatinine

If endogenous production of creatinine remains constant, the amount of it excreted in the urine each day becomes constant and the plasma [creatinine] will then be inversely proportional to creatinine clearance. The reference range of

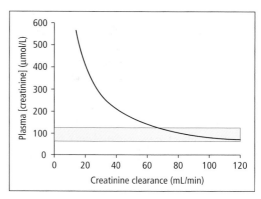

Figure 4.1 Relationship between plasma [creatinine] and creatinine clearance.

serum [creatinine] in adults is 55–120µmol/L. However, individual subjects maintain their [creatinine] within much tighter limits than this. The consequence of this and the form of the relationship between [creatinine] and creatinine clearance is that a raised plasma [creatinine] is a good indicator of impaired renal function, but a normal [creatinine] does not necessarily indicate normal renal function (Figure 4.1). If a patient's 'personal' reference range is low within the overall population reference range, [creatinine] may not be elevated until the GFR has fallen by as much as 50%. However, a progressive rise in serial creatinine measurements, even within the reference range, indicates declining renal function.

Creatinine clearance or plasma [creatinine]?

Measurement of plasma [creatinine] is more precise than creatinine clearance, as there are two extra sources of imprecision in clearance measurements, that is, timed measurement of urine volume and urine [creatinine]. Accuracy of urine collections is very dependent on patients' co-operation and the care with which the procedure has been explained or supervised. The combination of these errors causes an imprecision (1 SD) in the creatinine clearance of about 10% under ideal conditions with 'good' collectors; this increases to 20–30%

under less ideal conditions. This means that large changes in creatinine clearance may not reflect any real change in renal function.

It will be apparent that creatinine clearance measurements are cumbersome and potentially unreliable. They have essentially been superseded by calculation of the eGFR (see p. 56).

Low plasma [creatinine]

A low [creatinine] is found in subjects with a small total muscle mass (Table 4.1). A low plasma [creatinine] may therefore be found in children, and values are, on average, normally lower in women than in men. Abnormally low values may be found in wasting diseases and starvation, and in patients treated with corticosteroids, due to their protein catabolic effect. Creatinine synthesis is increased in pregnancy, but this is more than offset by the combined effects of the retention of fluid and the physiological rise in GFR that occur in pregnancy, so plasma [creatinine] is usually low.

High plasma [creatinine]

Plasma [creatinine] tends to be higher in subjects with a large muscle mass (Table 4.1). Other non-renal causes of increased plasma [creatinine] include the following:
• A high meat intake can cause a temporary increase.
• Transient, small increases may occur after vigorous exercise.
• Some analytical methods are not specific for creatinine. For example, plasma [creatinine] will be overestimated by some methods in the presence of high concentrations of acetoacetate or cephalosporin antibiotics.
• Some drugs (e.g. salicylates, cimetidine) compete with creatinine for its tubular transport mechanism, thereby reducing tubular secretion of creatinine and elevating plasma [creatinine].

If non-renal causes can be excluded, an increased plasma [creatinine] indicates a fall in GFR, which can be due to pre-renal, renal or post-renal causes, as follows:

Table 4.1 Causes of an abnormal plasma [creatinine]

Reduced plasma [creatinine]	
Physiological	Pregnancy
Pathological	Reduced muscle bulk (e.g. starvation wasting diseases, steroid therapy)
Increased plasma [creatinine]	
No pathological significance	High meat intake, strenuous exercise
	Drug effects (e.g. salicylates)
	Analytical interference (e.g. due to cephalosporin antibiotics)
Pathological	Renal causes, i.e. any cause (acute or chronic) of a reduced GFR

• Impaired renal perfusion (e.g. reduced blood pressure, fluid depletion, renal artery stenosis).
• Loss of functioning nephrons (e.g. acute and chronic glomerulonephritis).
• Increased pressure on the tubular side of the nephron (e.g. urinary tract obstruction due to prostatic enlargement).

Plasma urea

Urea is formed in the liver from ammonia released by deamination of amino acids. Over 75% of non-protein nitrogen is excreted as urea, mainly by the kidneys; small amounts are lost through the skin and the GI tract. Urea measurements are widely available, and have come to be accepted as giving a measure of renal function. However, as a test of renal function, plasma [urea] is inferior to plasma [creatinine], since 50% or more of urea filtered at the glomerulus is passively reabsorbed through the tubules, and this fraction increases if urine flow rate decreases, such as in dehydration. It is also more affected by diet than [creatinine].

Low plasma [urea]

Less urea is synthesised in the liver if there is reduced availability of amino acids for deamina-

Table 4.2 Causes of an abnormal plasma [urea]

Reduced plasma [urea]	Low protein diet, severe liver disease, water retention
Increased plasma [urea]	
Pre-renal causes	High protein diet, GI haemorrhage ('meal' of blood)
	Any cause of increased protein catabolism (e.g. trauma, surgery, extreme starvation)
	Any cause of impaired renal perfusion (e.g. ECF losses, cardiac failure, hypoproteinaemia)
Renal causes	Any cause (acute or chronic) of a reduced GFR
Post-renal causes	Any cause of obstruction to urine outflow (e.g. benign prostatic hypertrophy, malignant stricture or obstruction, stone)

tion, as in the case of starvation or malabsorption (Table 4.2). However, in extreme starvation, plasma [urea] may rise, as increased muscle protein breakdown then provides the major source of fuel. In patients with severe liver disease (usually chronic), urea synthesis may be impaired leading to a fall in plasma [urea].

Plasma [urea] may fall as a result of water retention associated with inappropriate vasopressin secretion or dilution of plasma with IV fluids.

High plasma [urea]

It is convenient to subdivide the causes of high plasma [urea] into pre-renal, renal and post-renal (Table 4.2).

- *Pre-renal uraemia* may develop whenever there is impaired renal perfusion, and is essentially the result of a physiological response to hypovolaemia or a drop in blood pressure. This causes renal vasoconstriction and a redistribution of blood such that there is a decrease in GFR, but preservation of tubular function. Stimulation of vasopressin secre-

tion and of the renin–angiotensin–aldosterone system causes the excretion of small volumes of concentrated urine with a low Na content. This reduced urine flow in turn causes increased passive tubular reabsorption of urea. Thus shock, due to burns, haemorrhage or loss of water and electrolytes (e.g. severe diarrhoea), may lead to increased plasma [urea]. Renal blood flow also falls in congestive cardiac failure, and may be further reduced if such patients are treated with potent diuretics. If pre-renal uraemia is not treated adequately and promptly by restoring renal perfusion, it can progress to intrinsic renal failure.

- Increased production of urea in the liver occurs on high protein diets, or as a result of increased protein catabolism (e.g. due to trauma, major surgery, extreme starvation). It may also occur after haemorrhage into the upper GI tract, which gives rise to a 'protein meal' of blood.
- Plasma [urea] increases relatively more than plasma [creatinine] in pre-renal uraemia. This is because tubular reabsorption of urea is increased significantly in these patients, whereas relatively little reabsorption of creatinine occurs.

- *Renal uraemia* may be due to acute or chronic renal failure, with reduction in glomerular filtration. Plasma [urea] increases until a new steady state is reached at which urea production equals the amount excreted in the urine, or continues to rise in the face of near-total renal failure. Although frequently measured as a test of renal function, it is always important to remember that plasma [urea] may be increased for reasons other than intrinsic renal disease (pre-renal and post-renal uraemia).

- *Post-renal uraemia* occurs due to outflow obstruction, which may occur at different levels (i.e. in the ureter, bladder or urethra), due to various causes (e.g. renal stones, prostatism, genitourinary cancer). Back-pressure on the renal tubules enhances back-diffusion of urea, so that plasma [urea] rises disproportionately more than plasma [creatinine].

Impaired renal perfusion and urinary tract obstruction, each in itself possible causes of uraemia, may in turn cause damage to the kidney and thus renal uraemia.

Estimated GFR and chronic kidney disease

Chronic kidney disease (CKD) affects up to 10% of the population and is often asymptomatic until renal function is severely reduced. Furthermore, mild CKD is a significant risk factor for cardiovascular disease. Detection of asymptomatic progressive CKD could allow patients to be actively treated to preserve renal function and reduce cardiovascular risk. However, it is apparent that creatinine clearance can be a reasonable measure of GFR, but is cumbersome and imprecise, whereas [creatinine] gives an indication of GFR and is readily performed, but can be misleading. In particular, [creatinine] is influenced by muscle mass (and hence by sex and age) as well as by GFR. A small elderly woman could lose a large proportion of her GFR and still have a [creatinine] within the population reference range and less than that of a young more muscular man, so a 'normal' [creatinine] can be misleading in such a patient.

eGFR is an estimate of GFR from a formula developed from a large study of patients with renal impairment (the Modification of Diet in Renal Disease (MDRD) study). A number of equations were derived in this study, but the four-variable MDRD equation is widely used in clinical laboratories. This uses [creatinine], age, sex and ethnic origin (for African-Caribbean people the eGFR should be multiplied by 1.212). This equation is not valid in people less than 18 years old, in acute renal failure, when [creatinine] is changing rapidly, pregnancy, muscle wasting diseases, malnutrition or amputees. The eGFR suffers from significant imprecision, and as GFR increases the precision and accuracy of eGFR decreases. Most laboratories therefore report eGFR >60 mL/min/1.73 m² as such, rather than as an exact number.

eGFR is the basis for the classification of CKD (Table 4.3). It should be emphasised that an eGFR >60 mL/min/1.73 m² should be regarded as normal in the absence of any other indication of kidney disease. This can be structural, such as polycystic kidney disease, or a urine abnormality, such as proteinuria or haematuria.

Tests of tubular function

Specific disorders affecting the renal tubules may affect the ability to concentrate urine or to excrete an appropriately acidic urine, or may cause impaired reabsorption of amino acids, glucose,

Table 4.3 Classification of CKD

Stage	eGFR mL/min/1.73 m²	Description	Treatment stage
1*	90+	Normal kidney function	Observation Control blood pressure
2*	60–89	Mildly impaired kidney function	Observation Control blood pressure and risk factors
3	30–59	Moderately impaired kidney function	Observation Control blood pressure and risk factors
4	15–29	Severely impaired kidney function	Planning for end-stage renal failure
5	<15	Established kidney failure	Treatment choices for renal replacement therapy

* In addition to eGFR results, the diagnosis of stage 1 or 2 CKD requires a structural abnormality of the kidneys (such as polycystic kidney disease) or a functional abnormality (such as persistent proteinuria or haematuria. In the absence of these an eGFR between 60 and 89 is not abnormal.

phosphate, etc. In some conditions, these defects occur singly; in others, multiple defects are present. Renal tubular disorders may be congenital or acquired, the congenital disorders all being very rare. Chemical investigations are needed for specific identification of these abnormalities and may include amino acid chromatography, or investigation of calcium and phosphate metabolism (Chapter 5), or an oral glucose tolerance test (OGTT) (p. 94). The functions tested most often are renal concentrating power and the ability to produce an acid urine.

The healthy kidney has a considerable reserve capacity for reabsorbing water, and for excreting H^+ and other ions, only exceeded under exceptional physiological loads. Moderate impairment of renal function may reduce this reserve, and this is revealed when loading tests are used to stress the kidney. Tubular function tests are only used when there is reason to suspect that a specific abnormality is present.

Urine osmolality and renal concentration tests

Urine osmolality varies widely in health, between 50 and 1250 mmol/kg, depending upon the body's requirement to produce a maximally dilute or a maximally concentrated urine.

The failing kidney loses its capacity to concentrate urine at a relatively late stage. A patient with polyuria due to chronic renal failure is unable to produce either a dilute or a concentrated urine. Instead, urine osmolality is generally within 50 mmol/kg of the plasma osmolality (i.e. between about 240 and 350 mmol/kg). This has important implications. To excrete the obligatory daily solute load of about 600 mmol requires approximately 2 L of water at a maximum urine osmolality of 350 mmol/kg, compared with 500 mL of the most concentrated urine achieved by the normal kidney. Hence, patients with CKD require a daily water intake of at least 2 L to maintain their water balance. On the other hand, a large intake of water can lead to dangerous hyponatraemia, since water excretion is limited by the inability to produce a sufficiently dilute urine.

Urine osmolality is directly proportional to the osmotic work done by the kidney, and is a measure of concentrating power. Urine specific gravity, which can be estimated using urinalysis dipsticks, is usually directly proportional to osmolality, but gives spuriously high results if there is significant glycosuria or proteinuria.

Renal concentration tests are not normally required in patients with established chronic renal failure, and indeed may be dangerous. However, the tests may be indicated in patients with polyuria in whom common causes (e.g. diabetes mellitus) have first been excluded. In a number of conditions, the kidney loses its ability to maintain medullary hyperosmolality, and hence to excrete a concentrated urine, but these should have been excluded before renal concentration tests are performed. Causes of failure to concentrate urine are shown in Table 4.4.

In patients with polyuria, measurement of the osmolality of early morning urine specimens should be made before proceeding to formal concentration tests. If urinary osmolality greater

Table 4.4 Causes of failure to concentrate urine

Causal mechanism	Examples of causes
Insufficient secretion of vasopressin	Lesions of the supraoptic–hypothalamic–hypophyseal tract (e.g. trauma, neoplasm)
Inhibition of vasopressin release	Psychogenic polydipsia, lesions of the thirst centre causing polydipsia
Inability to maintain renal medullary hyperosmolality	Chronic renal failure, hydronephrosis, lithium toxicity, hypokalaemia, hypercalcaemia, renal papillary necrosis (e.g. analgesic nephropathy)
Inability to respond to vasopressin	Renal tubular defects (e.g. nephrogenic diabetes insipidus, Fanconi syndrome)
Increased solute load per nephron	Chronic renal failure, diabetes mellitus

than 800 mmol/kg is observed in any specimen, as should be the case in most patients who can concentrate urine normally, there is no need to perform further tests of concentrating ability.

Formal tests of renal concentrating power measure the concentration of urine produced in response either to fluid deprivation or to intramuscular (IM) injection of 1-deamino,8-D-arginine vasopressin (DDAVP), a synthetic analogue of vasopressin. If the patient is receiving drugs that affect the renal concentrating ability (e.g. carbamazepine, chlorpropamide, DDAVP), these should be stopped for at least 48 h before testing. A fluid deprivation test is performed first. If the patient is unable to concentrate the urine adequately following fluid deprivation, then a DDAVP test follows immediately.

Fluid deprivation test

This test is effectively a bioassay of vasopressin, which is itself difficult to measure. The test can be hazardous in a patient excreting large volumes of dilute urine, and requires close supervision. There are a number of ways of performing a fluid deprivation test, differing in detail but all involving fluid deprivation over several hours, ensuring that the patient under observation takes no fluid, and that excessive fluid losses do not occur. Local directions for test performance should be followed. For instance, beginning at 10 pm, the patient is told not to drink overnight, and urine specimens are collected while the patient continues not to drink between 8 am and 3 pm the next day. During the test, the patient should be weighed every 2 h, and the test should be stopped if weight loss of 3–5% of total body weight occurs. Blood and urine specimens are collected for measurement of osmolality.

Normally, there is no increase in plasma osmolality (reference range 285–295 mmol/kg) over the period of water deprivation, whereas urine osmolality rises to 800 mmol/kg or more. A rising plasma osmolality and a failure to concentrate urine are consistent with either a failure to secrete vasopressin or a failure to respond to vasopressin at the level of the distal nephron. When this pattern of results is obtained, it is usual to proceed immediately to perform the DDAVP test.

DDAVP test

The patient is allowed to drink a moderate amount of water at the end of the fluid deprivation test, to alleviate thirst. An IM injection of DDAVP is then given, and urine specimens are collected at hourly intervals for a further 3 h and their osmolality measured.

Interpretation of tests of renal concentrating ability

These tests are of most value in distinguishing among hypothalamic–pituitary, psychogenic and renal causes of polyuria (Table 4.4).

- Patients with diabetes insipidus of hypothalamic–pituitary origin produce insufficient vasopressin; they should therefore not respond to fluid deprivation, but should respond to the DDAVP. As a rule, these patients show an increase in plasma osmolality during the fluid deprivation test, to more than 300 mmol/kg, and a low urine osmolality (200–400 mmol/kg). There is a marked increase in urine osmolality, to 600 mmol/kg or more, in the DDAVP test.
- Polyuria of renal origin may be due to inability of the renal tubule to respond to vasopressin, as in nephrogenic diabetes insipidus. In this condition, there is failure to produce a concentrated urine in response either to fluid deprivation or to DDAVP injection, the urinary osmolality usually remaining below 400 mmol/kg; in these patients, plasma osmolality increases as a result of fluid deprivation.
- Patients with psychogenic diabetes insipidus should respond to both fluid deprivation and DDAVP. In practice, however, renal medullary hypo-osmolality often prevents the urine osmolality from reaching 800 mmol/kg after fluid deprivation or DDAVP injection in these tests, as normally performed. Also, the chronic suppression of the physiological mechanism that con-

trols vasopressin release may impair the normal hypothalamic response to dehydration. These patients have a plasma osmolality that is initially low, but which rises during the tests. However, fluid deprivation may have to be continued for more than 24 h in these patients before medullary hyperosmolality is restored; only then do they show normal responses to fluid deprivation or to DDAVP injection.

Urinary acidification tests

Urine is normally acidic, compared with plasma, in healthy subjects on a meat-containing diet. An alkaline urine may be found in vegans, in patients ingesting alkali or in patients with urinary tract infections. Urinalysis using dipsticks can be used to give a rough estimate of urine pH over the range 5–9. It is important to measure urine pH on freshly voided urine specimens.

Urine acidification is a function of the distal nephron, which can secrete H^+ until the limiting intraluminal pH of approximately 5.0 or less is reached. Acidification occurs as a result of the kidney reabsorbing the large amounts of the HCO_3^- that were filtered at the glomerulus, and excreting H^+ produced as non-volatile acids during tissue metabolism. The amount of H^+ that can be secreted into the tubules before the limiting intraluminal pH is reached depends on the presence of urine buffers. The H^+ in urine is only partly eliminated as such, and it is mostly excreted as H^+ combined with buffer ions, principally inorganic phosphate (Figures 3.1 and 3.2).

It is possible to assess the capacity of the kidney to produce an acid urine after a metabolic acidosis has been induced by administering ammonium chloride (NH_4Cl). In response to the NH_4Cl load, urine pH normally falls to below 5.3 in at least one specimen. It is essential to check that a satisfactory acidosis was induced, and this is assumed to have occurred if plasma [total CO_2] falls by about 4 mmol/L after NH_4Cl ingestion. More elaborate tests of urinary acidification (e.g. determining the renal threshold for HCO_3^-) are needed to differentiate between proximal and distal renal tubular acidosis.

Renal tubular acidosis

At least two distinct tubular abnormalities may give rise to conditions in which there is acidosis of renal origin but little or no change in plasma [creatinine], or other measure of the GFR. The impaired ability to excrete H^+ means that when Na^+ is reabsorbed in the distal tubule, there is an increased loss of K^+, resulting in K^+ depletion and hypokalaemia. This combination of metabolic acidosis and hypokalaemia is an unusual one, since hyperkalaemia is more commonly seen in acidosis.

• *Distal renal tubular acidosis* (type I) is the more common type. It is due to an inability to maintain a gradient of [H^+] across the distal tubule and collecting ducts. It is usually caused by an inherited abnormality, but may occur in certain forms of acquired renal disease. Bone disease, commonly osteomalacia, results from the buffering of H^+ by bone, and there is often hypercalciuria and nephrocalcinosis. Loss of Na^+ and K^+ in the urine and hypokalaemia are common. Urinary pH rarely falls below 6.0 and never below 5.3 in the ammonium chloride test of urinary acidification.

• *Proximal renal tubular acidosis* (type II) is much less common. It is due to proximal tubular loss of HCO_3^- caused by a low renal threshold for HCO_3^-. This means that if the [HCO_3^-] is low, HCO_3^- may be completely reabsorbed, resulting in the excretion of normal amounts of acid, but at the expense of a continuing systemic acidosis. [HCO_3^-] rarely falls below about 15 mmol/L. Occasionally, this is an isolated abnormality. More often, it occurs as one of the features in some patients with Fanconi syndrome (see below). If these patients are given enough NH_4Cl to reduce plasma [total CO_2] below the renal threshold for HCO_3^-, urinary pH may fall below 5.3. Diagnosis requires assessment of the renal threshold for HCO_3^-.

Glycosuria

Glucose is most commonly found in the urine in patients with diabetes, when the plasma [glucose] exceeds the renal threshold. Glycosuria in the presence of a normal plasma [glucose] occurs in proximal tubular malfunction causing a reduced renal threshold. This can be a benign isolated abnormality, may occur during pregnancy or may be part of a more generalised disorder (the Fanconi syndrome, see below).

The amino acidurias

Amino acids can be categorised into four groups – the neutral, acidic and basic amino acids, and the imino acids proline and hydroxyproline. Each has its own specific mechanism for transport across the proximal tubular cell. Normally, the renal tubules reabsorb all the filtered amino acids except for small amounts of glycine, serine, alanine and glutamine. Amino aciduria may be due to disease of the renal tubule (renal or low threshold type), or to raised plasma [amino acids] (generalised or overflow type).

Renal amino aciduria may be due to impairment of one of the specific transport mechanisms. For example, in cystinuria there is a hereditary defect in the epithelial transport of cystine and the basic amino acids lysine, ornithine and arginine; it is a rare cause of renal (cystine) stones. Renal amino aciduria may also occur as a non-specific abnormality due to generalised tubular damage, together with reabsorption defects affecting glucose or phosphate, or both.

The overflow types of amino aciduria result when the renal threshold for amino acids is exceeded, due to overproduction or to accumulation of amino acids in the body (e.g. PKU, p. 295; acute hepatic necrosis).

Fanconi syndrome

Fanconi syndrome may be inherited (e.g. in cystinosis) or secondary to a number of other disorders (e.g. heavy metal poisoning, multiple myeloma). The syndrome comprises multiple defects of proximal tubular function. There are excessive urinary losses of amino acids (generalised amino aciduria), phosphate, glucose and sometimes HCO_3^-, which gives rise to a proximal renal tubular acidosis. Distal tubular functions may also be affected. Sometimes globulins of low molecular mass may be detectable in urine, in addition to the amino aciduria.

Renal handling of sodium and potassium

Sodium excretion

The kidneys are essential for maintaining sodium balance, normally filtering about 21 000 mmol Na^+/day through the glomeruli. On a diet of 100 mmol Na^+, and in the absence of any pathological loss of Na^+, the kidney matches this intake with an excretion of 100 mmol Na^+, which represents about 0.5% of the filtered Na^+ load.

As the GFR declines in chronic renal failure, the proportion of the filtered Na^+ that is excreted needs to increase progressively to maintain Na^+ balance. The limit cannot generally exceed 20–30% of the filtered Na^+ load. Once this is reached, any further reduction in GFR, or an increase in dietary Na^+, leads to Na^+ retention. Most patients with chronic renal failure tolerate normal levels of dietary Na^+ if the GFR is more than 10 mL/min. However, if the GFR falls below this level, Na^+ retention occurs, leading to expansion of the ECF, weight gain and worsening hypertension. In the presence of other Na^+-retaining states (e.g. congestive cardiac failure or cirrhosis), Na^+ retention will be even more pronounced. Treatment depends upon Na^+ restriction and careful use of diuretic therapy.

In chronic renal failure, excessive Na^+ loss may also occur. The capacity of the kidneys to adapt to changes in Na^+ intake is limited, and a requirement to conserve Na^+ (e.g. in response to excessive use of diuretics or if the patient has severe diarrhoea) may not be met by the damaged kidneys. This leads on to a further fall in GFR. In chronic pyelonephritis and other disorders primarily affecting the renal tubules, large amounts of Na^+ may be lost in the urine, and severe Na^+ and water depletion can occur.

Potassium excretion

About 90% of K^+ in the glomerular filtrate is normally reabsorbed in the proximal tubules, the distal tubules regulating the amount of K^+ excreted in the urine. The rate of secretion of K^+ by the distal tubules is influenced by the transtubular potential and by the tubular cell $[K^+]$, and is usually maintained adequately, provided the daily urine flow rate is greater than 1 L.

In the presence of a normal GFR, about 550 mmol K^+ is filtered daily at the glomerulus. An average dietary intake of K^+ is about 80 mmol/day, and external K^+ balance is normally achieved by excreting about 15% of the filtered K^+. A reduction in GFR to about 10 mL/min requires an increase in the proportion of the filtered K^+ that is excreted to 150%. Distal tubular secretion of K^+ is needed to achieve this. Generally, the normal daily intake of K^+ can be tolerated if the GFR is 10 mL/min. At a GFR of about 5 mL/min, however, the limit of adaptation is reached, leading to K^+ retention and hyperkalaemia. The ability of the GI tract to increase excretion of K^+ helps to delay the onset of hyperkalaemia.

In chronic renal disease, excessive renal losses of K^+ are rare, but the Na^+ depletion that sometimes develops in renal disease may be associated with secondary aldosteronism, which in turn causes excessive loss of K^+.

Measurement of urinary K^+ output can prove helpful in patients suspected of losing abnormal amounts of K^+. Persistence of a relatively high urinary K^+ output in the presence of hypokalaemia strongly suggests that the kidney is unable to conserve K^+ adequately.

Renal failure

Acute renal failure

By definition, this is renal disease of acute onset, severe enough to cause failure of renal homeostasis. Often oliguric, diuretic and recovery phases can be recognised, although a few patients maintain a normal urine output throughout the course of the illness. Chemical investigations help to determine the severity of the disease and to follow its course, but do not help much in determining the cause. eGFR calculations are not valid in acute renal failure or when [creatinine] is changing rapidly. Proteinuria is present, and haem pigments from the blood may make the urine dark.

Oliguric phase

In this phase, less than 400 mL of urine is produced each day; if the renal failure is due to outflow obstruction, there may be anuria. The oliguria is mainly due to a fall in GFR. The urine that is formed usually has an osmolality similar to plasma and a relatively high $[Na^+]$, since the composition of the small amount of glomerular filtrate produced is little altered by the damaged tubules.

Plasma $[Na^+]$ is usually low due to a combination of factors, including intake of water in excess of the amount able to be excreted, increase in metabolic water from increased tissue catabolism and possibly a shift of Na^+ from ECF to ICF. Plasma $[K^+]$, on the other hand, is usually increased due to the impaired renal output and increased tissue catabolism, which is aggravated by the shift of K^+ out of cells that accompanies the metabolic acidosis that develops due to failure to excrete H^+ and also due to the increased formation of H^+ from tissue catabolism.

Retention of urea, creatinine, phosphate, sulphate and other waste products occurs. The rate at which plasma [urea] rises is affected by the rate of tissue catabolism; this, in turn, depends on the cause of the acute renal failure. In renal failure due to trauma (including renal failure developing after surgical operations), plasma [urea] tends to rise more rapidly than in patients with renal failure due to medical causes such as acute glomerulonephritis.

To differentiate the low urinary output of suspected acute renal failure from that due to severe circulatory impairment with reduced blood volume, the tests summarised in Table 4.5 may be helpful. However, none of these tests can be completely relied upon to make the important and urgent distinction between renal failure and hypovolaemia. Careful assessment of the patient's fluid status, possibly including measure-

Table 4.5 Investigation of low urinary output

Investigation	Simple hypovolaemia	Acute renal failure
Urine osmolality	Usually >500 mmol/kg	Usually <400 mmol/kg
Urine [urea] : plasma [urea]	Usually >10	Usually <5
Urine [Na$^+$]	Usually <20 mmol/L	Usually >40 mmol/L

ment of the central venous pressure, is also required.

For monitoring patients in the oliguric phase of acute renal failure, plasma [creatinine] or [urea] and plasma [K$^+$] are particularly important, and need to be determined at least once daily. Decisions to use haemodialysis are reached at least partly on the basis of the results of these tests. The volume of urine and its electrolyte composition (and the volume and composition of any other measurable sources of fluid loss) should also be assessed in order to determine fluid and electrolyte replacement requirements.

Diuretic phase

With the onset of this phase, urine volume increases, but the clearance of urea, creatinine and other waste products may not improve to the same extent. Plasma [urea] and [creatinine] may therefore continue to rise, at least at the start of the diuretic phase. Large losses of electrolytes may occur in the urine and require to be replaced orally or parenterally. Measurement of these losses is needed so that correct replacement therapy can be given; this requires urine collections, for urine [Na$^+$] and [K$^+$] measurement, and calculation of daily outputs.

Plasma [K$^+$] tends to fall as the diuretic phase continues, due to the shift of K$^+$ back into the cells and to marked losses in urine resulting from impaired conservation of K$^+$ by the still-damaged tubules. Usually, Na$^+$ deficiency also occurs, due to failure of renal conservation. Throughout the diuretic phase, therefore, it is important to measure plasma [creatinine] and both plasma [Na$^+$] and [K$^+$] at least once daily, and to monitor the output of Na$^+$ and K$^+$ in the urine.

Chronic renal failure

Most of the functional changes seen in chronic renal failure can be explained in terms of a full solute load falling on a reduced number of normal nephrons. The GFR is invariably reduced, associated with retention of urea, creatinine, urate, various phenolic and indolic acids, and other organic substances. The progress and severity of the disease are usually monitored by measuring plasma [creatinine] and [urea], and by calculating the eGFR.

Sodium, potassium and water

The renal handling of Na$^+$, K$^+$ and water by normal kidneys and in chronic renal failure has already been considered above (p. 60).

Acid–base disturbances

The total excretion of H$^+$ is impaired, mainly due to a fall in the renal capacity to form NH$_4^+$. Metabolic acidosis is present in most patients, but its severity remains fairly stable in spite of the reduced urinary H$^+$ excretion. There may be an extrarenal mechanism for H$^+$ elimination, possibly involving buffering of H$^+$ by calcium salts in bone; this would contribute to the demineralisation of bone that often occurs in chronic renal failure.

Calcium and phosphate

Plasma [calcium] tends to be low, often due, at least partly, to reduced plasma [albumin]. Plasma [phosphate] is high, mainly due to the reduction of GFR.

Virtually all patients with chronic renal failure have secondary or, much less often, tertiary hyperparathyroidism, and they may develop osteitis fibrosa. Plasma [calcium], which is decreased or close to the lower reference value in patients with secondary hyperparathyroidism, increases later if tertiary hyperparathyroidism develops. Many patients with a low plasma [calcium] have reduced activity of renal cholecalciferol 1α-hydroxylase, the enzyme responsible for the synthesis of the most active form of vitamin D. They can potentially develop osteomalacia or rickets, but this would be uncommon in adequately treated patients. A few patients show a third type of bone abnormality: increased bone density (osteosclerosis). It is not clear why any particular one of these various types of renal osteodystrophy should develop in an individual patient (p. 84).

Other laboratory abnormalities

Other findings in chronic renal failure may include impaired glucose tolerance (IGT) and raised plasma [magnesium]. These may need appropriate treatment, but are of no particular diagnostic significance. Impaired renal erythropoietin synthesis contributes to the anaemia which is often present in patients with chronic renal failure. Biosynthetic erythropoietin can be used to treat this.

Proteinuria

Glomerular filtrate normally contains about 30 mg/L protein; this corresponds to a total filtered load of about 5 g/24 h. Since less than 200 mg of protein is normally excreted in the urine each day (half of which is Tamm–Horsfall mucoprotein, secreted by tubular cells), tubular reabsorption and catabolism are very efficient in health.

Proteinuria is described as glomerular proteinuria if the glomerulus becomes abnormally leaky, or as tubular proteinuria when tubular reabsorption of protein becomes defective. Abnormally large amounts of some plasma proteins may lead to an overflow proteinuria. Protein may also enter the urinary tract distal to the kidneys (e.g. due to inflammation), leading to post-renal proteinuria; if

post-renal proteinuria is suspected, urine microscopy (including cytology) and culture should be carried out. Electrophoresis of a concentrated urine specimen may help to distinguish these forms of proteinuria. In tubular proteinuria, the proteins are mainly of low molecular weight, having been filtered through the glomerulus but not reabsorbed. In glomerular proteinuria, larger proteins that have filtered through the defective glomeruli are also present.

Dipstick testing of urine for protein should be part of the full clinical examination of every patient. These tests detect albumin at concentrations greater than 200 mg/L, but are less sensitive to other proteins, and in particular fail to detect the Bence Jones proteins that may be excreted in multiple myeloma. If the presence of proteinuria is confirmed, it should be quantified as a protein: creatinine ratio, or in a timed (usually 24 h) urine collection, and simple tests of renal function performed. If the renal function tests are normal and the protein excretion is less than about 500 mg/24 h, it is probably not necessary to subject the patient to further investigation, although follow-up should be arranged. If the protein excretion is greater than this, or renal function is impaired, further investigation is necessary, and may include imaging techniques and biopsy.

Overflow proteinuria

Several conditions may give rise to abnormal amounts of low molecular mass proteins (i.e. less than about 70 kDa) in plasma and in urine. These proteins are filtered at the glomerulus and may then be neither reabsorbed nor catabolised completely by the renal tubular cells. The principal examples are listed in Table 4.6.

Glomerular proteinuria

Table 4.7 classifies glomerular proteinuria separately from tubular proteinuria, but many patients show features of both glomerular and tubular protein loss. Where quantitative measurements of urine protein loss are required (e.g. when monitoring treatment for the nephrotic syndrome), side-

Table 4.6 Overflow proteinuria

Protein	Molecular mass (kDa)	Cause
Amylase	45	Acute pancreatitis
Bence Jones protein	44	Multiple myeloma
Hb	68	Intravascular haemolysis
Lysozyme	15	Myelomonocytic leukaemia
Myoglobin	17	Crush injuries

Table 4.7 Glomerular and tubular proteinuria

Classification	Examples of causes
Glomerular proteinuria	
May or may not be of pathological significance	Orthostatic proteinuria, effort proteinuria, febrile proteinuria
Of pathological significance	Glomerulonephritis, all forms; pathological causes of altered haemodynamics (e.g. renal artery stenosis)
Tubular proteinuria	Chronic nephritis and pyelonephritis, acute tubular necrosis, renal tubule defects (e.g. renal tubular acidosis), heavy metal poisoning, renal transplantation

room tests are insufficiently precise; laboratory measurements are required.

Some patients, typically with protein excretion rates of less than 1 g/24 h, have benign or functional proteinuria. This probably results from blood flow changes through the glomeruli, and is found in association with exercise, fever and congestive cardiac failure. Amongst these conditions, it is particularly important to recognise orthostatic proteinuria.

Nephrotic syndrome

In the nephrotic syndrome, large amounts of protein are lost in the urine, and hypoproteinae-mia and oedema (due to the low (albumin) and secondary hyperaldosteronism) develop. Usually, the protein losses in the urine are over 5 g/24 h. More than this is filtered at the glomerulus, but most is catabolised in the tubules and is therefore lost from the circulation, but does not appear in the urine. The amount of proteinuria does not correlate well with the severity of the renal disease. Patients with nephrotic syndrome may also have a secondary hyperlipidaemia.

Causes of nephrotic syndrome include glomerulonephritis, systemic lupus erythematosus and diabetic nephropathy.

Glomerulonephritis

This is the most common group of causes of persistent proteinuria. Plasma proteins escape in varying amounts, depending on their molecular mass, on the amount of glomerular damage and on the capacity of the renal tubule cells to reabsorb or metabolise the proteins that have passed the glomerulus.

The degree of proteinuria does not provide an index of the severity of renal disease. However, it is convenient to distinguish mild or moderate proteinuria, in which the loss is not sufficient to cause protein depletion, from severe proteinuria, in which the protein loss exceeds the body's capacity to replace losses by synthesis (usually 5–10 g/24 h). Severe, persistent proteinuria is one feature of the nephrotic syndrome, in which urinary protein loss is sometimes more than 30 g/24 h.

Orthostatic proteinuria

This is usually a benign condition that affects children and young adults, who exhibit proteinuria only after they have been standing up. For orthostatic (or postural) proteinuria to be diagnosed, protein is not detectable in an early morning urine specimen when tested by normal side-room methods (i.e. urine contains <100 mg/L). The patient is instructed to empty the bladder just before going to bed, and the test for protein is performed on a specimen of urine passed the following morning, collected immediately after getting up.

Orthostatic proteinuria is usually observed in only some of the urine specimens passed when up and about, and for these individuals the prognosis is good. It is less so for those in whom proteinuria is always detected.

Tubular proteinuria

This may be due to tubular or interstitial damage resulting from a variety of causes. The proteinuria is due to failure of the tubules to reabsorb some of the plasma proteins filtered by the normal glomerulus, or possibly due to abnormal secretion of protein into the urinary tract. The proteins excreted in tubular proteinuria mostly have a low molecular mass, for example β_2-microglobulin (11.8 kDa) and lysozyme (15 kDa). The loss of protein is usually mild, rarely more than 2 g/24 h.

Urinary β_2-microglobulin excretion is normally very small (<0.4 mg/24 h). Its measurement has been used as a sensitive test of renal tubular damage. However, the test is of limited value for this purpose, if there is evidence of impaired renal function, for example increased plasma [creatinine].

Renal stones

Physicochemical principles govern the formation of renal stones, and are relevant to the choice of treatment aimed at preventing progression or recurrence. Stones may cause renal damage, often progressive.

The solubility of a salt depends on the product of the activities of its constituent ions. Frequently, the solubility product in urine is exceeded without the formation of a stone, provided there is no 'seeding' by particles present in urine, such as debris or bacteria, which promote crystal formation. Formation of stones can also be prevented by inhibitory substances that are normally present in the urine, such as citrate, which can chelate calcium, keeping it in solution.

People living or working in hot conditions are liable to become dehydrated, and show a greater tendency to form renal stones, as the urine becomes more concentrated. There are also several metabolic factors that can cause stones to form in the renal tract. However, in many patients, no cause can be found to explain why stones have formed. The main types of renal stones are listed in Table 4.8.

Hypercalciuria

Stones in the upper renal tract occur in 5–10% of adults in western Europe and the USA. These are mostly either pure calcium oxalate or a mixture of calcium oxalate and phosphate. Not every patient with renal stones, however, has hypercalciuria, since there is considerable overlap between the 24-h urinary calcium excretion of healthy individuals on their normal diet (up to 12 mmol/24 h) and the urinary calcium excretion of stone-formers.

Table 4.8 Renal stones

Type of stone	Frequency in UK (%)	Metabolic cause or relevant factors
Calcium oxalate stones and mixed (calcium oxalate and phosphate stones)	80–55	Hypercalciuria (see text), excessive absorption of dietary oxalate, primary hyperoxaluria
Triple phosphate stones	5–10	Urinary tract infection (fall in [H⁺])
Urate stones	5–10	Gout, myeloproliferative disorders, high protein diet, uricosuric drugs
Cystine stones	~1	Cystinuria
Xanthine stones	<1	Xanthinuria

Increased urinary calcium excretion may be associated with hypercalcaemia, for instance, in primary hyperparathyroidism (p. 76), vitamin D overdosage and hypersensitivity to vitamin D (p. 79), or with normocalcaemia, as in idiopathic hypercalciuria, prolonged immobilisation and renal tubular acidosis. In many patients with what was previously considered to be 'idiopathic' hypercalciuria, the underlying disorder is an increase in intestinal calcium absorption.

Up to 10% of renal calculi, depending on the series, have been attributed to primary hyperparathyroidism (p. 76). It is important to investigate patients with recurrent renal calculi for primary hyperparathyroidism, as this condition can be cured.

phate and urate. Occasionally, assessment of urinary excretion of oxalate, cystine or xanthine may be required, or urinary acidification tests.
• Renal function tests plasma [creatinine] and/or plasma [urea].
In addition to chemical tests, microbiological examination of urine is usually performed. Radiological investigations of the urinary tract will be required to localise the stone.

Reference

Cockcroft, D.W. and Gault, M.H. (1976) Prediction of creatinine clearance from serum creatinine. *Nephron*, 16, 41.

Oxalate, cystine and xanthine excretion

The majority of urinary calculi contain oxalate, but excessive excretion of oxalate is primarily responsible for the formation of stones in only a small percentage of cases. Other occasional causes of stone formation include cystinuria and xanthinuria.

Primary hyperoxaluria is a rare condition in which there is increased excretion of oxalate and of glyoxylate, the latter due to deficiency of the enzyme responsible for converting glyoxylate to glycine. Patients with disease of the terminal ileum may have an increased tendency to form oxalate stones, due to the hyperoxaluria caused by increased absorption of dietary oxalate.

Chemical investigations on patients with renal stones

Stones should be analysed for some or all of the constituents listed in Table 4.7, as this can be helpful. The following tests may also be helpful in reaching a diagnosis:
• Plasma calcium, albumin, phosphate, total CO_2 and urate concentrations, and ALP activity. Full acid–base assessment is rarely needed.
• Urine dipstick testing (pH and protein), and measurement of 24-h excretion of calcium, phos-

Keypoints

• The GFR is the best single measure of the number of functioning nephrons, and measured by endogenous creatinine clearance, although this overestimates true GFR at low levels of GFR.
• Plasma [creatinine] is a more precise measurement than creatinine clearance, and is usually sufficient for following the progress of patients with renal disease. However, GFR may decline by as much as 50% before plasma [creatinine] exceeds the upper limit of the reference range.
• GFR can be estimated (eGFR) from the plasma [creatinine] and other variables including age and sex, and thereby avoids some of the circumstances where [creatinine] can be misleading. The eGFR suffers from significant imprecision, but is the basis for the classification of chronic kidney disease.
• Plasma [urea] is a less valuable test of renal function than [creatinine], since it is reabsorbed by the tubule at low urine flow rates, as in pre-renal uraemia.
• Fluid deprivation or urinary acidification tests of tubular function are less often used.
• Chemical tests are of value in following the progress of both acute and chronic renal failure, but not in determining the aetiology.
• Side-room testing for urinary protein should form a part of all full clinical examinations.
• Renal stones have a variety of causes, but it is important to investigate for hyperparathyroidism.

Case 4.1

An elderly man was struck by a car while crossing the road, and received multiple injuries. He was admitted to a hospital, where he underwent emergency surgery. After 24 h, he was observed to be clinically dehydrated, hypotensive and only to have passed 400 mL of urine. Results of biochemical investigations were as follows:

Serum	Result	Reference range
Urea	23.2	2.5–6.6 mmol/L
Na$^+$	143	135–145 mmol/L
K$^+$	4.8	3.6–5.0 mmol/L
Creatinine	225	60–120 µmol/L

Urine	Result	Reference range
Urea	492	170–600 mmol/24 h
Na$^+$	6	100–200 mmol/24
Osmolality	826	mmol/kg

Comments: The patient has pre-renal uraemia due to inadequate fluid replacement. He has passed a small volume of concentrated urine that is low in sodium. This is a normal physiological response by the kidney to impaired perfusion, due in this case to hypovolaemia. The [urea] has increased relatively more than the [creatinine] due to passive tubular reabsorption, and possibly also due to increased tissue catabolism as part of the response to trauma.

The biochemical features that distinguish pre-renal uraemia from established renal failure are listed in Table 4.5, although in practice there may be some overlap. The prerequisite for using these values is the presence of oliguria, when the presence of concentrated low-sodium urine is a reliable indication of pre-renal uraemia. Dilute sodium-containing urine is not only characteristic of intrinsic renal failure in the presence of oliguria, but is also found in well-hydrated healthy individuals. The biochemical values for making this distinction are all invalidated by the use of diuretics, and osmolalities are invalidated by the use of X-ray contrast media.

Case 4.2

A 58-year-old man, a patient with known manic depression who was being treated with lithium, was admitted to a hospital psychiatric ward with a recent history of lethargy and confusion. On examination, he was found to be very dehydrated, and the results of biochemical investigations were

Serum	Result	Reference range
Urea	16.1	2.5–6.6 mmol/L
Na$^+$	197	135–145 mmol/L
K$^+$	3.6	3.6–5.0 mmol/L
Glucose	6.2	mmol/L

Urine	Result	
Osmolality	209	mmol/kg

(continued on p. 68)

Case 4.2 *(continued)*

Comments: The value for the calculated plasma osmolality, using the formula given on p. 16, is 423 mmol/kg. This high value accords with the findings on clinical examination. The kidneys would have been expected to produce a very concentrated urine, and the low urinary osmolality (lower than the plasma value) indicates either that vasopressin is not being secreted (leading to cranial diabetes insipidus), or that the kidneys are not responding to vasopressin (nephrogenic diabetes insipidus). It was not known whether or not the patient felt thirsty, but patients with any kind of diabetes insipidus, if unable or unwilling to respond to the thirst stimulus, rapidly become dehydrated.

Lithium is a known cause of nephrogenic diabetes insipidus and can also cause hypothyroidism and hypercalcaemia. Lithium has a narrow therapeutic : toxic ratio, and its dosage should be reviewed periodically and renal function, electrolytes, [Ca^{2+}] and thyroid function checked.

Case 4.3

A previously healthy 32-year-old bricklayer was admitted to a hospital in shock, with severe crush injuries to his legs caused by the collapse of a wall under which he had been trapped for several hours. The following results were obtained on specimens collected 3 days later:

Serum	Result	Reference range
Urea	42	2.5–6.6 mmol/L
Na^+	131	135–145 mmol/L
K^+	6.8	3.6–5.0 mmol/L
Total CO_2	12	22–30 mmol/L
Osmolality	330	280–296 mmol/kg

Urine	Result	Reference range
Volume	36	mL/24 h
Urea	280	170–600 mmol/24 h
Na^+	62	100–200 mmol/24 h
Osmolality	330	mmol/kg

Comments: This man has developed acute renal failure as a result of his crush injury. The combination of hypovolaemia with the release of myoglobin from the crushed muscles has caused acute impairment of renal function, with a high plasma [urea]. The plasma [K^+] is increased as a result of the acute renal failure; there might also be significant K^+ leakage from damaged cells contributing to this increase. The low plasma [total CO_2] reflects the metabolic acidosis that is a feature of acute renal failure.

The urine volume is very low, as glomerular filtration has almost completely ceased. This low volume is accompanied by a urine with a composition inappropriate for someone who is severely volume depleted, i.e. it is dilute and contains a relatively high [Na^+]. Vasopressin and aldosterone levels would both be expected to have been high in this patient, leading to urine that was both concentrated and low in [Na^+].

In general terms, the formation of a urine that is both dilute and containing relatively high [Na^+], in a patient with an acute increase in plasma [urea], favours an acute failure of renal function rather than pre-renal uraemia (where renal function may be intrinsically normal). A urine osmolality >500 mmol/kg and a urine [Na^+] <20 mmol/L would tend to favour a pre-renal (reversible) cause for the uraemia, whereas a urine osmolality <400 mmol/kg and a urine [Na^+] >40 mmol/L would tend to favour a renal cause for the uraemia.

Case 4.4

A 62-year-old man visited his GP and complained of malaise, tiredness and weight loss over the previous 6 months. His only other complaint was of passing more urine than usual, especially at night, when he had to get up three or four times. He appeared pale, was hypertensive, with a blood pressure of 182/114. Urinalysis revealed protein, but no glucose.

The results of simple initial investigations were as follows

Serum or blood	Result	Reference range
Urea	38.2	2.5–6.6 mmol/L
Creatinine	635	60–120 µmol/L
Sodium	129	135–145 mmol/L
Potassium	5.4	3.6–5.0 mmol/L
Total CO_2	17	22–30 mmol/L
Glucose	5.2	mmol/L
Calcium	1.88	2.1–2.6 mmol/L
Phosphate	2.38	0.8–1.4 mmol/L
ALP	226	40–125 U/L
Hb	92	130–180 g/L

Comments: The lengthy history suggests the onset of a slowly progressive illness, rather than an acute one. The symptoms of weight loss, tiredness and polyuria might suggest the onset of diabetes, but the lack of glycosuria, backed up by the normal random [glucose], rules this out. The results are typical of chronic renal failure. This is supported by the anaemia and the raised ALP (due to renal osteodystrophy), neither of which is a specific finding, but which are more consistent with chronic than with acute renal failure. Chronic renal failure is also supported by the presence of hypertension, and by the finding of small kidneys if the patient goes on to receive an abdominal ultrasound examination.

Case 4.5

A 6-year-old boy developed marked oedema over a period of a few days, and his parents had noted that his urine had become frothy. His GP detected proteinuria, and arranged admission to a hospital, where the following results were obtained:

Serum	Result	Reference range
Urea	3.4	2.5–6.6 mmol/L
Creatinine	48	60–120 µmol/L
Sodium	131	135–145 mmol/L
Potassium	4.0	3.6–5.0 mmol/L
Total CO_2	27.0	22–30 mmol/L
Calcium	1.65	2.1–2.6 mmol/L
Albumin	14	35–50 g/L
Total protein	34	60–80 g/L
Cholesterol	11	mmol/L
Triglyceride	15	0.2–1.6 mmol/L
24-h urine protein	12	0.03–0.10 g/24 h

(continued on p. 70)

Case 4.5 *(continued)*

Comments: The nephrotic syndrome is the combination of oedema, hypoproteinaemia and proteinuria, as seen in this child. The oedema is the consequence of the hypoproteinaemia causing a redistribution of ECF from the vascular compartment to the interstitial fluid, often exacerbated by a consequent secondary hyperaldosteronism causing sodium retention and potassium depletion. Proteins other than albumin are also depleted, including anti-thrombin III, immunoglobulins (Igs) and complement. Conversely, some large proteins are present in high concentrations, fibrinogen and apolipoproteins being examples. These changes can predispose patients to infection and to venous thrombosis.

In nephrotic syndrome, the GFR may be low, normal or high. In the age group of this patient, the most common cause of nephrotic syndrome is minimal change nephropathy. The GFR is often high, as reflected by the observed low urea and creatinine. These patients usually respond satisfactorily to steroids, and the prognosis is good.

Chapter 5

Disorders of calcium, phosphate and magnesium metabolism

Calcium is the most abundant mineral in the body, there being about 25 mol (1 kg) in a 70 kg man. Approximately 99% of the body's calcium is present in the bone, mainly as the mineral hydroxyapatite, where it is combined with phosphate. About 85% of the body's phosphate content is in the bone.

In this book, 'calcium' is used as a composite term that embraces ionised calcium, protein-bound calcium and complexed calcium, whereas 'Ca^{2+}' means that only calcium ions are being considered. The total concentration of calcium in serum or urine is shown as serum or urine [calcium], whereas plasma [Ca^{2+}] refers specifically (and solely) to the concentration of ionised calcium.

Both hypercalcaemia and hypocalcaemia are relatively common biochemical abnormalities, as are abnormalities in serum [phosphate]. Abnormal serum [calcium] measurements often arise from alterations in serum [albumin], the major calcium-binding protein in serum. Other cases result from an increase or decrease in the unbound or ionised calcium. It is important to identify the latter group, since pathological levels of ionised calcium may be life threatening and

the conditions themselves are amenable to treatment.

In this chapter, the hormonal regulation of plasma [Ca^{2+}] is described, followed by a consideration of the causes of hypercalcaemia and hypocalcaemia and their investigation. Abnormalities in serum [phosphate] and [magnesium] are also briefly discussed.

Calcium homeostasis

Calcium balance

In adults, calcium intake and output are normally in balance (Figure 5.1). External balance is largely achieved through the body normally matching net absorption over 24 h closely with the corresponding 24-h urinary excretion; this varies with the diet. On a normal diet, urinary calcium excretion in healthy adults may overlap with the output in some patients who are renal stone-formers. In infancy and childhood, there is normally a positive balance, especially at times of active skeletal growth. In older age, calcium output may exceed input, and a state of negative balance then exists; this negative external balance is particularly marked in women after menopause, and is important in the development of post-menopausal osteoporosis. In women, the mother loses calcium to the foetus during pregnancy, and by lactation.

Lecture Notes: Clinical Biochemistry, 8e. By G. Beckett, S. Walker, P. Rae & P. Ashby. Published 2010 by Blackwell Publishing.

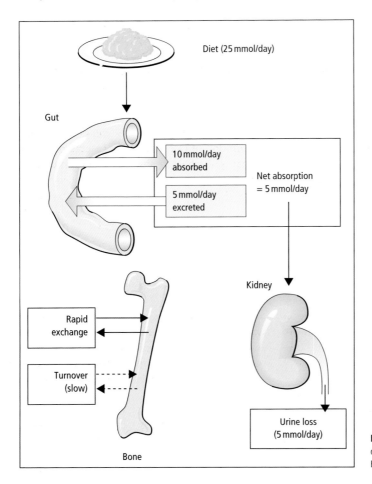

Figure 5.1 Summary of the typical daily movements of calcium between ECF, gut, bone and kidney.

Biological function of calcium

Calcium is a major mechanical constituent of the bone. Bone by itself is a specialised mineralised connective tissue containing cellular elements (bone-forming osteoblasts and bone-resorbing osteoclasts), organic matrix (type I collagen, proteoglycan, etc.) and the calcium-containing mineral hydroxyapatite. Calcium salts in bone have a mechanical role, but are not metabolically inert. There is a constant state of turnover in the skeleton associated with deposition of calcium in sites of bone formation and release at sites of bone resorption (~5% per year of the adult skeleton is remodelled). Calcium in the bone also acts as a reservoir that helps to stabilise ECF [Ca^{2+}].

Maintenance of extracellular [Ca^{2+}] within narrow limits is necessary for normal excitability of nerve and muscle. An increase in [Ca^{2+}] raises the threshold for the nerve action potential, and vice versa. The ion is also required in the activation of the clotting and complement cascades.

While the ECF [Ca^{2+}] is approximately 1 mmol/L (10^{-3} M), cytosolic [Ca^{2+}] is much lower, approximately 100 nmol/L (10^{-7} M). Cells possess a number of transport mechanisms for Ca^{2+} that allow maintenance of this large gradient across the cell membrane.

An increase in cytosolic [Ca^{2+}] serves as a signal for several cell processes, which include cell shape change, cell motility, metabolic changes, secretory activity and cell division. Many intercellular signals, including several hormones, bring about an increase in cytosolic [Ca^{2+}] by opening plasma membrane Ca^{2+} channels, or by releasing intracellular stores of Ca^{2+}, or by a combination of these effects.

Control of calcium metabolism

Calcium is present in plasma in three forms (Table 5.1), in equilibrium with one another. Plasma [Ca^{2+}] is the physiologically important component, and is closely regulated in humans by PTH and 1:25-dihydroxycholecalciferol (DHCC): both act to increase plasma [Ca^{2+}] and hence plasma [calcium]. The body's responses to a fall in plasma [Ca^{2+}], in terms of changes in PTH and 1:25-DHCC production, are shown in Figure 5.2. Growth hormone (GH), glucocorticoids (e.g. cortisol), oestrogens, testosterone and thyroid hormones (thyroxine (T4) and tri-iodothyronine (T3)) also influence calcium metabolism.

Parathyroid hormone (PTH)

PTH is the principal acute regulator of plasma [Ca^{2+}]. Plasma PTH levels exhibit a diurnal rhythm, being highest in the early hours of the morning and lowest at about 9 am. The active hormone is secreted in response to a fall in plasma [Ca^{2+}], and its actions are directed to increase plasma [Ca^{2+}]. An increase in plasma [Ca^{2+}] suppresses PTH secretion.

- *In bone*, PTH stimulates bone resorption by osteoclasts, with a requirement for osteoblasts to mediate this effect. Biochemical measures of both increased osteoblast activity (e.g. increased serum

Table 5.1 The components of calcium in plasma

Calcium component	Percentage of plasma [calcium]
Ionised calcium, Ca^{2+}	50–65
Calcium bound to plasma proteins – mainly albumin	30–45
Calcium complexed with citrate, etc.	5–10

ALP activity) and increased osteoclast activity (e.g. raised urinary hydroxyproline and deoxypyridinoline excretion) may be evident. In severe hyperparathyroidism, radiological demineralisation may be seen, including subperiosteal resorption of the terminal phalanges, bone cysts and pepper skull.

- *In the kidney*, PTH increases the distal tubular reabsorption of calcium. It also reduces proximal tubular phosphate reabsorption and promotes activity of the 1α-hydroxylation of calcidiol (see below). Renal loss of HCO$_3^-$ also increases, which may lead to a mild metabolic acidosis. Formation of 1:25-DHCC indirectly increases the absorption of calcium from the small intestine.

1:25-Dihydroxycholecalciferol (1:25-DHCC, or calcitriol)

Most vitamin D$_3$ (cholecalciferol) is synthesised by the action of ultraviolet light on the vitamin D precursor 7-dehydrocholesterol in the skin. Vitamin D$_3$ is also present naturally in food (a rich source is fish oils), while vitamin D$_2$ (ergosterol) is added to margarine.

Endogenous synthesis of vitamin D$_3$ is important. Vitamin D deficiency can develop if exposure to sunlight is inadequate, or because of inadequate dietary intake, but is usually a result of the combined effects of these two factors. In the body, vitamin D$_3$ and vitamin D$_2$ undergo two hydroxylation steps before attaining full physiological activity (Figure 5.3):

- *25-Hydroxylation* This occurs in the liver, with the production of 25-hydroxycholecalciferol (25-HCC, or calcidiol). Other inactive metabolites are formed, but are excreted in the bile. The main form of vitamin D circulating in the plasma is 25-HCC, bound to a specific transport protein; it is carried to the kidney for further metabolism. Plasma [25-HCC] shows marked seasonal variation, with levels highest in summer.
- *1α-Hydroxylation of 25-HCC* This takes place in the kidney, with the production of 1:25-DHCC, biologically the most active naturally occurring derivative of vitamin D. The kidney also contains other hydroxylases, such as 24-hydroxylase,

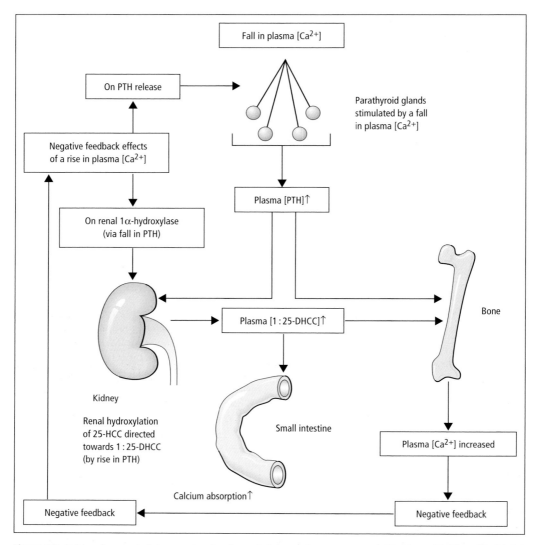

Figure 5.2 Calcium homeostasis in man showing the main hormonal responses to a fall in plasma [Ca²⁺], and indicating the places where the negative feedback mechanism operates if plasma [Ca²⁺] becomes high. The effect of PTH on the renal tubules, causing increased reabsorption of calcium, is not shown.

which converts 25-HCC to 24:25-DHCC. Renal 1α-hydroxylation is increased by low plasma [phosphate], high [PTH] and where there is a tendency to hypocalcaemia, whatever the cause. The reverse circumstances direct metabolism of 25-HCC towards the formation of 24:25-DHCC, which has no clearly established physiological function.

The principal action of 1:25-DHCC is to induce synthesis of a Ca²⁺-binding protein in the intestinal epithelial cell necessary for the absorption of calcium from the small intestine. Deficiency of 1:25-DHCC leads to defective bone mineralisation. Maintenance of both ECF [Ca²⁺] and ECF [phosphate] by 1:25-DHCC may be a key factor in normal mineralisation.

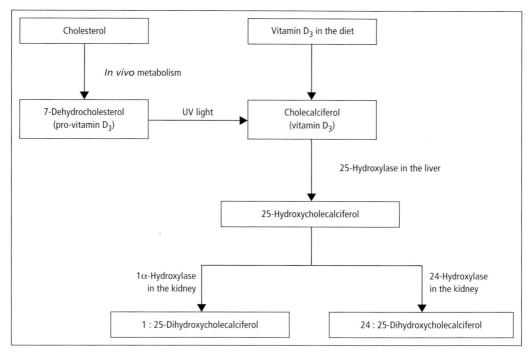

Figure 5.3 The formation of 1:25-DHCC, the most active form of vitamin D_3, from pro-vitamin D_3 (normally the main source of the vitamin in man) and from dietary vitamin D_3. Vitamin D_2 (ergosterol) undergoes similar hydroxylations. By the action of ultraviolet (UV) light, pro-vitamin D_3 is converted in the dermis into pre-vitamin D_3 (not shown) in which the B-ring of the steroid skeleton has been opened; pre-vitamin D_3 then rearranges spontaneously to give vitamin D_3. The factors that influence the hydroxylation of 25-HCC in the direction of 1:25-DHCC or 24:25-DHCC are described in the text.

Calcitonin

Although calcitonin can decrease plasma $[Ca^{2+}]$ by reducing osteoclast activity and decreasing renal reabsorption of calcium and phosphate, its actions are transient, and chronic excess or deficiency is not associated with disordered calcium or bone metabolism. Its use as a tumour marker is discussed elsewhere (p. 251).

Investigation of abnormal calcium metabolism

Measurement of serum calcium and albumin, inorganic phosphate and ALP, and sometimes magnesium, PTH and vitamin D metabolites, underlie the diagnosis of most disorders of calcium metabolism.

Serum [calcium] (reference range 2.10–2.60 mmol/L)

Because of technical difficulties associated with the measurement of $[Ca^{2+}]$, clinical biochemistry laboratories only measure serum [calcium] routinely, even though the physiologically important fraction is plasma $[Ca^{2+}]$.

Effects of serum [albumin]

Because albumin is the principal binding protein for calcium, a fall in serum [albumin] will lead to a fall in bound calcium and a decrease in total [calcium] (and vice versa). Under these circumstances, the unbound plasma $[Ca^{2+}]$, the physiologically important fraction, will be maintained at normal levels by PTH . Modest but potentially misleading increases in serum [calcium] may also result from abnormal calcium binding, due to raised serum [albumin]. This is often due to faulty or non-standardised venepuncture technique (p. 242). To avoid misdiagnosis of hypocalcaemia or hypercalcaemia, serum [albumin] should always be measured at the same time as serum [calcium]. The serum [calcium] (in mmol/L) can be approximately 'corrected' to take account of an abnormal albumin (in g/L) using a formula such as

$$\text{'Corrected'} \, [\text{calcium}] = \text{measured} \, [\text{calcium}] + 0.02 \times (40 - [\text{albumin}])$$

Effects of plasma H⁺

In acidosis, the protonation of albumin reduces its ability to bind calcium, leading to an increase in unbound $[Ca^{2+}]$, and vice versa, without any change in total [calcium]. Thus, hyperventilation with respiratory alkalosis can reduce plasma $[Ca^{2+}]$, with the development of tetany. In chronic states of acidosis or alkalosis, PTH acts to readjust the plasma $[Ca^{2+}]$ back to normal.

Serum [phosphate] (reference range 0.8–1.4 mmol/L)

Serum [phosphate] shows considerable diurnal variation, especially following meals; the reference range relates to the fasting state. Different ranges should be used for different age groups. About 85% of serum phosphate is free and 15% protein bound.

Alkaline phosphatase (ALP)

Reference ranges for serum ALP activity are very method dependent. For physiological reasons, there are also considerable variations in this enzyme's activity in childhood, adolescence and pregnancy. The bone isoenzyme of ALP activity is increased in serum from patients with diseases in which there is increased osteoblastic activity, for example hyperparathyroidism, Paget's disease, rickets and osteomalacia, and carcinoma with osteoblastic metastases.

Hypercalcaemia

Increased plasma $[Ca^{2+}]$ is a potentially serious problem that can lead to renal damage, cardiac arrhythmias and general ill-health. The clinical features are listed in Table 5.2. The most common causes (Table 5.3) are primary hyperparathyroidism and malignant disease, although the likelihood of these diagnoses will vary depending on the patient population. In asymptomatic ambulatory patients with hypercalcaemia, primary hyperparathyroidism may account for up to 80% of cases whereas in sick hospitalised hypercalcaemic patients, malignancy-associated hypercalcaemia is more likely.

Primary hyperparathyroidism

Autonomous overproduction of PTH occurs typically from a single, parathyroid adenoma. Diffuse hyperplasia (involving all four glands) or, rarely, parathyroid carcinoma may be responsible.

The excess PTH leads to a raised $[Ca^{2+}]$, with the potential for clinical problems (Table 5.2). Both serum [calcium] and [albumin] should be measured, and may need to be repeated, since the hypercalcaemia can be intermittent. Serum [phosphate] is sometimes low as a result of the phosphaturic effect of PTH, though this is not a reliable finding. A mild metabolic acidosis may be present, since PTH increases urinary HCO_3^- losses. Some patients develop bony problems as a consequence of the high plasma [PTH], especially if the problem becomes chronic. Markers of increased osteoblast and osteoclast activity may be increased (p. 82).

Table 5.2 Clinical consequences of high $[Ca^{2+}]$

Neurological symptoms (inability to concentrate, depression, confusion)
Generalised muscle weakness
Anorexia, nausea, vomiting, constipation
Polyuria with polydipsia
Nephrocalcinosis, nephrolithiasis
ECG changes (shortened Q–T interval), with bradycardia, first-degree block
Pancreatitis, peptic ulcer

Table 5.3 The causes of hypercalcaemia

Category	Examples
Common	
Parathyroid disease	Hyperparathyroidism, primary and tertiary; multiple endocrine neoplasia syndromes, MEN I and MEN IIa
Malignant disease	Lytic lesions in bone: myeloma, breast carcinoma
	PTHrP: carcinoma of lung, oesophagus, head and neck, renal cell, ovary and bladder
	Ectopic production 1:25-DHCC by lymphomas
Uncommon	
Endogenous production of 1:25-DHCC	Sarcoidosis and other granulomatous diseases
Excessive absorption of calcium	Vitamin D overdose (including self-medication); milk–alkali syndrome
Bone disease	Immobilisation
Drug induced	Thiazide diuretics, lithium
Miscellaneous (mostly rare)	
	Familial hypocalciuric hypercalcaemia
	Hypercalcaemia in childhood (p. 292)
	Thyrotoxicosis
	Addison's disease
Artefact	Poor venepuncture technique (excessive venous stasis)

Table 5.4 'First-line' biochemical tests for investigating suspected hyperparathyroidism

Plasma or serum	Comments
Calcium	If increased [calcium], supports the diagnosis
Albumin	Should be performed as a check on plasma [calcium]
Phosphate (fasting)	If decreased [phosphate], supports the diagnosis
ALP	If enzymic activity increased, supports the diagnosis
Total CO_2	If decreased, supports the diagnosis
Creatinine and/or urea	Simple tests of renal function, needed in all patients with suspected abnormalities of calcium metabolism PTH

Table 5.4 summarises the results of first-line chemical tests for the investigation of suspected hyperparathyroidism.

PTH assay

The single most important test in the differential diagnosis of hypercalcaemia is the measurement of serum PTH (Figure 5.4). Immunometric ('sandwich') assays that measure serum [intact PTH] (reference range 10–55 ng/L) are now in widespread use. They have a high diagnostic sensitivity, and up to 90% of patients with primary hyperparathyroidism have an elevated level. Approximately 10% of patients with primary hyperparathyroidism may have serum [intact PTH] in the upper part of the reference range. However, in the setting of persistent hypercalcaemia, such levels are considered to be inappropriately high since serum [intact PTH] should be suppressed if hypercalcaemia is unrelated to increased parathyroid activity. If serum [intact PTH] is within reference limits or is only marginally elevated in an asymptomatic hypercalcaemic patient, the diagnosis of familial benign hypocalciuric hypercalcaemia (FBHH) should also be considered (see below).

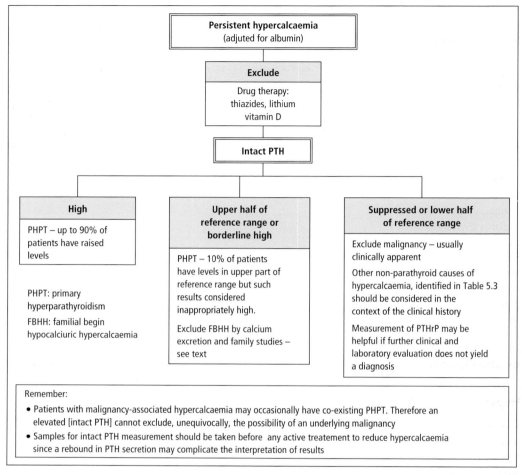

Figure 5.4 Biochemical investigation of persistent hypercalcaemia.

Sometimes PTH assays are required for the investigation of patients who also require urgent therapeutic intervention to reduce marked hypercalcaemia. Under these circumstances, it is important to obtain a sample for PTH analysis before treatment is initiated, since an acute fall in plasma [Ca^{2+}] may trigger a rebound in PTH secretion and complicate the interpretation of the result.

Occasionally, in patients with proven hyperparathyroidism who have undergone an unsuccessful neck exploration, PTH assay on samples collected during selective venous catheterisation may be used to localise the source of PTH. A sestamibi parathyroid imaging scan may also be useful in this setting.

Management of primary hyperparathyroidism

In view of the technical difficulty often associated with parathyroid surgery, it is not unusual for the operation to be deferred in patients with asymptomatic hyperparathyroidism if their serum [calcium] is less than 3.0 mmol/L. As symptoms may develop insidiously, these patients must be followed up with regular further measurements of serum [calcium] and careful clinical reassessment. Indications for parathyroidectomy include (1) the presence of symptoms; a urine calcium excretion over 9 mmol/24 h; (2) cortical radial bone density over 2 SD below normal; (3) reduced creatinine clearance (if no other cause identified); and (4) age under 50 years. In general, it is advisable to proceed to parathyroidectomy early rather than late.

After parathyroidectomy, serum [calcium] falls rapidly, and it should be measured several times on the first post-operative day and at least daily for the next few days. If the serum [calcium] falls below normal, calcium gluconate should be given and treatment with 1:25-DHCC or 1α-HCC should be started.

Multiple endocrine neoplasia (MEN) syndromes

Primary hyperparathyroidism may be one of the abnormalities in the so-called MEN syndrome. Three types of MEN syndrome have been described, all of them familial. Further details are discussed elsewhere (p. 251).

Hypercalcaemia of malignancy

Several factors are responsible for the hypercalcaemia of malignancy. These vary, depending on the type of tumour and on whether or not there are bone metastases:

- Solid tumours that have metastasised to bone may cause hypercalcaemia by paracrine activation of osteoclasts. The tumour cells may also increase bone resorption directly.
- Some solid tumours (e.g. carcinoma of the lung, head and neck), in the absence of bony metastases, may give rise to hypercalcaemia. An important factor in this humoral hypercalcaemia of malignancy is PTH-related protein (PTHrP), a peptide with marked sequence homology with PTH that also acts through the PTH receptor. PTHrP may also be secreted by some tumours that metastasise to bone, so that humoral and local osteolytic mechanisms may combine to produce hypercalcaemia. True ectopic production of PTH appears to be rare.

- In multiple myeloma, hypercalcaemia appears to result from the release of local cytokines that promote local bone resorption. Lymphomas may also cause hypercalcaemia.

Serum [intact PTH] is usually suppressed in patients with malignancy-associated hypercalcaemia, although it sometimes falls within the lower part of the reference range. Assays for PTHrP are available in specialist laboratories and may occasionally be helpful in the investigation of patients with unexplained hypercalcaemia.

Other causes of hypercalcaemia

The history of the patient's illness, the findings on clinical examination and various investigations as suggested by the provisional diagnosis will usually mean that the other conditions (Table 5.3) can be recognised. These will be briefly considered here.

Vitamin D excess

Increased serum [1:25-DHCC] and hypercalcaemia may result from excessive vitamin D intake or if overdosage with 25-HCC, 1α-HCC or 1:25-DHCC occurs. Measurement of serum [25-HCC] or [1:25-DHCC] confirms the diagnosis.

Drugs

A mild degree of hypercalcaemia may develop during treatment with thiazide diuretics; these interfere with renal calcium excretion. Long-term lithium therapy may also be a cause, possibly by stimulating PTH secretion. Serum [calcium] should be monitored on a regular basis in patients receiving lithium therapy.

Sarcoidosis

About 10–20% of patients with sarcoidosis may have hypercalcaemia, often only intermittently. More often, they have hypercalciuria. The unregulated conversion of 25-HCC to 1:25-DHCC (and consequently increased intestinal absorption of calcium) by sarcoid tissue macrophages is responsible. Hypercalcaemia may show seasonal variation in parallel with the production of vitamin D_3 in the skin in response to sunlight.

Tertiary hyperparathyroidism

This description refers to the development of parathyroid hyperplasia as a complication of previously existing secondary hyperparathyroidism. This diagnosis needs to be considered in patients with renal failure or intestinal malabsorption if they develop hypercalcaemia that is not attributable to treatment with vitamin D or one of its hydroxylated derivatives (usually 1α-HCC or 1:25-DHCC). Serum [calcium] is almost always increased and serum [PTH] inappropriately high. Unlike primary hyperparathyroidism, however, fasting serum [phosphate] may be increased, especially if tertiary hyperparathyroidism develops in a patient with renal failure.

Familial benign hypocalciuric hypercalcaemia (FBHH)

This is an autosomal dominant disorder that is usually asymptomatic and may have a population prevalence of up to 1 : 16 000. It arises from a mutation in the calcium-sensing receptor gene in the parathyroid gland, kidney and other organs, and results in a high plasma $[Ca^{2+}]$ that is sensed as 'normal', with normal or marginally elevated plasma [PTH]. It is important that FBHH is distinguished from primary hyperparathyroidism since parathyroidectomy does not reduce plasma $[Ca^{2+}]$, and no active treatment is indicated. While there is no single biochemical test that can always distinguish, unequivocally, FBHH from primary hyperparathyroidism, in patients with FBHH, urinary calcium is usually low and serum [magnesium] tends to be high normal. Therefore, a combination of family studies and the measurement of calcium excretion together with serum [magnesium] is helpful in identifying the condition. Calcium excretion is measured on a second void spot urine and blood sample obtained after an overnight fast, and is calculated by multiplying the urine calcium : creatinine ratio (both in mmol/L) by the serum creatinine (in μmol/L). Calcium excretion less than 14 μmol/L of glomerular filtrate suggests FBHH.

Endocrine disorders

Hypercalcaemia has been reported occasionally in association with hypoadrenalism, phaeochromocytoma and thyrotoxicosis.

Milk–alkali syndrome

Milk consumption may be excessive in patients with symptoms of peptic ulceration; calcium intake is correspondingly increased. If this is accompanied by excessive intake of alkali (e.g. $NaHCO_3$), as an antacid, hypercalcaemia may develop. The alkali is thought to reduce urinary calcium excretion and to be important in the pathogenesis of the condition.

Other bone-related causes

Causes other than malignant disease include Paget's disease in association with immobilisation.

Hypocalcaemia

If potentially misleading hypocalcaemia due to either contamination of the sample with EDTA (from a full blood count tube) or decreased serum [albumin] is first excluded, then the hypocalcaemia must be pathological and must result from a decrease in plasma $[Ca^{2+}]$.

Tetany is the symptom that classically suggests the presence of a low plasma $[Ca^{2+}]$. It may occur in any of the pathological conditions listed in Table 5.5, and may also be caused by a rapid fall in plasma $[H^+]$ (e.g. acute respiratory alkalosis produced by hyperventilation or IV infusion of $NaHCO_3$). Occasionally it is due to a low plasma $[Mg^{2+}]$ in the absence of low plasma $[Ca^{2+}]$, and rarely it is due to a sudden increase in plasma [phosphate]. Neuropsychiatric symptoms and cataract are other possible consequences of hypocalcaemia (Table 5.6).

This section considers the underlying pathological processes that may lead to the development of hypocalcaemia.

Table 5.5 The causes of hypocalcaemia

Category	Examples
Artefact	EDTA contamination of sample
Hypoproteinaemia	Low serum [albumin] (p. 75)
Renal disease	Hydroxylation of 25-HCC impaired
Inadequate intake of calcium	Deficiency of calcium or vitamin D, or of both; intestinal malabsorption (p. 217)
Magnesium depletion	See below (p. 86)
Hypoparathyroidism	Autoimmune, post-surgical, magnesium deficiency, infiltrative disease
Pseudohypoparathyroidism	Target organ resistance to PTH
Neonatal hypocalcaemia	(p. 291)
Acute pancreatitis	Calcium soaps in the abdominal cavity?
Critical illness	Mixed pathology – not clearly defined

Table 5.6 Clinical consequences of hypocalcaemia

Enhanced neuromuscular irritability (positive Chvostek's sign and Trousseau's sign); tetany
Numbness, tingling (fingers, toes, circumoral)
Muscle cramps (legs, feet, lower back)
Seizures
Irritability, personality changes
ECG changes (prolonged Q–T interval)
Basal ganglia calcification; subcapsular cataracts (especially with low PTH)

Vitamin D deficiency

The most common pathological cause of hypocalcaemia is defective calcium absorption due to inadequate plasma levels of 1:25-DHCC. Deficiency of 1:25-DHCC may result from lack of vitamin D or failure at any stage in its conversion to 1:25-DHCC (Figure 5.3); rarely, the action of 1:25-DHCC is defective at the receptor level. In malnutrition, the effects of vitamin D deficiency are accentuated by inadequate dietary calcium.

Defective absorption of calcium ultimately leads to a low plasma $[Ca^{2+}]$ accompanied by increased PTH secretion in response to the low ECF $[Ca^{2+}]$ (i.e. secondary hyperparathyroidism). Serum [phosphate] is often low, partly through impaired absorption, but also as a result of the secondary hyperparathyroidism (renal disease is an exception). Serum ALP activity is often increased, reflecting increased osteoblastic activity. However,

its measurement is of limited diagnostic value in childhood because of the marked physiological variations in activity that normally occur in this age group. Urinary calcium excretion is nearly always low or very low.

Confirmation of the diagnosis of vitamin D deficiency depends on measurement of serum [25-HCC] or (less widely available) serum [1:25-DHCC]. Serum [25-HCC] assays provide a reasonable indication of the overall vitamin D status of the patient if renal function is normal and renal 1α-hydroxylase activity can be assumed to be normal. There is a seasonal variation in serum [25-HCC] that can make interpretation of single results difficult. Measurement of serum [25-HCC] is also of value in monitoring patients who are being treated for vitamin D deficiency by dietary supplementation.

The main causes of hypocalcaemia due to lack of vitamin D or of disturbances of its metabolism will be briefly considered here.

• *Nutritional deficiency of vitamin D* Poor diet, inadequate exposure to sunlight or a combination of these can lead to vitamin D deficiency with development of hypocalcaemia and osteomalacia (see section on Metabolic bone disease below). This has largely been eliminated in developed countries with vitamin D supplementation of food, but the elderly are still at risk (as they may be immobile indoors with an inadequate diet). Cultural and geographical factors are probably important in the susceptibility to vitamin D deficiency of the immigrant Asian community in Northern Europe.

• *Malabsorption of vitamin D* This may be due to coeliac disease, or may occur as a result of fat malabsorption due to pancreatic disease, biliary obstruction or as a complication of gastric or intestinal surgery (e.g. intestinal bypass or resection). Biliary obstruction is much more likely to lead to vitamin D deficiency (through malabsorption) than the theoretical possibility of 25-HCC deficiency in parenchymal liver disease.

• *Renal disease* Destruction of the renal parenchyma leads to loss of 1α-hydroxylase activity, reduced formation of 1:25-DHCC and consequent malabsorption of calcium. Serum [phosphate] is likely to be high in renal failure, and this may interfere with the 1α-hydroxylation step.

Specific deficiency of 1α-hydroxylase may be the cause of hypocalcaemia in vitamin D-resistant rickets, type I, a rare inherited disorder. In vitamin D-resistant rickets, type II, there is end-organ unresponsiveness to 1:25-DHCC.

Hypoparathyroidism

Primary hypoparathyroidism is rare. The combination of a reduced serum [calcium] and an increased [phosphate] in a patient who does not have renal disease suggests the diagnosis of hypoparathyroidism; serum ALP activity is usually normal. Measurement of [intact PTH] confirms the diagnosis; levels are reduced and are sometimes undetectable even by the most sensitive assays.

Failure to secrete PTH may be a complication of surgery, or it may be familial or sporadic in origin. Also, the parathyroid glands may be destroyed by an autoimmune process, or as a result of infiltration by carcinoma of the thyroid or other neoplasms.

• *Secondary hypoparathyroidism* may occasionally be observed in patients with magnesium deficiency (see below).

• *Pseudohypoparathyroidism* is a rare but interesting condition, in which the end-organ receptors in the bone and kidneys fail to respond normally to PTH. Patients with pseudohypoparathyroidism have increased serum [PTH].

Other causes of hypocalcaemia are listed in Table 5.5.

Metabolic bone disease

Generalised defects in bone mineralisation, frequently associated with abnormal calcium or phosphate metabolism, are sometimes grouped together under the term 'biochemical or metabolic bone diseases'. The most common are osteoporosis, rickets and osteomalacia, and Paget's disease.

In many examples of metabolic bone disease, patients show features of two or more of these conditions, and it can be difficult to define the pathological process fully, even with the aid of radiological examination and bone biopsy. Results of biochemical investigations (Table 5.7) must be interpreted in relation to all the available evidence. For example, in renal osteodystrophy, a combination of osteomalacia, hyperparathyroidism and other metabolic abnormalities contributes to the metabolic bone disease. Various other conditions, often rare, may produce generalised bone disease, with or without biochemical changes.

Markers of bone turnover

Biochemical markers of bone turnover can be divided into those which reflect bone formation and those which reflect bone resorption (Table 5.8). The formation markers include enzymes and peptides released by the osteoblast at the time of bone formation, whereas the resorption markers are typically a measure of the breakdown products of type 1 collagen. While bone markers cannot reveal how much bone is present in the skeleton and cannot substitute for the measurement of bone mineral density, they have the potential to be used in the assessment of fracture risk and may be used to monitor the response of patients with osteoporosis to anti-resorptive and anabolic therapies. However, the clinical utility of routine bone marker measurements has not yet been fully established and these assays remain available in specialist centres only.

Table 5.7 Metabolic bone disease: chemical investigations on blood specimens

Diagnosis	Calcium	Phosphate (fasting)	PTH	Alkaline phosphatase	Ca²⁺
Hyperparathyroidism					
Primary	↑ (or N)	↓ or N	↑ or N*	N or ↑	↑ (or N)
Secondary	↓ or N	↑ or N	↑	↑ or N	N
Tertiary	↑ or N	↑ or N	↑	↑ or N	↑
Rickets and osteomalacia					
Deficient intake	↓ or N	↓ or N	↑ (or N)	↑	N (or ↓)
Renal failure	↓ or N	↑ or N	↑	↑	N
Fanconi syndrome*	↓ or N	↓ or N	N	↑	N
Osteoporosis	N	N	N	N	N
Paget's disease	N (or ↑)	N	N	↑	N

N = normal; ↑ = increased; ↓ = decreased. N* indicates that plasma [PTH] is sometimes within the upper reference range, i.e. it is inappropriately high in primary hyperparathyroidism and not suppressed, as would normally be expected, in the presence of hypercalcaemia.

* Included as an example of proximal renal tubular defects.

Table 5.8 The most sensitive biochemical markers of bone turnover

Formation	Resorption
Serum	
Bone alkaline phosphatase	C-telopeptide cross-links (CTX)
Osteocalcin	
Procollagen type 1	
N-terminal propeptide	
(P1NP)	
Urine	N-telopeptide cross-links (NTX)
	Deoxypyridinoline

Rickets and osteomalacia

Patients who have vitamin D deficiency or disturbed metabolism of vitamin D are all liable to suffer from the bone disease osteomalacia or, in children, from rickets. These patients have bone pain, with local tenderness, and may have a proximal myopathy. Skeletal deformity may be present, particularly in rickets. Mineralisation of osteoid is defective, with absence of the calcification front.

Other causes of rickets or osteomalacia, unrelated to vitamin D deficiency or defects in its metabolism, have also been described. An inherited defect in the tubular reabsorption of phosphate, hypophosphataemic vitamin D-resistant rickets, leads to similar bone deformities, but without muscle weakness; there is a low serum [phosphate] and phosphaturia. In Fanconi syndrome (p. 60), tubular phosphate loss may also lead to low serum [phosphate] associated with rickets or osteomalacia.

Hypophosphatasia is a hereditary disease in which vitamin D-resistant rickets is the most prominent finding. Tissue and serum ALP activities are usually low, and excessive amounts of phosphoryl ethanolamine are present in the urine.

Osteoporosis

This is a very common disorder that affects about one in four women. It is characterised by low bone mass and susceptibility to vertebral, forearm and hip fractures in later life. Results of routine chemical investigations are usually all normal.

Table 5.9 lists some of the risk factors for the development of osteoporosis. The diagnosis should exclude primary hyperparathyroidism, thyrotoxi-

Table 5.9 Risk factors for osteoporosis

Unmodifiable
Age (1.4- to 1.8-fold increase per decade)
Genetic (Caucasians and Orientals > Blacks and Polynesians)
Sex (female > male)
Modifiable (environmental)
Nutritional calcium deficiency
Physical inactivity
Smoking
Alcohol excess; drugs (e.g. glucocorticoids, anti-convulsants)
Modifiable (endogenous)
Endocrine (oestrogen or androgen deficiency, hyperthyroidism)
Chronic diseases (gastrectomy, cirrhosis, rheumatoid arthritis)

cosis, corticosteroid excess, multiple myeloma and hypogonadism.

Paget's disease

This is a common disorder of the bone, affecting up to 5% of the population over 55 years old in the UK. Bone turnover is focally increased, with disordered bone remodelling. Serum [calcium] and [phosphate] are usually normal, although hypercalcaemia can develop, especially as a result of immobilisation. The increased bone turnover leads to a high serum ALP activity and an increase in indices of osteoclast activity.

Renal osteodystrophy

The pathophysiology of renal osteodystrophy is complex. The bone changes in it are varied, and derive from one or more of the following mechanisms:

• *Vitamin D metabolism* There is ineffective conversion of 25-HCC to 1:25-DHCC due to loss of renal 1α-hydroxylase. This causes defective calcium absorption and osteomalacia in adults, or rickets in children. It may be corrected by treatment with 1α-HCC or 1:25-DHCC.

• *Phosphate retention* There is increased plasma [phosphate], and this, by complexing with Ca^{2+} and combined with defective calcium absorption, tends to make plasma $[Ca^{2+}]$ fall. This leads to secondary hyperparathyroidism, which tends to restore plasma [phosphate] and plasma [calcium] towards normal. Phosphate retention can further inhibit the renal 1α-hydroxylase. Osteitis fibrosa, if it develops, may require parathyroidectomy.

• *Phosphate binders* Failure of the secondary hyperparathyroidism to maintain normal plasma [phosphate] as renal disease progresses leads to treatment of patients with oral phosphate binders, usually aluminium hydroxide. Excess absorption of aluminium may cause osteomalacia and dialysis dementia. Plasma [aluminium] should be measured periodically.

• *Dialysis fluid composition* The fluid [calcium] must be carefully controlled; if it is too low, osteoporosis often develops. If fluid [calcium] is too high, extraskeletal calcification may occur. Care is also needed to ensure that dialysis fluid [aluminium] is sufficiently low.

In order to control and treat these various abnormalities, all patients with chronic renal failure require biochemical monitoring. Serum creatinine, urea, Na^+, K^+, total CO_2, albumin, calcium and phosphate concentrations and ALP activity should all be measured regularly. The main objective of treatment with 1α-HCC or 1:25-DHCC is to increase plasma [calcium] to normal and to reverse bone disease due to parathyroid overactivity. If treatment is successful, serum PTH falls to normal. When treatment is first started, it may be difficult to adjust the dose of 1α-HCC or 1:25-DHCC satisfactorily, and hypercalcaemia, possibly with extraskeletal calcium deposition, may occur if too much is given.

Phosphate metabolism

Eighty-five percent of body phosphorus is located in the mineral phase of bone. The remainder is present outside bone, largely in an intracellular location as phosphate compounds. In the ECF, phosphate is mostly inorganic, where it exists as a mixture of HPO_4^{2-} and $H_2PO_4^-$ at physiological pH.

Intracellular phosphate has vital functions in macromolecular structure (e.g. in DNA), energy metabolism (e.g. energy-rich phosphates such as ATP), cell signalling and enzyme activation by phosphorylation. Intracellular phosphate is largely organic as a component of phospholipids, phosphoproteins, nucleic acids and nucleotides (e.g. ATP).

Hypo- and hyperphosphataemia

Phosphate and calcium homeostasis are inextricably linked, and several of the factors that influence serum [phosphate] have already been discussed earlier in this chapter. The causes of hypophosphataemia and hyperphosphataemia are summarised in Table 5.10.

A serum [phosphate] below 0.4 mmol/L may be associated with widespread cell dysfunction and even death. Muscle pain and weakness, including respiratory muscle weakness, associated with a raised CK, are possible. Urgent phosphate supplementation is required. Dietary deficiency is unusual (phosphate occurs widely in food), but antacids may bind phosphate. Movement of phosphate into the cell occurs with metabolic and respiratory acidosis. Hypophosphataemia in DKA may be worsened when insulin is administered (insulin promotes cellular uptake of glucose and phosphate). Hyperalimentation or re-feeding starved patients is also accompanied by cellular utilisation of phosphate and the potential for serious hypophosphataemia in the absence of appropriate supplementation.

Magnesium metabolism

Magnesium is the second most abundant intracellular cation. It is essential for the activity of many enzymes, including the phosphotransferases. Bone contains about 50% of the body's magnesium; a small proportion of the body's content is in the ECF.

Dietary intake of magnesium is normally about 12 mmol (300 mg) daily. Green vegetables, cereals and meat are good sources. Significant amounts are contained in gastric and biliary secretions. Factors concerned with the control of magnesium absorption have not been defined, but may involve active transport across the intestinal mucosa by a process involving vitamin D. Renal conservation of magnesium is at least partly controlled by PTH and aldosterone. When the dietary intake is restricted, renal conservation mechanisms are normally so efficient that depletion, if it develops at all, only comes on very slowly.

Plasma [magnesium] is normally kept within narrow limits, which implies close homeostatic

Table 5.10 Causes of hyperphosphataemia and hypophosphataemia

Hyperphosphataemia		Hypophosphataemia	
Increased intake	IV therapy	Decreased intake/ absorption	Vitamin D deficiency (see also below)
	Phosphate enemas		Malabsorption
			Oral phosphate binders
Reduced excretion	Acute/chronic renal failure	Increased excretion	Primary PTH excess
	Low PTH or resistance to PTH		Secondary PTH excess (e.g. vitamin D deficiency)
	Vitamin D toxicity		Post-renal transplant
			Re-feeding starved patients
Redistribution	Tumour lysis	Redistribution	Hyperalimentation
	Rhabdomyolysis		Recovery from diabetic ketoacidosis
	Heat stroke		Alkalosis (respiratory)

control. Marked alterations in the body's content can occur with little or no change detectable in serum [magnesium]. In this respect, magnesium is very much like potassium. The serum [magnesium] may be normal although a state of intracellular depletion exists.

Hypomagnesaemia and magnesium deficiency

Magnesium deficiency (Table 5.11) rarely occurs as an isolated phenomenon. Usually it is accompanied by disorders of potassium, calcium and phosphorus metabolism. It may therefore be difficult to identify signs and symptoms that can be specifically attributed to magnesium deficiency. However, muscular weakness, sometimes accompanied by tetany, cardiac arrhythmias and CNS abnormalities (e.g. convulsions), may all be due to magnesium deficiency.

Normal levels of magnesium are not only necessary for PTH release but may also be required to ensure an adequate end-organ response to PTH. Therefore, magnesium deficiency should be suspected in patients who present with hypocalcaemia and/or hypokalaemia without an obvious cause or who fail to respond to treatment of these abnormalities. Serum [magnesium] is usually below 0.5 mmol/L in patients with symptoms directly attributable to magnesium deficiency; its level should be measured before treatment with magnesium salts is instituted.

Serum [magnesium] may not reflect the true state of the body's reserves, particularly in chronic disorders. Other tests have been advocated (e.g. erythrocyte [magnesium], muscle [magnesium], magnesium loading tests), but there is no general agreement on the best test to use. Urinary excretion of magnesium is relatively easy to measure, and it is useful in distinguishing renal losses of magnesium from the other causes of hypomagnesaemia and magnesium deficiency. Renal excretion of magnesium often falls below 0.5 mmol/24 h in non-renal causes of magnesium deficiency.

Table 5.11 Magnesium deficiency

Causes	Examples
Abnormal losses	
GI tract	Prolonged aspiration, persistent diarrhoea, malabsorptive disease, fistula, jejuno-ileal bypass, small-bowel resection
Urinary tract	
Renal disease	Renal tubular acidosis, chronic pyelonephritis, hydronephrosis
Extrarenal	Conditions that modify renal function (e.g. primary and secondary hyperaldosteronism, diuretics, osmotic diuresis) Conditions affecting transfer of magnesium from cells to bone (e.g. primary and tertiary hyperparathyroidism, ketoacidosis)
Reduced intake	If severe and prolonged, protein-energy malnutrition
Mixed aetiology	Chronic alcoholism, hepatic cirrhosis

Hypermagnesaemia

This is most often due to acute renal failure or the advanced stages of chronic renal failure. Its presence is readily confirmed by measuring serum [magnesium]. There may be no symptoms. However, if serum [magnesium] exceeds 3.0 mmol/L, nausea and vomiting, weakness and impaired consciousness may then develop, but these symptoms may not necessarily be caused solely by the hypermagnesaemia.

Hypermagnesaemia may rarely be caused by IV injection of magnesium salts, and adrenocortical hypofunction may cause a slight increase in serum [magnesium].

Keypoints

- Calcium is the most abundant body mineral, largely present in bone. In addition to this major mechanical function, extracellular calcium is necessary for normal neuromuscular function, blood clotting and complement activation. Intracellular calcium is a key signal for many important cellular events (contraction, motility, secretion and cell division).
- About 50% of plasma calcium is bound to albumin, the rest being mostly ionised (the physiologically active fraction). Changes in serum [albumin] may alter serum total [calcium] without any pathological change in the ionised fraction ([Ca^{2+}]).
- PTH is a key regulatory hormone of plasma [Ca^{2+}]. A fall in [Ca^{2+}] stimulates PTH, which increases Ca^{2+} release from bone, renal reabsorption of Ca^{2+} and loss of phosphate in the urine. 1:25-DHCC is essential for intestinal absorption of calcium (and phosphate) and the longer term maintenance of plasma [Ca^{2+}] and [phosphate].
- True hypercalcaemia (increase in [Ca^{2+}]) is most commonly due to primary hyperparathyroidism or malignant disease. True hypocalcaemia (decrease in [Ca^{2+}]) is most often the result of low 1:25-DHCC levels (renal disease, vitamin D deficiency, malabsorption), and less often to hypoparathyroidism.
- Defects in bone mineralisation (biochemical bone disease) include rickets and osteomalacia, renal osteodystrophy (both associated with abnormalities in [Ca^{2+}] and [phosphate]) and osteoporosis and Paget's disease (typically without effect on these measurements).
- Magnesium deficiency is usually associated with other electrolyte deficiencies. Hypermagnesaemia is most often found in acute or chronic renal failure.

Case 5.1

A 47-year-old secretary was admitted as an emergency with left-sided ureteric colic. She had had one similar episode 3 years before, when she had passed a small calculus spontaneously. In addition, she had been receiving treatment with cimetidine for the previous 6 months, for dyspepsia. Physical examination only revealed slight tenderness in the left loin and on palpating the abdomen. Side-room tests on urine showed a trace of blood, and a plain X-ray of the abdomen showed a small opacity in the line of the left ureter. Blood investigations were performed, with the following results:

Serum	Result	Reference range
Creatinine	150	60–120 µ mol/L
Na$^+$	141	135–145 mmol/L
K$^+$	4.2	3.6–5.0 mmol/L
Total CO_2	20	22–30 mmol/L
Urea	8.1	2.5–6.6 mmol/L
Albumin	40	35–50 g/L
Calcium	3.49	2.10–2.60 mmol/L
Phosphate	0.60	0.8–1.4 mmol/L
ALP activity	160	40–125 U/L

What was the likely cause of this patient's urinary calculi? What further chemical investigations would you have requested in order to confirm the diagnosis? What treatment would you have instituted after initiating these further investigations?

(continued on p. 88)

Case 5.1 *(continued)*

Comments: The most likely diagnosis is primary hyperparathyroidism; the history of recurrent renal calculi and peptic ulceration are highly suggestive, and strongly supported by the results for the serum calcium, phosphate and ALP measurements, and by the presence of a mild metabolic acidosis.

The diagnosis in this patient was confirmed by measuring serum [PTH]; results for this analysis are most readily interpreted if the blood specimen is collected at a time when the serum [calcium] is increased, i.e. before any calcium-lowering treatment is instituted. This patient's serum [calcium] was sufficiently high to warrant urgent attempts to lower it, after an IV urogram had been performed to make sure that the calculus was not causing obstruction. Treatment would consist of fluids to correct dehydration, and might require a loop diuretic (frusemide). This patient then proceeded to parathyroidectomy for removal of a solitary adenoma.

Case 5.2

A 64-year-old retired shop assistant with Crohn's disease (regional ileitis) had had her condition well controlled by means of oral prednisolone until 2 or 3 months before her regular follow-up outpatient appointment. Latterly, she had had severe pain in the back, and radiological examination showed a compression fracture of the fourth lumbar vertebra. Chemical investigations on a blood specimen gave the following results:

Serum	Result	Reference range
Albumin	26	35–50 g/L
Calcium	1.72	2.10–2.60 mmol/L
Phosphate, fasting	0.8	0.8–1.4 mmol/L
ALP activity	170	40–125 U/L
Total protein	50	60–80 g/L
Creatinine	110	60–120 μmol/L
Urea	5.8	2.5–6.6 mmol/L
Na+	136	135–145 mmol/L
K+	3.5	3.6–5.0 mmol/L
Total CO_2	21	22–30 mmol/L

Comment on these results. What further investigations might be indicated?

Comments: The long-term use of steroids may lead to the development of osteoporosis. However, in uncomplicated osteoporosis, the serum [calcium] would be expected to be normal. In this patient the serum [calcium] is low, and lower than can be accounted for in terms of the low serum [albumin]. The combination of a low serum [calcium] with a low normal serum [phosphate] and elevated ALP activity is consistent with a diagnosis of osteomalacia. The low serum [total protein] and [albumin], and the low [total CO_2], indicative of a mild metabolic acidosis, suggest that chronic diarrhoea with intestinal malabsorption could be the cause of the osteomalacia.

A diagnosis of osteomalacia can be confirmed by bone biopsy. However, this is seldom required if the history is suggestive and the results of chemical investigations and radiological examination (generalised rarefaction of bones, Looser's zones) are characteristic. Measurement of 25-HCC in serum might be considered worthwhile, and responses to a therapeutic trial of vitamin D might be helpful as a means of making a diagnosis of osteomalacia retrospectively.

Case 5.3

A 73-year-old man with no significant medical history was admitted as an emergency. He had been unwell over the past 2 weeks and there had been episodes of vomiting and diarrhoea. On admission he was confused and clinically dehydrated. His diet had been poor for some time and he regularly consumed half a bottle of whisky a day. The results of initial biochemical investigations were as follows:

Serum	Result	Reference range
Urea	18.3	2.5–6.6 mmol/L
Creatinine	150	60–120 µmol/L
Na$^+$	141	135–145 mmol/L
K$^+$	2.3	3.6–5.0 mmol/L
Total CO$_2$	35	22–30 mmol/L
Calcium	1.10	2.10–2.60 mmol/L
Albumin	30	35–50 g/L
Phosphate	0.9	0.8–1.4 mmol/L
ALP activity	106	40–125 U/L

Comment on these results. What further investigations are indicated?

Comments: These data reveal significant disturbances in renal function and in calcium and potassium homeostasis. The modest increase in serum [urea], which is disproportionately greater than the increase in serum [creatinine], is consistent to a moderate degree of renal impairment in a dehydrated patient (p. 55).

The marked reduction in serum [calcium] is not due to specimen contamination with EDTA (from a full blood count tube) since the serum [potassium] would be increased under these circumstances. After correction of the serum [calcium] for the low serum [albumin] (p. 75), the adjusted calcium remains very low at 1.30 mmol/L. Consideration of the clinical history suggested that the hypocalcaemia was likely to relate to magnesium depletion and the serum [magnesium] was subsequently shown to be <0.10 mmol/L. Magnesium depletion may develop following long-term alcohol abuse as a result of a renal leak of magnesium and poor nutritional intake, and in this patient losses in diarrhoea fluid may have been a contributing factor. Patients with magnesium deficiency develop secondary hypoparathyroidism and end-organ resistance to the effects of PTH. Serum [intact PTH] on admission was subsequently shown to be 63 ng/L (reference range 10–55 ng/L). Although elevated, the observed value was much lower than expected in such a markedly hypocalcaemic patient. In view of the poor nutritional history, 25OH vitamin D$_3$ was also measured and found to be undetectable, indicating that vitamin D deficiency may have contributed to the hypocalcaemia. The reduction of serum [potassium] may have been related to poor intake, vomiting (p. 27) with an associated mild alkalosis suggested by the increased serum [bicarbonate] and to magnesium depletion which induces renal potassium loss.

The patient was treated with IV fluids containing magnesium and potassium, together with oral calcium supplements. On the day after admission, the serum [magnesium] had risen to 0.9 mmol/L and the [intact PTH] to 320 ng/L. Within 5 days, all biochemical parameters had returned to normal.

Chapter 6

Diabetes mellitus and hypoglycaemia

Diabetes is the most common metabolic disorder, and its incidence is increasing. Biochemical measurements are particularly important in detecting it, monitoring its control and treating its metabolic complications. Hypoglycaemia occurs in insulin-treated diabetic patients, but is otherwise rare. However, it is an important diagnosis to make because of its possible consequences. Other disorders of carbohydrate metabolism are uncommon.

In this chapter, we consider diabetes and hypoglycaemia. Some of the inherited disorders of carbohydrate metabolism are considered in Chapter 21.

Glucose homeostasis

Blood [glucose] is maintained within a narrow range imposed at the lower limit by the undesirable effects of hypoglycaemia, and at the upper limit by the potential for loss in the urine if the renal threshold is exceeded. The liver plays a key role in maintaining blood [glucose]. After a carbohydrate-containing meal, it removes about 70% of the glucose load that is delivered via the portal circulation. Some of the glucose is oxidised and some is converted to glycogen for use as a fuel under fasting conditions. Glucose in excess of these

requirements is partly converted by the liver to fatty acids and triglycerides, which are then incorporated into very low density lipoproteins (VLDLs) and transported to adipose tissue stores.

In the fasting state, blood [glucose] is maintained by glycogen breakdown in the liver in the short term, while glycogen stores last, and then by gluconeogenesis (from glycerol, lactate and pyruvate and from the gluconeogenic amino acids), occurring mostly in the liver, but also in the kidneys. Glucose is spared, under fasting conditions, by the ability of muscle and other tissues to adapt to the oxidation of fatty acids, and by the ability of the brain and some other organs to utilise ketone bodies that are formed under these conditions.

The hormones mainly concerned with regulating glucose metabolism in the fed and fasting states are insulin, glucagon, GH, adrenaline and cortisol. Of these, insulin has the most marked effects in humans (Table 6.1), and is the only hormone that lowers blood [glucose]. Glucagon, GH, adrenaline and cortisol all tend, in general, to antagonise the actions of insulin (Table 6.2).

Insulin secretion

Insulin is synthesised in the β-cells of the islets of Langerhans in the pancreas. It is formed as preproinsulin, which is rapidly cleaved to pro-insulin. The pro-insulin is packaged into secretory granules

Lecture Notes: Clinical Biochemistry, 8e. By G. Beckett, S. Walker, P. Rae & P. Ashby. Published 2010 by Blackwell Publishing.

Table 6.1 The effects of insulin on cellular metabolism

Tissue	Processes activated by insulin	Processes inhibited by insulin
Liver	Uptake of amino acids and glycerol Synthesis of glycogen, proteins, triglycerides and VLDLs	Glycogenolysis Gluconeogenesis Ketone body formation
Muscle	Uptake of glucose and amino acids Synthesis of glycogen	Triglyceride utilisation Lipolysis
Adipose	Uptake of chylomicrons and VLDLs and of glucose Utilisation of glucose	

Table 6.2 The effects on glucose metabolism of hormones that antagonise the actions of insulin

Tissue and hormone	Effects of the various hormones on glucose metabolism			
	Gluconeogenesis	Glycogenolysis	Glycolysis	Glucose uptake
Liver				
Adrenaline	Increased	Increased	Decreased	
Cortisol	Increased			Decreased
Glucagon	Increased	Increased		
Growth hormone		Increased	Increased	Decreased
Muscle				
Adrenaline		Increased	Increased	
Cortisol				Decreased
Growth hormone				
Short term			Increased	
Long term			Decreased	
Adipose				
Cortisol			Decreased	

in the Golgi apparatus and cleaved to insulin and C peptide. Insulin and C peptide are later released into the circulation in equimolar amounts.

A rise in blood [glucose] is the main stimulus for insulin secretion. Some amino acids (e.g. leucine), fatty acids and ketone bodies also promote insulin secretion. Vagal stimulation also promotes insulin release. The release of insulin in response to hyperglycaemia is enhanced by the presence of incretin hormones released from the gastrointestinal tract (glucagon-like polypeptide-1 (GLP-1) and glucose-dependent insulinotropic polypeptide (GIP)). Incretins explain the larger release of insulin that occurs in response to an oral glucose load, compared with the same dose of glucose given intravenously. GLP-1 and GIP are inactivated in the circulation by the enzyme dipeptidyl peptidase-4 (DPP-4). Some new drugs for the treatment of type 2 diabetes enhance glucose-dependent endogenous insulin secretion by targeting this system. Both GLP-1 agonists and DPP-4 inhibitors are available.

The insulin receptor is located on the cell surface and is internalised after insulin binding. Within different organs, target enzymes have been identified that serve to explain the known effects of insulin on intermediary metabolism. For instance, activation of glucose transport, induction of hexokinase (or glucokinase) and activation of phosphofructokinase, pyruvate kinase and pyruvate dehydrogenase in the liver are all consistent with the actions of insulin in promoting increased glucose uptake and glycolytic breakdown. Stimulation of glycogen synthase accords with the effects of insulin on glycogen formation in the liver.

Diabetes mellitus

Diabetes is common, affecting 1–2% of Western populations, and population screening programmes reveal that many patients are previously unrecognised. It results in chronic hyperglycaemia, usually accompanied by glycosuria and other biochemical abnormalities, expressed as a wide range of clinical presentations ranging from asymptomatic patients with relatively mild biochemical abnormalities to patients admitted to hospitals with severe metabolic decompensation of rapid onset that has led to coma. Long-term complications may develop, including retinopathy, neuropathy and nephropathy. It is a major risk factor for cardiovascular disease.

Diabetes may be a secondary consequence of other diseases. For example, in diseases of the pancreas, such as pancreatitis or haemochromatosis, there is a reduction in insulin secretion. In some endocrine disorders, such as acromegaly or Cushing's syndrome, there is antagonism of insulin action by abnormal secretion of hormones with opposing activity. Several drugs adversely affect glucose tolerance. Table 6.3 summarises these different causes. Secondary diabetes is, however, not common.

Most cases of diabetes are not associated with other conditions, but are primary, and fall into two distinct types. In type 1 diabetes, there is essentially no insulin secretion, whereas in type 2 diabetes insulin is secreted, but in amounts that are inadequate to prevent hyperglycaemia, or there is resistance to its action.

• *Type 1 diabetes* usually presents acutely over a period of days or a few weeks in young non-obese subjects, but can occur at any age. In addition to polyuria, thirst and glycosuria, there is often marked weight loss and ketoacidosis. Insulin is required for its treatment. Type 1 diabetes is an autoimmune condition with genetic and environmental precipitating factors in its pathogenesis. Islet-cell antibodies that react with the β-cells of

Table 6.3 Examples of causes of secondary diabetes or of IGT

Category of cause	Examples
Drugs	Oestrogen-containing oral contraceptives, corticosteroids, salbutamol and some other catecholaminergic drugs, thiazide diuretics
Endocrine disorders	Acromegaly, Cushing's syndrome and Cushing's disease, glucagonoma, phaeochromocytoma, prolactinoma, thyrotoxicosis (occasionally)
Insulin receptor abnormalities	Autoimmune insulin receptor antibodies, congenital lipodystrophy
Pancreatic disease	Chronic pancreatitis, haemochromatosis, pancreatectomy

the pancreas have been demonstrated in serum from over 90% of patients with newly diagnosed type 1 diabetes. They have also been demonstrated occasionally in serum several years before clinical and biochemical features of diabetes were developed. Most of the islet-cell antibodies are directed against the enzyme glutamic acid decarboxylase (GAD). Individuals with certain human leucocyte antigens (HLAs) have been shown to have a particularly high risk of developing type 1 diabetes. There is a well-recognised association between type 1 diabetes and other autoimmune endocrinopathies, such as hypothyroidism and Addison's disease, and also with pernicious anaemia.

• *Type 2 diabetes* generally presents in a less acute manner in older (>40 years) patients who are obese; many patients have clearly had the condition for some time (even years) before diagnosis. Rarely does type 2 diabetes occur in young patients. Measurable levels of insulin are present, and the metabolic defect appears to lie either in defective insulin secretion or in insulin resistance. In general, insulin is not required for the prevention of ketosis, as these patients are relatively resistant to its development. However, insulin may be needed to correct abnormalities of blood [glucose]. There appears to be no association between type 2 diabetes and either the HLA system or the development of autoimmunity. However, there is a strong genetic element to the disorder.

In established diabetic patients who become pregnant, poor blood glucose control is associated with a higher incidence of intrauterine death and foetal malformation. In addition, abnormal glucose tolerance or diabetes mellitus may develop during pregnancy, a condition referred to as 'gestational diabetes mellitus'.

Monogenic forms of diabetes may account for 1–2% of cases of diabetes. Clinical features may overlap with those of type 1 or type 2 diabetes. Forms include:

• *Neonatal diabetes* is diabetes diagnosed within the first 6 months of life, and may be transient or permanent. Up to 60% of patients with permanent neonatal diabetes have a mutation in one of the potassium channel genes, which results in failure of insulin production. This is an important diagnosis since 90% of these patients can stop insulin and achieve good control on sulphonylureas.

• *Maturity onset diabetes of the young (MODY)* may be better called familial diabetes and may be suspected in a patient with a strong family history of diabetes or when apparent type 2 diabetes occurs at a relatively young age, or in the absence of typical type 2 features such as insulin resistance. Patients may be on insulin. A number of subtypes are recognised, the more common ones being caused by mutations in:

  • Glucokinase. This often causes mild asymptomatic hyperglycaemia typically only picked up during screening. Diabetic complications are very unusual and treatment can usually be stopped.

  • Hepatic nuclear factor 1 alpha (HNF-1α). This is the most common cause of MODY. [Glucose] deteriorates with age and becomes symptomatic in adolescence or young adulthood. Diabetic complications occur, so treatment is needed. Low dose sulphonylureas achieve excellent [glucose] lowering and in patients less that 45 years old may even replace insulin if that has been started before the correct diagnosis was made.

Diagnosis

The diagnosis of diabetes mellitus has serious consequences. It confers a risk of long-term diabetic complications, including blindness, renal failure and amputations, as well as an increased risk of cardiovascular disease. It also means a lifetime of dietary restriction and medications and can seriously curtail lifestyle and employment prospects. The diagnosis may be suggested by the patient's history, or by the results of dipstick tests for glucose on urine specimens. However, urine glucose measurements by themselves are inadequate for diagnosing diabetes. They potentially yield false-positive results in subjects with a low renal threshold for glucose, and in a patient with diabetes they may yield false-negative results if the patient is fasting. A provisional diagnosis of diabetes mellitus must always be confirmed by glucose measurements on blood specimens.

The most recent criteria for the diagnosis of diabetes mellitus have been laid down by the World Health Organization (WHO) in 2006, and by the American Diabetes Association in 2003. These are broadly similar but differ in some details. It is likely that the precise requirements for the diagnosis of diabetes and the states of impaired glucose regulation will continue to evolve as knowledge of the relationship between glucose regulation and the future development of complications accumulates. The following descriptions adhere to the WHO recommendations. Separate criteria are described depending on whether venous or capillary whole blood, or venous or capillary plasma specimens are used. In practice, results for this important diagnosis will usually come from a clinical laboratory and use venous plasma. According to the criteria, a random venous plasma [glucose] of 11.1 mmol/L or more, or a fasting plasma [glucose] of 7.0 mmol/L or more, establishes the diagnosis. A single result is sufficient in the presence of typical hyperglycaemic symptoms of thirst and polyuria. In their absence, a venous plasma [glucose] in the diabetic range should be detected on at least two separate occasions on different days. Where there is any doubt, an OGTT should be performed (see below), and if the fasting or random values are not diagnostic, the 2-h value should be used. In practice, the diagnosis is often obvious clinically, and [glucose] is only needed for confirmation and is unequivocally high. The diagnosis should never be made on the basis of a single test in a patient without symptoms.

A raised glycated haemoglobin (HbA$_{1c}$) should not be used to make a diagnosis of diabetes since it is influenced by red cell lifespan as well as by [glucose].

Blood and plasma glucose

Most laboratory instruments measure plasma [glucose], but some use whole blood. Plasma [glucose] is 10–15% higher than whole blood [glucose], since red cells contain less water per unit volume than plasma. The discrepancy can be greater than this if [glucose] changes rapidly, because glucose will not have reached equilibration across the red cell membrane. Plasma, therefore, yields more reliable results. At normal plasma [glucose], there is little difference between results obtained on capillary and venous blood. However, at hyperglycaemic levels, capillary plasma [glucose] may be significantly higher than venous plasma [glucose]. These factors are important in the interpretation of glucose tolerance tests.

If there is likely to be any delay in measuring [glucose] in blood specimens, it is essential either to separate the plasma immediately or to inhibit glycolysis in blood by using a sodium fluoride-containing collection tube. This stabilises the [glucose] for several hours. Measurements of blood [glucose] that are to be performed using a 'stick' test must be carried out without delay on specimens that do not contain sodium fluoride.

Oral glucose tolerance test (OGTT)

The OGTT remains the 'gold standard' for the diagnosis of diabetes and should be performed when random [glucose] falls into a range where the diagnosis is uncertain. Several precautions must be taken in preparing for and performing the test. It should not be performed on patients suffering from an intercurrent infection or the effects of trauma, or those recovering from a serious illness.

Drugs such as corticosteroids and diuretics may impair glucose tolerance and should be stopped before the test if possible. The patient should have been on an unrestricted diet containing at least 150 g of carbohydrate/day for at least 3 days, and should not have indulged in unaccustomed amounts of exercise. The patient must not smoke before or during the test, nor eat or drink anything other than as specified below.

An OGTT is usually performed after an overnight fast, although a fast of 4–5 h may be enough. The patient is allowed to drink water during the fast. A standard dose of glucose (82.5 g of glucose monohydrate or 75 g of anhydrous glucose) dissolved in 250–300 mL of water is given by mouth over a 5-min period. Smaller amounts of glucose (1.92 g of glucose monohydrate or 1.75 g of anhydrous glucose/kg body weight) are given to children. During the test, the patient should be sitting up or lying down on the right side so as to facilitate rapid emptying of the stomach. Blood specimens are collected before giving the glucose load and after 2 h.

Table 6.4 summarises the criteria for identifying healthy adults, patients with diabetes mellitus and individuals with IGT for blood and plasma [glucose], and for venous and capillary specimens.

Impaired fasting glucose (IFG) and impaired glucose tolerance (IGT)

The current WHO criteria define two conditions of impaired glucose homeostasis intermediate between normality and diabetes. These are the states of IFG and IGT. They cannot be considered as distinct clinical entities but in both there is an increased risk of development of cardiovascular (macrovascular) disease, but not the microvascular complications of diabetes. Both also increase the risk of developing diabetes in the future.

Monitoring the treatment of diabetic patients

There is now excellent evidence that in both type 1 and type 2 diabetes, the incidence of long-term complications such as retinopathy can

Table 6.4 Diagnostic criteria for diabetes mellitus and their dependence on the nature of the specimens collected for analysis. Clinical laboratory analysis will usually give results for venous plasma (bold)

	Glucose concentration (mmol/L)		
	Fasting		**2 h post-75 g glucose**
Normal individuals			
Venous plasma	**<6.1**		**<7.8**
Venous blood	<5.6		<6.7
Capillary blood	<5.6		<7.8
Diabetes mellitus			
Venous plasma	**≥7.0**	**or**	**≥11.1**
Venous blood	≥6.1	or	≥10.0
Capillary blood	≥6.1	or	≥11.1
IGT			
Venous plasma	**<7.0**	**and**	**≥7.8 and <11.1**
Venous blood	<6.1	and	≥6.7 and 10.0
Capillary blood	<6.1	and	≥7.8 and 11.1
IFG			
Venous plasma	**≥6.1 and <7.0**		**<7.8**
Venous blood	≥5.6 and <6.1		<6.7
Capillary blood	≥5.6 and <6.1		<7.8

be reduced by achieving tight control, albeit at the expense of an increased frequency of hypoglycaemic episodes. This level of control requires meticulous monitoring of glycaemic control.

Home blood glucose monitoring

In order to achieve this level of control, in type 1 patients, insulin doses need to be frequently and carefully adjusted on the basis of multiple daily blood [glucose] measurements. In patients in whom this level of control is unrealistic or is not needed, this requirement can be relaxed. In such patients, and in patients with type 2 diabetes, less frequent blood [glucose] measurements can be made, preferably covering different times of the day, although the frequency should be increased at times of illness or when control appears to have deteriorated.

Glycated haemoglobin

Blood glucose measurements made at the clinic only indicate the [glucose] at that time, and may be unrepresentative of overall control. Measurement of the extent of the non-enzymatic glycation of Hb allows assessment of diabetic control over a longer period.

Glucose reacts spontaneously and non-enzymatically with free amino groups on proteins to form covalent glycated proteins. The extent of glycation depends on the average [glucose] to which the protein is exposed and on the half-life of the protein. Thus, long-lived structural proteins (e.g. lens protein) may be damaged as a result of the abnormal increase in protein glycation found in diabetics. Indeed, it has been suggested that glycation of structural proteins might be responsible for some of the long-term complications of diabetes. Shorter half-life proteins such as Hb also undergo excessive glycation in diabetes.

Several glycated derivatives of Hb exist, derived from the reaction of Hb with glucose, glucose-6-phosphate, etc. These are collectively known as HbA_1. The principal complex is the one formed with glucose itself, HbA_{1c}, which normally forms about 5% of circulating Hb.

Once formed, the HbA_{1c} stays within the red cell for its lifetime. Since the half-life of the red cell is about 60 days, the HbA_{1c} value reflects the average level of blood [glucose] over the previous 1–2 months, with higher levels indicating poor diabetic control. The reliable interpretation of HbA_{1c} levels does however depend on the red cell half-life being normal. Artefactually low results will be obtained in any condition where the lifespan of the red cell is shortened. These conditions include haemolytic and some other anaemias, some haemoglobinopathies and repeated venesection, for example in the treatment of haemochromatosis.

A number of landmark trials have established the association between better glycaemic control, lower [HbA$_{1c}$] and lower incidence of diabetic complications. These trials have demonstrated that achieving lower levels of HbA$_{1c}$, ideally towards or into the non-diabetic range, reduces the incidence of micro- and macrovascular complications. However, this is at the expense of an increase in episodes of hypoglycaemia. For an individual patient, the balance between preventing future complications and avoiding hypoglycaemia will determine the goals of treatment, as judged by the HbA$_{1c}$ achieved. In a young patient with type 1 diabetes and no pre-existing complications, the goal will be low and as close to the normal range as possible, or even into it, with the hope of achieving many years of complication-free survival. In an elderly patient with type 2 diabetes and multiple other problems, the aim of treatment may simply be the avoidance of symptoms of hyperglycaemia, and the HBA$_{1c}$ goal will be correspondingly higher.

Standardisation of HbA$_{1c}$ assays has been a problem because of the lack both of a gold standard reference method and of preparations of absolutely known concentration to use as calibrators. Both of these issues have been solved on behalf of the International Federation for Clinical Chemistry (IFCC). Assays calibrated against these new standards give results slightly lower than previously, since there is a lack of interference from other species. International agreement has been reached that from 2009 the new 'IFCC' HbA$_{1c}$ is reported alongside the old HbA$_{1c}$ for a period, before the old HbA$_{1c}$ is phased out. In order to avoid potential confusion the units will change from the current % to mmol/mol.

Glycated plasma proteins

Measurement of glycated plasma proteins (the major component of these proteins being albumin)

can also be used to monitor diabetic control. The shorter half-life of albumin means that this test reflects control of blood [glucose] over the previous 10–15 days. Plasma fructosamine is a measure of glycated plasma proteins, but the widespread adoption of [HbA$_{1c}$] as the accepted marker of glycaemic control means that fructosamine measurements are not widely available. Fructosamine measurement has a use in patients with haemoglobinopathies, in whom [HbA$_{1c}$] can be difficult to measure and interpret.

Microalbumin

Urinary 'microalbumin' is a term that refers to urinary albumin loss that is greater than normal, but which remains below the threshold of detection by the urinalysis dipstick tests widely used for detecting the presence of urinary protein. The more sensitive tests required to detect 'microalbuminuria' are usually performed in the laboratory, although dipstick tests are also available. There is no analytical difficulty in measuring these low levels of albumin, but there is some variation in the type of sample to use and how best to express the results. Overnight timed urine collections are possibly most satisfactory, but random urine samples are usually used for convenience. Results are expressed on timed collections as an albumin excretion rate, or on a random sample as an albumin : creatinine ratio.

Up to 50% of type 1 diabetics may develop nephropathy, and the detection of microalbuminuria has been shown to signal an eventual progression to diabetic nephropathy. With the benefit of the early warning provided by the detection of microalbuminuria, there is some evidence that meticulous control of diabetes and hypertension, and the use of ACE inhibitors, delays the progress of the nephropathy.

Metabolic complications of diabetes mellitus

Patients with diabetes can develop severe metabolic derangements potentially leading to coma.

The causes can be classified as follows:

- Hyperglycaemia, with or without ketoacidosis.
- Lactic acidosis, with or without hyperglycaemia.
- Hypoglycaemia, due to insulin excess.
- Uraemia, for example due to diabetic nephropathy.

Diabetic ketoacidosis (DKA)

Diabetic ketoacidosis may be the presenting feature in a patient not previously recognised as having diabetes. In a patient with known diabetes, it may be precipitated by omitting insulin doses, or by the insulin dose becoming inadequate because of an increase in hormones with opposing action, due to intercurrent infection, trauma, or unusual physical or psychological stress. The clinical features are dehydration, ketosis and hyperventilation ('air hunger'). The degree of hyperglycaemia does not correlate with the severity of the metabolic disturbance in DKA, and in some patients it may not be very high (e.g. in children, pregnant women, malnourished or alcoholic patients).

Ketoacidosis is due to insulin deficiency, accompanied by raised plasma concentrations of the counter-regulatory hormones (adrenaline, cortisol, GH and glucagon). The changes in these circulating hormones result in hyperglycaemia and in mobilisation of free fatty acids from adipose tissue, and subsequent increased ketone body production in the liver (Figure 6.1).

The major metabolic abnormalities result from hyperglycaemia or ketoacidosis, or both. Hyperglycaemia causes extracellular hyperosmolality, which in turn leads to intracellular dehydration as well as to an osmotic diuresis. The osmotic diuresis causes loss of water, Na$^+$, K$^+$, calcium and other inorganic constituents, and leads to a fall in circulating blood volume. Ketone bodies stimulate the chemoreceptor trigger zone, so vomiting may exacerbate all these effects. The increased production of ketone bodies causes a metabolic acidosis with associated hyperkalaemia. Lactic acidosis and pre-renal uraemia may also be present.

Ketone bodies

Acetoacetate, 3-hydroxybutyrate (β-hydroxybutyrate) and acetone are collectively described as the 'ketone bodies', although 3-hydroxybutyrate is not in fact a ketone. They are most commonly found in the blood in excessive amounts in uncontrolled diabetes. The levels of ketone bodies also

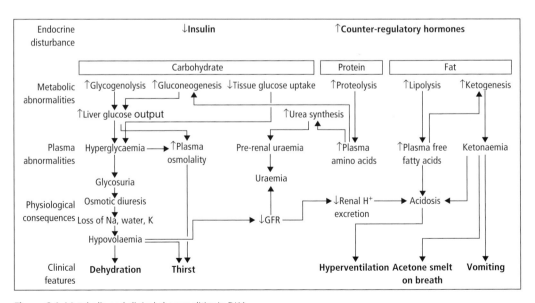

Figure 6.1 Metabolic and clinical abnormalities in DKA.

increase during starvation, since ketone bodies form an important energy source for many tissues when carbohydrate intake or metabolism is limited. Ketone bodies are synthesised in the liver from acetyl-coenzyme A (CoA), itself derived from the oxidation of free fatty acids. Some of the acetoacetate may then be reduced to 3-hydroxybutyrate or decarboxylated with the formation of acetone and CO_2.

Acetoacetic acid and 3-hydroxybutyric acid production give rise to metabolic acidosis, since the liver and other tissues cannot, in general, completely metabolise the increased amounts of these ketone bodies that are being formed. The acidosis is partly compensated by hyperventilation, with reduction in P_{CO_2}. The acidosis causes H^+ to move into cells and K^+ to move out. Increased plasma $[K^+]$ often results from the combined effects of the acidosis and the lack of insulin action that normally promotes K^+ entry into cells.

'Ketones' can be detected in serum or urine using a number of semi-quantitative point of care stick tests. The tests that have been most widely used in fact detect acetoacetate and do not react with β-hydroxybutyrate. Newer versions specific for β-hydroxybutyrate are now available.

Laboratory assessment and management of diabetic ketoacidosis

An initial diagnosis is usually made on the basis of the history, clinical examination and dipstick testing of urine for glucose and ketone bodies, and testing of blood [glucose]. Laboratory-based tests on blood are needed to evaluate the severity of the condition more precisely, and to monitor progress during treatment. It is rarely necessary, and indeed may be positively dangerous, to wait for laboratory results before starting emergency treatment. However, further treatment should be based on regular clinical assessment and on chemical measurements in the laboratory.

Plasma glucose, urea, Na^+ and K^+ concentrations are measured on venous blood. Plasma $[Na^+]$ may be normal or low initially. Plasma $[K^+]$ is usually increased, but may be normal. Plasma [urea] is usually increased due to dehydration. Acid–base status is assessed by measurement of venous [total CO_2] or by measurement of arterial 'blood gases' ($[H^+]$, P_{CO_2}, $[HCO_3^-]$ and P_{O_2}). Plasma [total CO_2] is nearly always reduced, often being less than 5 mmol/L in severe cases. Results of blood gas analysis indicate a metabolic acidosis with compensatory reduction in P_{CO_2}.

Treatment aims to replace fluid and electrolyte deficits, and to correct the metabolic abnormality by infusion of insulin. Knowledge of the fluid and electrolyte deficits likely to be present helps in planning appropriate therapy. The deficits may be as much as 5–10 L of water, 500 mmol of Na^+, 250–800 mmol of K^+ and 300–500 mmol of base (e.g. $[HCO_3^-]$) in patients with severe acidosis. Fluid replacement is usually given initially as isotonic saline. The rate of infusion will depend on the clinical circumstances, but should usually be rapid, at least initially, with careful monitoring of fluid status, often including the use of measurement of central venous pressure.

Most hospitals will have a protocol for the treatment of DKA, and this should be followed. However, a typical infusion regimen might entail isotonic saline infused at a rate of 1 L/h for the first 2 h, then 500 mL/h for the next 2 h. Potassium replacement is usually started early, in the knowledge that the patient has almost certainly developed a large K^+ deficit, and insulin will rapidly cause K^+ to enter the cells from the ECF. Serious hypokalaemia can develop fairly quickly in the absence of early corrective action.

The use of $NaHCO_3$ to correct the acidosis is not required or beneficial, since restoring normal renal perfusion allows excretion of H^+ and regeneration of $[HCO_3^-]$, and the return of metabolism to normal reduces H^+ production. In very severe acidoses (arterial $[H^+]$ >100 nmol/L) which do not rapidly begin to resolve with treatment it may be considered, but can be hazardous. It can cause:

● Hypokalaemia, as rapid correction of the acidosis augments K^+ influx into cells

● A paradoxical rise in CSF $[H^+]$ rather than a fall, since CO_2 diffuses more rapidly into the CSF than HCO_3^-.

● Na^+ overload.

- Shift of the oxy-haemoglobin saturation curve to the left, impairing oxygen delivery.

Insulin is usually given as a constant IV infusion, a typical starting rate being 6 U/h. If the [glucose] does not fall in the first hour, the rate of infusion may need to be increased. Plasma [glucose] is monitored, and once it has fallen to between 10 and 15 mmol/L, dextrose is added to the IV fluids (e.g. 10% dextrose at an infusion rate of 100 mL/h), and it may be possible to decrease the rate of insulin infusion to maintain euglycaemia. This is continued until it is possible to re-establish the patient on oral food and water and a conventional subcutaneous insulin regimen.

The frequency and timing of repeat analyses depend on the severity and nature of the ketoacidosis, and on the method of treatment. For most patients, it is advisable to repeat some of the initial analyses, particularly plasma [K+], after 1 h and thereafter at longer intervals if treatment is progressing satisfactorily.

Non-ketotic, hyperglycaemic coma

These patients are usually older than the ketotic group and typically have type 2 diabetes. Insulin deficiency has the same effects on carbohydrate metabolism as in DKA, but the presence of at least some insulin allows suppression of ketogenesis. In addition, there may be poorer renal function in older patients, leading to greater losses of water and electrolytes. Severe hyperglycaemia (often >50 mmol/L) can develop with profound dehydration and a very high plasma osmolality (>320 mosm/kg), but no ketosis and minimal acidosis. This condition is often referred to as hyperosmolar non-ketotic hyperglycaemia. It should be noted that patients with ketoacidosis may also have a raised osmolality, although this is not so marked.

Treatment of patients with non-ketotic hyperglycaemia is similar to the treatment of ketotic hyperglycaemic patients, with administration of fluids and insulin. Because of the hypertonicity, hypotonic saline replacement may be used, although it is important that the osmolality does not fall too quickly. Once the acute illness has resolved, most patients will not require continuing insulin, but will

be managed on diet, with or without oral hypoglycaemic agents. There is an increased risk of thrombotic episodes in these patients, and treatment with anti-coagulants is generally considered advisable.

Lactic acidosis

If tissue perfusion is affected by extreme dehydration (hyperosmolality), or by the factors that precipitated the original metabolic decompensation (e.g. severe infection, myocardial infarction), tissue anoxia may lead on to lactic acidosis.

Hypoglycaemia

The plasma [glucose] at which hypoglycaemic symptoms appear is very variable, often related more to the rate of fall of blood [glucose] than to the absolute value observed. Arbitrarily, a venous plasma [glucose] below 2.2 mmol/L is the biochemical definition of hypoglycaemia. It is convenient to distinguish between the hypoglycaemia that occurs after several hours of fasting and the hypoglycaemia that is due to some other stimulus (reactive hypoglycaemia), including the stimulus of a meal. It is often possible to distinguish these two categories on the basis of the patient's history.

Fasting hypoglycaemia

Fasting hypoglycaemia only occurs after some hours without food and may be precipitated by exercise. It always indicates an identifiable underlying disease. Failure to maintain a normal blood [glucose] in the fasting state is a feature of a number of endocrine conditions. It may be due to drugs (e.g. insulin overdose, accidental or deliberate; sulphonylureas; salicylate overdose in children, but not adults) or poisons (e.g. some toadstools), inborn errors of metabolism (e.g. galactosaemia, hereditary fructose intolerance) or alcohol. It may be brought about by excess alcohol intake. Causes of fasting hypoglycaemia are summarised in Table 6.5, subdivided into causes of enhanced glucose utilisation and defective glucose production. An alternative classification is into causes of excess insulin-like activity (including insulinomas, administration of insulin or sulphonylureas, and as

Table 6.5 Fasting hypoglycaemia

Cause	Examples
Enhanced glucose utilisation	
Endogenous overproduction of insulin	Hyperinsulinism of childhood (nesidioblastosis), insulinoma, pancreatitis, pancreatic tumours (as part of MEN I syndrome)
Defective glucose production	
Endocrine disorders	Adrenocortical insufficiency and hypothyroidism (in both cases, primary and secondary), growth hormone deficiency
Liver disease	Severe portal cirrhosis, acute hepatic necrosis, hepatic tumours
Renal disease	End-stage renal failure
Miscellaneous	Severe malnutrition, starvation, inherited metabolic disorders (e.g. glycogen storage disease type 1)

a paraneoplastic phenomenon in some malignancies, see below) and causes of non-insulin-induced hypoglycaemia (including severe hepatic dysfunction, ethanol, and deficiency of cortisol or GH).

Reactive or postprandial hypoglycaemia

Reactive or postprandial hypoglycaemia occurs 2–5 h after meals and does not occur during a fast. It may occur after meals in patients who have undergone gastric surgery, or in early, usually type 2, diabetes.

Insulinoma

This is usually a small, solitary, benign adenoma of the pancreatic islets that secretes inappropriate amounts of insulin. Occasionally, multiple pancreatic adenomas may be associated with adenomas in other endocrine organs as part of the MEN I syndrome (pp. 79, 251 and Table 16.8). The symptoms may be bizarre, and laboratory investigations play a major part in diagnosis.

Most patients develop symptomatic hypoglycaemia after a fast of 24–36 h, but in a few the fast may have to last for up to 72 h before symptomatic hypoglycaemia develops. Blood specimens are collected when hypoglycaemic symptoms develop, or after three overnight fasts. Most patients with an insulinoma will have unequivocal hypoglycaemia in one of these specimens, even if they were asymptomatic. The diagnostic finding in patients suspected of having an insulinoma is a fasting plasma [insulin] that is inappropriately high in relation to the low plasma [glucose].

It can be difficult to demonstrate fasting hypoglycaemia satisfactorily in some patients. In these cases, it may still be possible to obtain support for a diagnosis of insulinoma by measuring plasma [C peptide] during an infusion of exogenous insulin sufficient to induce hypoglycaemia. Exogenous insulin contains little or no C peptide, and continuous detection of plasma [C peptide] shows that endogenous insulin release is not suppressed, as it should be in response to hypoglycaemia. This finding is strongly suggestive of insulinoma.

As stated above, therapeutic insulin preparations contain little or no C peptide. Accidental or deliberate overdose of insulin, giving rise to hypoglycaemia, can therefore be distinguished from insulinoma by measuring both plasma [insulin] and plasma [C peptide].

Other causes of fasting hypoglycaemia

Deficiency of hormones that antagonise insulin activity is an uncommon cause of hypoglycaemia. Some non-pancreatic tumours are associated with hypoglycaemia, mainly in patients with advanced malignant disease. Some of the larger tumours may consume excessive amounts of glucose, but there is also evidence for the production of hormonal insulin-like substances, as a paraneoplastic phenomenon. One cause of this is the excessive production of a large unprocessed form of insulin-like growth factor-2 (big IGF-2) by the tumour. Because of defective binding to IGF-binding proteins in the circulation, it is able to pass across capillary walls, reach insulin target tissues and exert its insulin-like effect.

Case 6.1

A 14-year-old boy was found by his mother in a drowsy and unco-operative state. When the GP arrived, she told her that her son had seemed to be unusually thirsty for the last 1–2 months, and she thought that he had lost weight. Recently, he had been complaining of abdominal pain and discomfort.

He was admitted to a hospital as an emergency. On examination he was semi-conscious, with deep sighing respiration, a pulse rate of 120/min, a blood pressure of 94/56 and cold extremities. Chemical investigations on blood after admission showed the following:

Serum	Result	Reference range
Urea	24.5	2.5–6.6 mmol/L
Na^+	128	135–145 mmol/L
K^+	6.9	3.6–5.0 mmol/L
Glucose	35.2	mmol/L

Blood gas analysis	Result	Reference range
H^+	82	37–45 nmol/L
P_{CO_2}	2.9	4.5–6.0 kPa
HCO_3^-	7.0	21–29 mmol/L
P_{O_2}	14.0	12–15 kPa

What is the probable diagnosis, and how would you confirm this quickly? What principles should guide the treatment of this patient?

Comments: The patient almost certainly had DKA with typical clinical and biochemical features. The tachycardia, hypotension and cold peripheries suggest marked depletion of ECF. The arterial sample shows that he has a metabolic acidosis, and the plasma sample contains a high concentration of glucose. The high urea is consistent with renal impairment or dehydration. Ketoacidosis was confirmed by testing a urine specimen for ketone bodies. If he had been too dehydrated to produce urine, a drop of plasma could have been used instead (note that only some people can smell acetone in patients' breath). The mainstays of treatment for patients with DKA are

(continued on p. 102)

Case 6.1 *(continued)*

- Fluid and electrolyte replacement, starting with saline (150 mmol/L) and containing added potassium chloride (40 mmol/L), usually as a standard regime (check local protocols, but one regimen would be 1 L in the first 30 min, 500 mL in the next 30 min, and then 2 L over the next 4 h, and 2 L over the next 8 h).
- Insulin infusion usually starting at a rate of 6 U/h.
- Frequent monitoring of the patient's plasma [glucose] and [K$^+$], and monitoring of the central venous pressure. As the treatment takes effect, plasma [K$^+$] is liable to fall rapidly due to the large whole-body K$^+$ deficit, despite the initially raised plasma [K$^+$].

Case 6.2

An elderly man was visited by his son and was found to be semi-conscious. He had last been seen by neighbours about 10 days previously, when he had seemed well. He was admitted to a hospital. On examination, he appeared extremely dehydrated. The results of biochemical investigations were as follows:

Serum	Result	Reference range
Urea	38	2.5–6.6 mmol/L
Na$^+$	151	135–145 mmol/L
K$^+$	4.8	3.6–5.0 mmol/L
Total CO$_2$	18	22–30 mmol/L
Glucose	61	mmol/L
Osmolality	417	280–290 mmol/kg

Comments: There is severe hyperglycaemia, resulting in a very high osmolality. The hyperglycaemia has driven an osmotic diuresis, resulting in loss of ECF and consequent reduction in the GFR and retention of urea. The sustained osmotic diuresis causes a loss of water in excess of sodium, explaining the hypernatraemia. The [total CO$_2$] is slightly reduced due to the impaired renal function, but is not as low as would be expected in a case of ketoacidosis with results as abnormal as these. The patient was too dehydrated to produce a urine sample to check for ketones, but a drop of plasma on the ketones square of a urine dipstick gave a negative result.

He had non-ketotic hyperglycaemia. This only occurs in patients with type 2 diabetes. The insulin concentration required to oppose the ketogenic actions of glucagon is lower than that required to prevent increased glucose production. These patients have sufficient circulating insulin to prevent the ketogenesis, but not enough to prevent the hyperglycaemia. Treatment is by replacement of fluid and electrolyte losses, and by insulin infusion to restore the [glucose]. Once the acute episode is over, insulin is unlikely to be needed.

When the patient recovered, he reported having experienced increasing thirst and polyuria over several weeks. In response to the thirst, he had been drinking several large bottles of lemonade every day.

Case 6.3

A 27-year-old man was referred to the local diabetes clinic. He had been diagnosed as having type 2 diabetes 3 years previously and his control was poor (HbA$_{1c}$ 9.6%) despite being on good doses of metformin. The GP was wondering whether he needed to start on insulin. Several close family members also had diabetes, he was slightly overweight with a BMI of 26, and he was normotensive.

Comments: In view of the strong family history of diabetes and the fact that he did not fit the typical phenotype of type 2 diabetes (he was relatively young, not obese and normotensive) the possibility of maturity onset diabetes of the young (MODY) was raised. Genotyping revealed a mutation in the *HNF1α* gene. Metformin was stopped and he achieved excellent control on a low dose of gliclazide.

Case 6.4

A 45-year-old woman who was unable to feed, wash or dress herself because of severe multiple sclerosis was being cared for in a nursing home. About 6 h after a visit by relatives, it was found that she could not be roused. On admission to a hospital, she was found to be profoundly hypoglycaemic ([glucose] 1.9 mmol/L), and required repeated IV infusions of glucose to maintain plasma [glucose] over the next 12–24 h. A sample of blood taken on admission was stored and subsequently analysed for insulin and C peptide. The results were inappropriately raised, considering the hypoglycaemia. Over the next few days, repeated overnight fasts failed to induce further hypoglycaemia. Eventually, after a prolonged fast of 4 days, [glucose] dropped to 2.5 mmol/L (not a hypoglycaemic level by strict criteria), at which time insulin and C peptide were undetectable.

Comments: The results on admission were suggestive of an insulinoma, with hypoglycaemia and inappropriately elevated insulin and C peptide levels. However, it proved difficult to induce a further episode of hypoglycaemia. Most patients with an insulinoma will be hypoglycaemic on one or more occasion after three overnight fasts, even if not symptomatic. Even a prolonged fast failed to induce true hypoglycaemia, and at that time the insulin level was appropriately low. Review of her history revealed no suggestions of previous hypoglycaemic episodes. The clinical staff were accordingly forced to reconsider the initial diagnosis.

The sample of blood taken at the time of admission was sent for toxicological analysis, and was found to contain high concentrations of the oral hypoglycaemic drugs chlorpropamide and glibenclamide. These drugs are sulphonylureas, which act by enhancing pancreatic insulin secretion in response to glucose. Both chlorpropamide and glibenclamide have long half-lives, making hypoglycaemia an occasional problem even when used therapeutically in patients with diabetes.

The patient would have been unable to obtain or take these drugs. It was likely that a relative, distressed by her condition, had administered them. The police were informed, but it was felt that there was insufficient evidence to proceed further.

Chapter 7

Disorders of the hypothalamus and pituitary

Endocrinology is the study of the biological systems in the body that communicate with each other through the release of hormones. The preceding two chapters have covered the endocrine systems that regulate calcium and glucose homeostasis. In this chapter the endocrine systems regulated through the hypothalamo-pituitary axis are discussed (Figure 7.1).

The diagnosis and management of endocrine diseases rely heavily on laboratory tests. In most cases a blood sample taken in the basal state is all that is required to aid diagnosis, but occasionaly stimulation or suppression testing need to be performed to uncover more subtle abnormalities. This chapter briefly describes the mechanisms that control the release of hormones by the hypothalamus and pituitary. Investigation of pituitary and hypothalamic function is often also intimately concerned with the investigation of the peripheral target glands which they control, and here we outline the methods commonly used to investigate suspected hypothalamo-pituitary dysfunction. Further information can be found in Chapters 8–10 concerning the thyroid, the adrenal and reproductive endocrinology.

Lecture Notes: Clinical Biochemistry, 8e. By G. Beckett, S. Walker, P. Rae & P. Ashby. Published 2010 by Blackwell Publishing.

The hypothalamus

The hypothalamus is derived from forebrain tissue on either side of the third ventricle and links the nervous system to the endocrine sytems through the pituitary gland. The hypothalamus is a complex region in the brain that co-ordinates many behavioural and circadian rhythms in addition to enforcing homeostatic mechanisms, on specific target glands. The hypothalamus must respond to many different external and internal signals by releasing a variety of factors that act on the pituitary. In order to accomplish such a complex process the hypothalamus is connected with many parts of the CNS (e.g. stress results in release of corticotrophin-releasing hormone (CRH)).

The hypothalamus secretes a number of hormones and other chemical agents that pass down the hypothalamo-hypophyseal portal blood vessels to the pituitary where they regulate the release of anterior pituitary hormones. The hormones produced by the target glands controlled by the anterior pituitary may exert negative feedback effects on the secretion of the corresponding hypothalamic or pituitary hormone. For example, plasma [free cortisol] primarily influences the output of hypothalamic CRH while plasma [free thyroxine (FT4)] inhibits the release of TSH from the pituitary. Table 7.1 list the various hypothalamic and pituitary hormones together with the

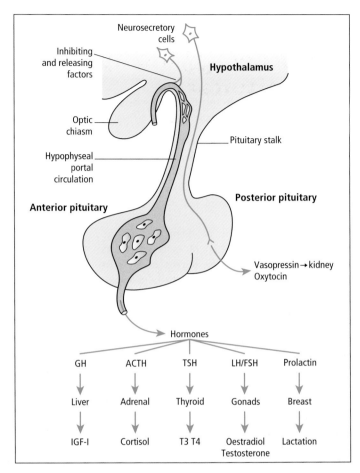

Figure 7.1 Factors which regulate the release of anterior pituitary hormones.

Table 7.1 Hypothalamic and anterior pituitary hormones and factors

Hypothalamic-stimulating hormone	Anterior pituitary hormone(s) released	Feedback control hormone or compound
CRH	ACTH, β-lipotrophin (LPH)	Cortisol
GHRH, GnRH	GH	Somatostatin
	FSH	Gonadal steroids and inhibin
GnRH	LH	Gonadal steroids
No stimulating factor identified	Prolactin	Dopamine
Thyrotrophin-releasing hormone (TRH)	TSH (and prolactin)	FT4, FT3

factors that regulate their release. Concentrations of hypothalamic hormones in peripheral blood for the most part do not reflect hypothalamic acyivity and are not considered to be of clinical relevance.

Anterior pituitary hormones

The pituitary gland comprises the embryologically and functionally distinct anterior pituitary (adenohypophysis) and posterior pituitary (neurohypophysis). The anterior pituitary hormones and their corresponding regulatory hormones/factors are described in detail below.

Corticotrophin-releasing hormone and adrenocorticotrophic hormone

Hypothalamic CRH is composed of 41 amino acids, and is the main stimulatory factor involved in the control of the pituitary–adrenal axis. Its release is subject to negative feedback control by [free cortisol] released from the adrenal cortex (Figure 9.2).

ACTH is a monomeric polypeptide hormone of 39 amino acids secreted by cells known as corticotrophs. The biological activity of ACTH is contained in the 24 amino acids at the N-terminal end. The major activity of ACTH is the stimulation of adrenal steroid synthesis, especially that of the glucocorticoid, cortisol, but it also plays a permissive role in the synthesis of aldosterone. ACTH also stimulates melanocytes to produce melanin. This is the cause of the increased pigmentation seen in patients with ACTH-driven causes of Cushing's syndrome, in adrenocortical hypofunction and in Nelson's syndrome, a rare disorder arising from an ACTH-secreting pituitary macroadenoma after a therapeutic bilateral adrenalectomy. ACTH shows a marked diurnal variation, with the highest concentrations being found at approximately 8 am and the lowest at midnight. Marked increases in ACTH also occur with stress. ACTH is unstable in blood or plasma unless frozen. Blood samples should be collected in EDTA on ice and the plasma separated within 30 min and then frozen immediately.

ACTH and β-lipotrophin (β-LPH) exist next to each other at the C-terminal end of a much larger precursor molecule, pro-opiomelanocortin. In ectopic ACTH production, it seems that there is abnormal processing of pro-opiomelanocortin which may result in the release of ACTH with a higher than normal molecular weight termed 'big ACTH'.

Gonadotrophin-releasing hormone and the gonadotrophins luteinising hormone and follicle-stimulating hormone

Gonadotrophin-releasing hormone (GnRH) is a decapeptide produced by the hypothalamus in pulses into the hypothalamic–hypophyseal portal circulation. GnRH stimulates the release of the gonadotrophins, luteinising hormone (LH) and follicle-stimulating hormone (FSH) from the gonadotroph. LH and FSH are dimeric glycopeptides and are released in pulses of approximately 90 min. This pulsatile release is essential for the gonadotrophins to exert their physiological actions. The release of GnRH is modified by oestrogens, progesterone, androgens and inhibins; these relationships are complex and are discussed in Chapter 10.

Thyrotrophin-releasing hormone and thyroid-stimulating hormone

Hypothalamic thyrotrophin-realeasing hormone (TRH) is a tripeptide that controls the secretion of thyrotrophin (TSH) by the thyrotroph cells of the anterior pituitary. Free thyroid hormones inhibit the release of TRH and TSH, but thyroid hormones exert their main negative feedback effects directly on TSH secretion (Figure 8.3).

TSH is a glycoprotein composed of an α-subunit that is common to LH, FSH and hCG, and a β-subunit specific to TSH. The place of TSH measurements in the investigation of thyroid function is discussed in Chapter 8.

Growth hormone-releasing hormone and growth hormone

The release of GH by the somatotrophs in the pituitary is stimulated by hypothalamic GHRH, a 44 amino acid peptide, and inhibited by hypothalamic somatostatin, a 14 amino acid peptide. The peptide hormone ghrelin also stimulates the release of GH, acting in concert with GHRH to control both the timing and magnitude of GH release. Gherelin is a 28 amino acid peptide

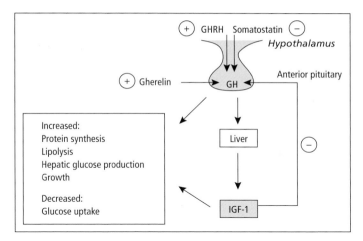

Figure 7.2 Factors which regulate the production and release of growth hormone (GH). In addition to the mechanisms shown, a regulatory effect on GH release is also achieved by insulin-like growth factor-1 (IGF-1) together with GH stimulating the release of somatostatin from the hypothalamus. In addition to GH promoting hepatic IGF-1 release, there is increasing evidence to suggest that GH may also promote the release of IGF-1 locally in target tissues, which then acts in a paracrine fashion. Gherelin also stimulates the release of GH, acting in concert with growth hormone-releasing hormone (GHRH) to control both the timing and magnitude of GH release. Gherelin is a 28 amino acid peptide released predominantly from epithelial cells lining the fundus of the stomach.

released predominantly from epithelial cells lining the fundus of the stomach. Gherelin also induces a feeling of hunger through action at the hypothalamus, and levels are very high in Prader–Willi syndrome patients who are obese and have voracious appetites. The release of GH is regulated to some extent by a negative feedback of IGF-1 on the pituitary to modify the action of GHRH and at the hypothalamus where IGF-1 together with GH stimulates the release of somatostatin, which in turn then downregulates GH release (Figure 7.2). GH release is suppressed by high doses of glucose, and this response is used in the investigation of suspected acromegaly and gigantism.

GH is a single polypeptide comprising 191 amino acids which circulates predominantly in a 22 kDa (75%) form, with the remainder circulating as a 20 kDa form or as glycosylated and sulphated derivatives. About half of the circulating GH is bound to a GH-binding protein, which is the cleaved extracellular domain of the GH receptor; the bound fraction has a longer half-life in plasma than free GH and as such the bound fraction has a prolonged bioactivity. GH is essential for normal growth, and originally it was thought that it acted mainly indirectly through stimulating the hepatic release of IGF-1 (also known as somatomedin C). In serum, IGF-1 circulates bound to six binding proteins (IGFBPs) with IGFBP3 being the most important. There is increasing evidence to suggest that GH may also promote the release of IGF-1 locally in target tissues, which in turn then acts in a paracrine fashion. The GH receptor is found in many tissues in the body, especially the liver. Stimulation of the receptor can give rise to activation of numerous signalling pathways which in turn allows GH to exhibit a wide variety of effects in different tissues.

Growth hormone deficiency

GH stimulates protein synthesis and growth, and also has metabolic effects that oppose the action of insulin, including increasing lipolysis and hepatic glucose production while decreasing tissue glucose uptake. It is now recognised that GH plays an important role in the adult as well as the child, and GH deficiency in the adult (most commonly caused by a pituitary tumour) is associated with significant morbidity and mortality. GH secretion occurs in pulses, mainly at night and lasting for approximately 1–2 h, giving rise to nocturnal peaks of approximately 12 µg/L. Only infrequent small pulses occur during the day, but exercise, stress, fasting, low blood [glucose] and ingestion of certain amino acids stimulate GH release, and this forms the basis of some of the stimulation tests used for the investigation of suspected GH deficiency. Measurement of basal [GH] is of little value since, during much of the day, levels are undetectable, but a low serum IGF-1 concentration is consistent with GH deficiency.

Prolactin

Prolactin is a single polypeptide (198 amino acids) secreted by the lactotrophs of the pituitary. The lactotrophs comprise 10% of the anterior pituitary cells in men but 30% in women. Prolactin acts via specific receptors which are widely distributed, but their main location is the mammary gland where their activation by prolactin stimulates lactation. Prolactin also has a role in the complex processes controlling gonadal function. High levels of prolactin can give rise to amenorrhoea, oligomenorrhoea, low libido and subfertility by impairing the pulsatile release of gonadotrophins.

Prolactin secretion is controlled by the inhibitory action of hypothalamic dopamine, but no hypothalamic stimulatory factor has been identified. There is a pulsatile release and diurnal rhythm of prolactin secretion, with the highest levels occurring during sleep and the lowest between 9 am and noon. Prolactin secretion increases in response to oestrogens, pregnancy, breastfeeding and stress. Certain drugs may also give rise to marked elevations in serum [prolactin].

A basal [prolactin] greater than 500 mU/L is regarded as being suspicious, but this should be confirmed on at least two or three occasions before follow-up investigations are initiated. There are many causes of hyperprolactinaemia other than pituitary disease (Table 7.2). Before collecting

Table 7.2 Causes of hyperprolactinaemia

Category of cause	Examples
Physiological	Pregnancy
	Breastfeeding
	Stress
Drugs	
Dopamine receptor-blocking agents	Phenothiazines
	Butyrophenones
	Tricyclic anti-depressants
	Metoclopramide
Dopamine-depleting drugs	Methyldopa
	Reserpine
Histamine receptor agonists	Cimetidine
Monoamine oxidase inhibitors	Phenelzine
Serotonin reuptake inhibitors	Paroxitine
Pathological	Prolactinoma
	Other pituitary tumours
	Idiopathic
	Chronic renal failure
	Primary hypothyroidism
	Macroprolactinaemia*

* Most studies suggest that macroprolactinaemia is not associated with a clinical disorder unless monomeric prolactin is increased.

blood for measuring [prolactin], it is particularly important to enquire about any medication that the patient is taking since many drugs can give rise to hyperprolactinaemia (Table 7.2).

Prolactin measurements should be performed in the investigation of amenorrhoea, oligomenorrhoea and subfertility, whether or not there is galactorrhoea (p. 159). It should also be measured in any patient with spontaneous inappropriate lactation. A significant proportion of subfertile female patients have hyperprolactinaemia, and may respond to treatment with dopamine agonists such as cabergoline and bromocriptine.

Macroprolactin is formed when normal (monomeric) prolactin combines with autoantibodies in a patient's serum to produce a prolactin–IgG complex (molecular weight 170 kDa), which is thought to be biologically inactive. The long half-life of the complex results in an elevated [total prolactin] being found in the serum. The clinical importance of macroprolactinaemia is controversial, with a few studies reporting clinical features typically associated with hyperprolactinaemia; however, most studies suggest that there is no associated clinical disorder. In view of this controversy, it is advisable to seek an endocrine opinion if macroprolactinaemia is found in symptomatic patients. All laboratories should assess whether a persistently elevated [total prolactin] is caused by macroprolactin. If macroprolactin is detected, the laboratory should estimate and report the concentration of normal (monomeric) prolactin that is present in the sample.

Anterior pituitary disease and its investigation

Causes

A wide range of conditions can affect the anterior pituitary and result in hypopituitarism either directly or through an effect on the hypothalamus (Table 7.3). The most common cause of hypopituitarism is a pituitary tumour. Failure may be total (panhypopituitarism) or partial, in which case secretion of one or more pituitary hormones is retained. Silent microadenomas are present in approximately 20% of the normal population, with clinically apparent tumours occurring in about 2 per 100 000. Pituitary tumours are usually either non-functional or secrete only one hormone. The following pituitary adenomas occur in decreasing order of frequency:

- non-functional
- prolactinoma
- GH secreting
- ACTH secreting
- TSH secreting
- LH/FSH secreting.

Therapeutic action such as the removal of a pituitary tumour or irradiation may also cause or exacerbate hypopituitarism.

Although most pituitary adenomas produce a single hormone in excess, pressure effects may decrease secretion of other pituitary hormones, so in all patients where the presence of an adenoma

Table 7.3 Causes of hypopituitarism

Category of cause	Examples
Tumours	Pituitary adenoma, craniopharyngioma, cerebral tumours
Trauma	
Vascular disease	Severe hypotension, cranial arteritis, infarction, especially of pre-existing tumour, postpartum necrosis (Sheehan syndrome)
Infection	Meningitis, especially tuberculous
Iatrogenic	Surgery, radiotherapy
Hypothalamic disorders	Tumours, functional disturbances as seen in starvation, anorexia nervosa, Cushing's syndrome
Granulomatous disease	Sarcoidosis

has been established, overall pituitary function should be assessed. Loss of pituitary hormones in progressive hypopituitarism usually occurs in a sequential and predictable manner. Secretion of LH, FSH and GH is usually lost first, followed by TSH and ACTH. Loss of prolactin production occurs only rarely and only when there is extensive pituitary damage. Because of this sequential loss, adults tend to have presenting symptoms that reflect loss of LH and GH which gives rise to infertility, menstrual disturbances, decreased libido and erectile dysfunction, with a reduction in muscle bulk and decreased body hair. A large expanding pituitary tumour may also give rise to headache, neuro-ophthalmological defects or facial pain. If the adenoma is functional, the presenting features will reflect which hormone is being oversecreted. For example, patients with prolactinoma may present with loss of libido, amenorrhoea and galactorrhoea.

Investigation

This requires the assessment of endocrine and neuro-ophthalmological function together with radiological investigations as appropriate. In the majority of cases, the measurement of basal pituitary hormones and primary target organ hormones in serum or plasma is sufficient. The investigation of suspected acromegaly (p. 111) and Cushing's syndrome (p. 136), however, requires the use of stimulation and/or suppression tests. Stimulation tests involving the IV administration of GnRH and TRH are now rarely used.

The following is a suggestion for the initial biochemical investigation of a patient with suspected pituitary disease. Further tests may be required, depending on the results and the clinical circumstances.

Basal hormone measurements

These provide useful diagnostic information, and should be performed first. A basal 9 am blood sample should be obtained for measurement of cortisol, FT4, TSH, testosterone or oestradiol depending on sex, LH, FSH and prolactin. ACTH can be measured but this hormone is labile and it may be inconvenient on the first occasion to organise the rapid centrifugation of the specimen. Serum and urine osmolalities should also be measured if there is clinical suspicion of posterior pituitary dysfunction. Measurement of [GH] in a basal sample is often unhelpful as undetectable GH is a common finding in normal individuals.

Interpreting basal hormone measurements
• Pituitary function can be assumed to be normal if the patient is of normal stature, there is no other clinical evidence of pituitary disease, the thyroid and gonadal axes and osmolalities are normal and plasma [cortisol] is greater than 400 nmol/L.
• If plasma [cortisol] at 9 am is below 100 nmol/L then adrenocortical deficiency is highly likely. If plasma [cortisol] is 100–400 nmol/L, then a Synacthen test should be carried out (p. 143) followed by an insulin stress test if the result is equivocal.
• The plasma [FT4] is low in all cases of secondary hypothyroidism but [TSH] is low in only approximately half of such patients; in the remainder [TSH] lies within reference limits or occasionally is slightly increased (p. 127).

• In the male, an early morning [total testosterone] of more than 14 nmol/L and a normal LH/FSH signifies adequate function of the pituitary–gonadal axis. If the patient has no other severe illness, gonadotrophin deficiency is diagnosed by a low [total testosterone] with low or inappropriately normal gonadotrophins. Many elderly males have a low-normal [total testosterone] with normal [LH] and [FSH], and it is still being debated if such patients have gonadal deficiency (p. 156).
• In the female, interpretation is complicated by the physiological changes that occur in LH/FSH and oestradiol during the normal menstrual cycle. Gonadotrophin deficiency is suggested by a persistently low level of gonadotrophins and oestradiol; however, oral contraceptives, stress and low BMI may also lead to suppression of these hormones (p. 161). The menopausal status of the women also needs to be considered. After the menopause most women will show a significant elevation in [LH] and [FSH], and an absence of such a response would indicate gonadotrophin deficiency.
• A [prolactin] which is persistently above 700 mU/L is suggestive of a pituitary tumour if other causes of a raised prolactin such as, drugs, renal failure, pregnancy etc (Table 7.2) can be excluded.

Further investigations

If there is strong clinical evidence for pituitary disease or there are basal deficiencies, an insulin stress test is often performed to assess ACTH and GH reserve. If thyroid and ACTH deficiencies have been identified on the basal sample, these should be treated with thyroxine and hydrocortisone, respectively, before any further investigation. Hypothyroidism reduces the ACTH and GH responses to an insulin stress test. If the insulin stress tests is contraindicated (e.g. cardiac disease and epilepsy) a Synacthen test and a glucagon stimulation test (1 mg IM) may be carried out. If the patient has acromegaly (where GH deficiency is not a consideration), a Synacthen test alone will often suffice (p. 143). A fluid deprivation test should be performed if symptoms or basal osmolalities suggest it is required.

Table 7.4 Hormone replacement in hypopituitarism

Pituitary deficiency	Replacement hormone
ACTH	Hydrocortisone
TSH	Thyroxine
LH/FSH male	Testosterone
LH/FSH female	Oestrogen
GH	GH
ADH	DDAVP
Prolactin	None required

Treatment

Hypopituitarism is treated by giving the appropriate hormone replacement (Table 7.4). Transspenoidal surgery is the usual first-line treatment for most pituitary adenomas although for prolactinoma, medical therapy with dopamine agonists is capable of successfully shrinking the tumour in more than 85% of cases.

Dynamic function tests

Insulin stress test

The insulin stress test was the traditional test for the assessment of GH reserve, as well as for the HPA axis. It is still used by some for the investigation of suspected hypopituitarism in adults and children. The test is contraindicated in patients with epilepsy or heart disease, untreated hypothyroidism or patients with a basal cortisol of less than 50 nmol/L.

Insulin is administered IV (typically 0.15 U/kg) to lower blood glucose to 2.2 mmol/L or less while monitoring serum cortisol and growth hormone. Samples for [glucose], [GH] and [cortisol] are taken basally (before insulin) and at 30, 45, 60 and 90 min after IV insulin injection. The test requires close supervision, with glucose available for immediate IV administration if symptoms of severe hypoglycaemia develop. Failure to achieve a glucose of 2.2 mmol/L invalidates the test, and repetition, with insulin incremented in steps of 0.05 U/kg, may be necessary.

Interpretation of results

Blood [glucose] must fall below 2.2 mmol/L and symptoms of hypoglycaemia must be present (i.e. sweating tachycardia, etc.). Serum [cortisol] normally reaches its maximum at 60 or 90 min, the level reached being at least 520 nmol/L, and serum [GH] exceeds 6 µg/L (20 mU/L). Patients with Cushing's syndrome, whatever the cause, do not respond normally to insulin-induced hypoglycaemia. There is often a high basal serum [cortisol] and usually little or no increase in serum [cortisol], despite the production of an adequate degree of hypoglycaemia.

In an attempt to avoid insulin stress tests, a number of other physiological and pharmacological tests of GH and ACTH secretion are used, especially in children. These include measurements of GH during the hours of sleep, or the response to standardised exercise or to administration of glucagon, clonidine or arginine. All these tests are associated with rather variable responses, and their choice depends on local preferences.

Acromegaly and gigantism

These disorders are usually caused by adenomas of the anterior pituitary and occasionally by ectopic secretion of GHRH. Gigantism results if the disorder occurs before closure of the epiphyses of the long bones, acromegaly if it occurs after their closure. Acromegaly has an insidious onset such that there is a mean delay of about 7 years prior to its diagnosis and in many cases the diagnosis is overlooked. Treatment aims to prevent the expanding tumour causing damage to the pituitary and optic nerves. Surgery is the usual first-line therapy but if this is unsuccessful, radiotherapy or medical intervention with somatostatin analogues (octreotide or lanreotide) or dopamine agonists are used. The GH antagonist pegvisomant appears to be very effective for treating the disease but requires daily injections and is very expensive.

Diagnosis

Diagnosis requires the measurement of [GH] and [IGF-1]. Random basal plasma [GH] is often very high in these patients, but the concentrations are too variable for accurate diagnosis and overlap with the range of [GH] found in some 'normal' individuals. However, a random GH of less than 0.5 μg/L essentially excludes a diagnosis of acromegaly *if* [IGF-1] is within the reference range, whilst an elevated [IGF-1] should prompt further investigation with a glucose tolerance tests (see below). Reference ranges for [IGF-1] are age and method specific and the local laboratory should provide these

Glucose tolerance test

The response of plasma [GH] to a glucose tolerance test remains the 'gold standard' for the diagnosis of acromegaly. The patient is fasted overnight and an IV cannula is inserted. Blood samples are taken at −30, 0, 30, 60, 90 and 120 min, with glucose being given (75 g of glucose in 100 mL of water) at time 0 min. Normally, plasma [GH] falls to less than 0.5 μg/L at some time during this test. However, in patients with acromegaly or gigantism, plasma [GH] does not fall in response to the stimulus of hyperglycaemia, and may even increase in about 30% of patients. The test is not specific for acromegaly and GH may fail to suppress in some patients who have poorly controlled diabetes mellitus, renal failure, anorexia or liver disease. In treated acromegalics, a GH of less than 0.5 μg/L is indicative of cure while a GH of less than 1.5 μg/L indicates satisfactory control. Measurement of [IGF-1] in the basal sample should also be carried out.

Hyperprolactinaemia and pituitary tumours

In females hyperprolactinaemia causes ammenhorea or oligomenorrhea, galactorrhoea, low libido and infertility. In males low libido and erectile dysfunction are the usual early symptoms. Serum [prolactin] greater than 700 mU/L (reference range 60–500 mU/L) may indicate the presence of a pituitary tumour. There are many causes of hyperprolactinaemia including pregnancy, lactation, pituitary tumours, renal failure and the use of drugs that have dopamine agonist effects (Table 7.2). The differential diagnosis of hyperprolactinaemia requires a careful and accurate history and, where possible, drug therapy to be discontinued. Drug withdrawal may be possible if the drug is an anti-emetic or tranquilliser. It may be impossible to withdraw anti-psychotic medication, although a change to an anti-psychotic with a less profound effect on prolactin may be possible (e.g. olanzapine). The measurement should be repeated on a number of occasions to confirm that the raised level is persistent, since there is some evidence that a high result may represent a response to stress.

Pituitary tumours may secrete prolactin directly (prolactinoma) or, alternatively, a non-prolactin-secreting tumour may give rise to hyperprolactinaemia because the tumour exerts pressure on the pituitary stalk and prevents dopamine from reaching the pituitary from the hypothalamus. Prolactin is the only hormone secreted by prolactinomas, although increased [prolactin] also occurs in some patients with acromegaly, when there is a tumour that secretes both GH and prolactin. Approximately one-third of prolactinomas are associated with only moderate increases in [prolactin], in the range 700–1000 mU/L, but, if other causes are excluded, persistent basal levels of [prolactin] greater than 1000 mU/L strongly suggest that a tumour is present. If, in addition, radiological abnormalities are visible in the pituitary fossa, this supports the diagnosis of prolactinoma rather than functional hyperprolactinaemia in these patients. Some rare ectopic hormone-secreting tumours produce prolactin.

Monitoring treatment in hypopituitarism

Following surgery or after pituitary irradiation for the treatment of a pituitary adenoma the residual pituitary function should be carefully monitored.

After surgery, transient diabetes insipidus is common. Glucocorticoid replacement is often given in the immediate post-operative period, but after 1 week the evening dose of hydrocortisone should be ommited and the morning 9 am plasma [cortisol] assessed. If the 9 am [cortisol] is less than 400 nmol/L therapy needs to be continued and further assessments carried out at a later period. If cortisol is more than 400 nmol/L, hydrocortisone therapy can be discontimued and further assessments made at follow-up. A Synacthen test can give misleading results until at least 2 weeks post-operatively. Basal [FT4], [TSH], [LH], [FSH] and [oestradiol] in females or [testosterone] in males should also be assessed 1 week post-surgery and again after after 1 month. Abnormalities in gonadotrophins and oestradiol may persist in females for 2–3 months after surgery.

After pituitary irradiation a slow decline in pituitary function may continue for many years, and long-term follow-up and monitoring is required.

Monitoring hormone replacement therapy

T4 should be given to achieve a plasma [FT4] in the upper third of the reference range. There is variability in practice with regards to monitoring hydrocortisone replacement, and random measurements of [cortisol] are of little value. Some assess serum [cortisol] throughout the day after each dose of hydrocortiosone is given, whilst others assess the urinary free cortisol profile. If testosterone replacement is required, monitoring depends on the mode of replacement therapy given. Plasma [total testosterone] should be measured a few days after an injection of testosterone ester depot followed by a repeat taken immediately before the next dose. If transdermal therapy is given, a similar protocol can be followed. For patients receiving oral testosterone undecanoate, serum [testosterone] can be misleading as low levels can be found when replacement is adequate; this is because of conversion of testosterone to dihydrotestosterone. Oestrogen replacement is difficult to assess biochemically since most hormone replacement pharmaceuticals for oestrogen contain synthetic or equine oestrogens that are not detected by the usual assays for oestradiol.

Endocrine changes in anorexia nervosa

Anorexia nervosa results in a number of abnormal endocrine findings that are reversed once normal eating patterns and normal weight have been restored. Many of these changes arise from altered hypothalamic responses. The secretion of GnRH is often impaired in women whose BMI falls below 20 kg/m², resulting in low serum levels of LH, FSH and oestradiol. The [FT4] often falls to low or low normal values, while [FT3] is nearly always subnormal. TSH concentrations and [prolactin] are usually normal but the TSH response to an injection of TRH (TRH test) is often delayed. Serum [cortisol] is usually raised as a consequence of both increased production and an increased half-life, and the usual diurnal variation is lost. GH levels are also often increased as a consequence of the starvation.

Posterior pituitary hormones

The posterior pituitary is an integral part of the neurohypophysis. It produces at least two hormones: arginine vasopressin (previously known as antidiuretic hormone (ADH)) and oxytocin. Both these hormones are synthesised in the hypothalamus as larger pro-hormones that are stored in neurosecretory granules. These granules migrate by axonal flow to the nerve terminals in the posterior pituitary from where they can be released into the circulation. During this migration the pro-hormones are cleaved to produce vasopressin and oxytocin together with neurophysin I and II. Uterine contraction and milk release from the lactating breast is controlled by oxytocin. Disorders of oxytocin secretion are uncommon and are not clinically important.

Vasopressin

Vasopressin is a nonapeptide that has an important role in the control of the tonicity of the ECF and hence water balance. It increases the water permeability of the distal tubules and collecting ducts of the kidney. The major stimulus to vasopressin release is a rise in plasma osmolality sensed by the osmoreceptors. A fall in ECF volume and blood pressure (sensed by baroreceptors) or stress can also trigger vasopressin release.

SIADH is defined as the excessive secretion of vasopressin in the absence of the normal major stimuli for vasopressin secretion. SIADH is considered in more detail on p. 22.

Diabetes insipidus

Deficiency of vasopressin gives rise to cranial diabetes insipidus. It is either primary (idio-pathic, familial) or secondary to disease or injury in or close to the pituitary. Deficiency of vaso-pressin may be the sole hormonal abnormality, or there may also be disturbances of anterior pituitary hormone production in patients with secondary vasopressin deficiency. Recognition of hyposecretion of vasopressin depends on mea-surement of urine and plasma osmolalities and the performance of urine concentration tests (p. 57).

Keypoints

- Pituitary function may initially be assessed by measuring basal cortisol, FT4, TSH, testosterone, oestradiol, LH, FSH and prolactin in serum or plasma. If these are all unequivocally normal, no further tests are usually needed, but if clinical suspicion is high or one or more abnormal results are found, stimulation tests may be necessary, for example the Synac-then test or insulin stress test.
- Posterior pituitary dysfunction should be investigated initially by measuring basal serum and urine osmolalities. A water deprivation test may be needed subsequently.
- In children with short stature, the insulin stress test should only be performed by experienced staff. A number of other tests of GH secretion can be used instead, including measurements of GH during sleep or in response to exercise, or to administration of glucagon, clonidine or arginine.
- In acromegaly, basal [GH] is often very high but the concentrations are too variable for accurate diagnosis. The failure of plasma [GH] to fall to less than $0.5\,\mu g/L$ in an OGTT is a more reliable test.
- Prolactin measurements help in the diagnosis of amenorrhoea, oligomenorrhoea and subfertility, and in spontaneous inappropriate lactation.
- A [prolactin] greater than $700\,mU/L$ may indicate the presence of a pituitary tumour, but it could also be due to stress, drugs or other causes.

Case 7.1

A 56-year-old bank manager complained to his GP of excessive sweating which was embarrassing him during meetings with clients. His GP had known him over many years, although he had not seen him recently, and thought that his facial features had become coarser over this period. Closer questioning revealed that he recently had to buy new shoes since his old ones were becoming tight, and that he had experienced problems with impotence over the past few months. Examination revealed hypertension and glucosuria. He was referred to an endocrine clinic with a presumptive diagnosis of acromegaly. Basal investigations on a sample taken at 9 am were as follows:

(continued on p. 115)

Case 7.1 (continued)

Serum	Result	Reference range
Cortisol	625	160–565 nmol/L
FT4	18	9–21 pmol/L
TSH	1.3	0.2–4.5 mU/L
Testosterone	7	10–30 nmol/L
LH	1.1	1.5–9.0 U/L
FSH	1.4	1.5–9.0 U/L
Prolactin	960	<500 mU/L

A GTT was performed:

Time (min)	Glucose (mmol/L)	GH (µg/L)
0	9.2	8.4
30	15.8	7.3
60	14.1	6.7
90	13.6	7.3
120	13.5	7.5

Visual fields were normal, and a magnetic resonance imaging (MRI) scan revealed the appearance of a small adenoma, confined within the pituitary gland.

Comments: The strong clinical suspicion of acromegaly is confirmed by the lack of suppression of GH during the GTT. The GTT also confirms the patient to have diabetes, due to the diabetogenic actions of GH. Abnormal glucose tolerance is seen in about a quarter of patients with acromegaly, IGT being slightly more common among these than frank diabetes.

Gonadotrophins and testosterone are low, confirming gonadal failure secondary to the pituitary lesion, rather than primary testicular failure.

The prolactin is elevated. Some GH-secreting adenomas also secrete prolactin. Alternatively, the adenoma may be interfering with the inhibitory control of prolactin secretion by dopamine.

The basal results suggest that the function of the adrenal and thyroid axes is normal.

Case 7.2

A 26-year-old woman attended an outpatient clinic with a complaint of galactorrhoea for several months. Her only other medical history was of troublesome migraines since childhood, for which she had taken a variety of medications whose names she could not remember. On examination, it was possible to express milk from her breasts.

Investigations were unremarkable apart from: prolactin 1127 mU/L (reference range <500 mU/L). What might be the cause of the galactorrhoea in this patient?

Comments: Closer questioning revealed that her migraine treatment had been changed some months previously to a preparation that combined an analgesic (paracetamol) and anti-emetic (metoclopramide). Metoclopramide can cause hyperprolactinaemia through its anti-dopaminergic activity.

The patient stopped this preparation, and took paracetamol alone. The galactorrhoea and hyperprolactinaemia resolved.

Case 7.3

A 58-year-old man saw his GP for review of his hypertension. He mentioned problems with impotence and decreased libido, which he ascribed to his anti-hypertensive medication (a β-blocker), having read the package insert containing information for patients. However, further questioning revealed that the patient was now shaving only once a week. Examination revealed pallor and loss of axillary and pubic hair. The results of baseline blood tests were as follows:

Serum	Result	Reference range
Cortisol	90	160–565 nmol/L
TSH	0.3	0.2–4.5 mU/L
FT4	8	9–21 pmol/L
Testosterone	4	10–30 nmol/L
LH	1.0	1.5–9.0 U/L
FSH	0.9	1.5–9.0 U/L
Prolactin	40	<500 mU/L

What do these results show? What further investigations are required?

Comments: The history, physical signs and hypofunction of multiple endocrine glands suggest hypopituitarism. In the presence of the other biochemical findings and the pallor, primary adrenal failure is unlikely to be the cause of the low plasma [cortisol]. This is due to ACTH deficiency. The thyroid function tests show insufficiency secondary to pituitary insufficiency, and the low gonadotrophins and testosterone confirm secondary gonadal failure.

The biochemical results are sufficiently informative, and further biochemical investigation are not needed, although plasma [ACTH] or a Synacthen test could be used to confirm ACTH deficiency. Radiological investigation of the pituitary using computed tomography (CT) or MRI scanning is indicated. The patient can be treated with cortisol and, in due course, thyroxine and testosterone. Although there is nothing in the history to suggest posterior pituitary insufficiency (diabetes insipidus), this may be unmasked by cortisol treatment. The patient may need investigation using a water deprivation test.

Case 7.4

A 20-year-old woman presented to her GP 9 months postpartum with persistent galactorrhoea despite never having breastfed. She also complained of agitation palpitations and weight loss. The following results were found in a random sample and confirmed in a second specimen taken 7 days later:

Serum	Result	Reference range
Cortisol	450	160–565 nmol/L
FT4	30	9–21 pmol/L
FT3	9.5	2.6–6.2 pmol/L
TSH	6.0	0.2–4.5 mU/L
LH	1.1	1.5–9.0 U/L
FSH	1.4	1.5–9.0 U/L
Prolactin	850	<500 mU/L
GH	<0.5	

There was no change in serum TSH 20 and 60 min after the injection of TRH (a TRH test).

Comment on these results.

(continued on p. 117)

Case 7.4 (continued)

Comments: The results are consistent with hyperthyroidism caused by a TSH secreting pituitary tumour (TSHoma) and hyperprolactinaemia due to hypothalamic disconnection causing loss of inhibitory dopamine reaching the pituitary. In end-organ resistance, the TSH response to TRH is normal or exaggerated while a flat or blunted response is seen in TSHoma. An MRI scan showed a 25 mm diameter mass arising in the pituitary fossa. The patient was treated by trans-phenoidal surgery to remove the tumour and post-operative pituitary radiotherapy was given. This rendered the patient euthyroid with normal prolactin and a resolution of her galactorrhoea. Histopathology of the resected tumour showed pituitary tumour cells that stained positive for TSH, prolactin and α-subunit but not for gonadotrophins or ACTH. TSHoma is rare with an incidence of 2 per 10^7, with most patients presenting with thyrotoxicosis and hyperprolactinaemia.

Chapter 8

Abnormalities of thyroid function

Thyroid hormones are essential for normal growth, development and metabolism, and their production is tightly regulated through the hypothalamic–pituitary–thyroid axis.

Thyroid disease is common, particularly in women, and the prevalence rises with age such that 10% of the population over 65 years of age may have some abnormality in thyroid function. Although primary diseases of the thyroid gland are the most common, pituitary disease and the use of certain drugs can also give rise to thyroid dysfunction. Once diagnosed, thyroid disease is easily treated, with an excellent long-term outcome for most patients.

This chapter outlines the pathways of thyroid hormone synthesis and metabolism. The tests used in diagnosis and management of thyroid disease are described, together with guidance on their interpretation.

Thyroid hormone synthesis, action and metabolism

Synthesis and metabolism

Thyroxine (T4) and small amounts of tri-iodothyronine (T3) and reverse T3 (rT3) are all synthesised in the thyroid gland (Figure 8.1) by a process involving:

- Trapping of iodide from plasma by a sodium iodine symporter in the thyroid.
- Oxidation of iodide to iodine by thyroid peroxidase.
- Incorporation of iodine into tyrosyl residues on thyroglobulin in the colloid of the thyroid follicle. Mono-iodotyrosine (MIT) and di-iodotyrosine (DIT) are formed.
- Production of T3 and T4 by coupling iodotyrosyl residues in the thyroglobulin molecule.
- Splitting off of T4 and T3 from thyroglobulin following its reabsorption from the colloid.
- Release of T4 and T3 into the circulation.

These stages are shown diagrammatically in Figure 8.2.

Thyroxine, a pro-hormone, is produced exclusively by the thyroid. The *biologically active hormone is T3*, and about 85% of plasma T3 is formed by outer-ring (5′) mono-deiodination of T4 in liver, kidneys and muscle (Figure 8.3). Thyroxine also undergoes inner-ring (5) mono-deiodination in non-thyroidal tissues, with the production of metabolically inactive rT3.

Plasma transport and cellular action

Thyroid hormones are transported in plasma almost entirely bound, reversibly, to plasma pro-

Lecture Notes: Clinical Biochemistry, 8e. By G. Beckett, S. Walker, P. Rae & P. Ashby. Published 2010 by Blackwell Publishing.

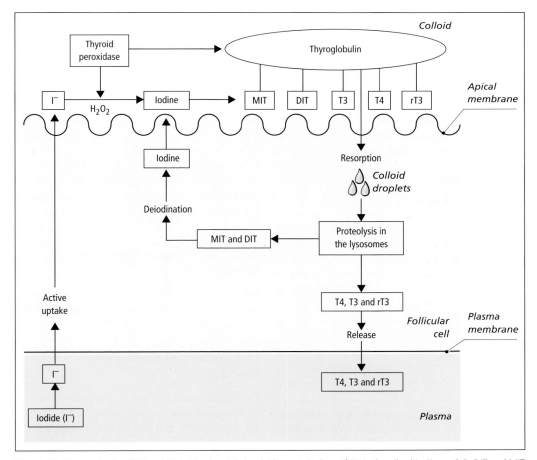

Figure 8.1 The structure of the thyroid hormones T4, T3 and reverse T3.

Figure 8.2 The synthesis of T3 and T4 in the thyroid gland. The metabolism of T4 is described in Figure 8.3. DIT and MIT are hormonally inactive.

teins. Thyroxine-binding globulin (TBG) is the major binding protein, binding about 70% of plasma T4 and 80% of plasma T3. Transthyretin (also called thyroxine-binding pre-albumin) and albumin also bind thyroid hormone such that more than 99.8% of thyroid hormones circulate bound to these three proteins.

Approximately 0.05% of plasma T4 and 0.2% of plasma T3 are free (i.e. unbound to protein). Only the free fractions can cross the cell membrane and affect intracellular metabolism. After binding to high-affinity binding sites on the plasma membrane, the hormones are actively transported into cells by specific energy-dependent transporters. In the cell T4 is metabolised to T3 which then binds to specific nuclear receptors that in turn activate T3-responsive genes. These gene products modify a wide range of cell function including basal metabolic rate and the metabolism of lipids, carbohydrates and proteins. High concentrations of thyroid hormone increase the basal metabolic rate and stimulate breakdown of protein and lipids. Low concentrations of thyroid hormone result in low metabolic rate, weight gain and poor physical and mental development in the child.

Regulation of thyroid function

The most important regulator of thyroid homeostasis is TSH (or thyrotrophin; Figure 8.3). The production of TSH is controlled by a stimulatory effect of the hypothalamic tripeptide, TRH (or thyroliberin), mediated by a negative feedback from circulating FT3 and FT4. It is thought that the hypothalamus, via TRH, sets the level of thyroid hormone production required physiologically, and that the pituitary acts as a 'thyroid-stat' to maintain the level of thyroid hormone production that has been determined by the hypothalamus.

Dopamine, somatostatin and glucocorticoids also appear to be involved in inhibiting the release of TSH, and these agents together with the interleukins may be important modifiers of TSH release in non-thyroidal illness (NTI).

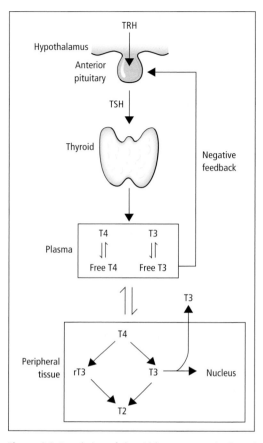

Figure 8.3 Regulation of thyroid hormone synthesis and metabolism.

Investigations to determine thyroid status

Measurement of TSH and thyroid hormones should be performed to determine the patient's thyroid status.

Thyrotrophin (reference range 0.5–4.5 mU/L)

The measurement of [TSH] in a basal blood sample by immunometric assay provides the single most sensitive, specific and reliable test of thyroid status in both overt and subclinical thyroid disease. In primary hypothyroidism, [TSH] is increased, while in primary hyperthyroidism, [TSH] is below

0.01 mU/L. There are exceptions to this, and both raised and undetectable [TSH] may be found in some euthyroid patients (Table 8.1).

Free T4 (reference range 10–21 pmol/L); free T3 (reference range 2.6–6.2 pmol/L)

Free thyroid hormone concentrations are independent of changes in the concentration and affinity of thyroid hormone-binding proteins and theoretically provide a more reliable means of diagnosing thyroid dysfunction than measurement of total hormone concentrations. Several assay techniques have been developed to measure free hormone concentrations. These methods produce results that show good agreement in most ambulant patients; however, in patients with NTI, results may not always correlate well with one another due to various assay artefacts.

Total T4 (reference range 70–150 nmol/L); total T3 (reference range 1.2–2.8 nmol/L)

Since more than 99% of T4 and T3 circulate in plasma bound to protein, any change in the concentration of these binding proteins, particularly [TBG], will be reflected in the concentrations of total T4 and total T3. However, [FT4] and [FT3] remain normal if pituitary–thyroid homeostasis is maintained. In practice [FT4] and [FT3] are more widely used than [total T4] and [total T3].

Selective use of thyroid function tests

Many laboratories measure basal [TSH] as the initial test of thyroid function. This strategy is not infallible, but it will detect both overt and subclinical primary thyroid disease. A normal [TSH] virtually excludes primary thyroid dysfunction. If an abnormal result is obtained, thyroid hormone measurements must be made to confirm that thyroid dysfunction is present, and to determine the severity of the disease.

Initial measurement of both TSH and FT4 together provides a more satisfactory method of assessing thyroid status, since in some situations a single TSH result may be misleading (Tables 8.1 and 8.2). If this strategy is followed, a significant number of cases will arise in which one test will be abnormal while the complementary test will be normal. It is thus essential to understand and appreciate the factors that can affect the results of thyroid function tests.

Table 8.1 Causes of an abnormal plasma [TSH] in some clinically euthyroid patients

Undetectable plasma [TSH]	Increased plasma [TSH]
Pregnancy, during the first 20 weeks	Subclinical hypothyroidism
Treated hyperthyroid patients – first 6 months	During recovery stage of NTI[1]
Ophthalmic Graves disease	
Various kinds of NTI*	
Non-toxic multinodular goitre	
Treatment with dopaminergic drugs	
Treatment with high-dose glucocorticoids	

The thyroid status of patients with subclinical hypothyroidism and need for treatment is controversial.

* NTI = non-thyroidal illness; discussed on p. 125.

Table 8.2 Situations in which first-line TSH is not ideal since it may give misleading results in some patients

First-line TSH not ideal	First-line TSH acceptable
Symptomatic patients – first presentation	Monitoring patients stabilised on thyroxine
Optimising treatment of hypothyroidism and hyperthyroidism – early months	Screening asymptomatic 'at risk' groups
Screening and monitoring in pregnancy	
Diagnosis and monitoring hypopituitarism	
Diagnosis of TSH secreting tumour and end organ resistance (rare)	

Screening and surveillance

Screening in the healthy asymptomatic population is not warranted. Thyroid function tests should be done however on:
- the elderly patient
- women who present to their primary care physician at the menopause
- patients presenting with diabetes or an autoimmune disorder
- any patient with features of a thyroid disorder.

Table 8.3 Suggested screening protocols for patients at high risk of thyroid dysfunction

Annual check
Patients with autoimmune disease
Turner's and Down's syndrome
Post-neck irradiation
Type 2 diabetes
6-monthly check
Amiodarone or lithium
At presentation
At menopause if vague symptoms
Elderly with vague symptoms

Patients with a *high risk of developing a thyroid disorder* should also be monitored annually using serum [TSH]. Such patients include type 1 and type 2 diabetes, Down's and Turner's syndrome, and post-neck irradiation. Patients taking lithium or aminodarone should be assessed before commencing treatment and 6-monthly thereafter (Table 8.3).

Interpreting results of thyroid function tests

Figures 8.4 and 8.5 provides a guide to the interpretation of thyroid function tests.

Hyperthyroidism

Overt primary hyperthyroidism (FT4 and FT3 high; TSH low)

[TSH] is nearly always below 0.01 mU/L, due to feedback inhibition on the pituitary. Free and total T4 and T3 concentrations are nearly always increased in overt hyperthyroidism. In a very small percentage of hyperthyroid patients, [total T4] and [FT4] are both normal, whereas both [total T3] and

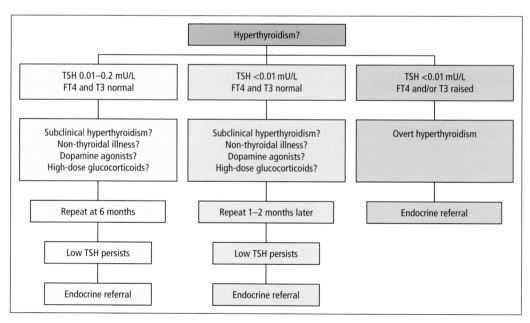

Figure 8.4 Interpretation of thyroid function tests in suspected hyperthyroidism.

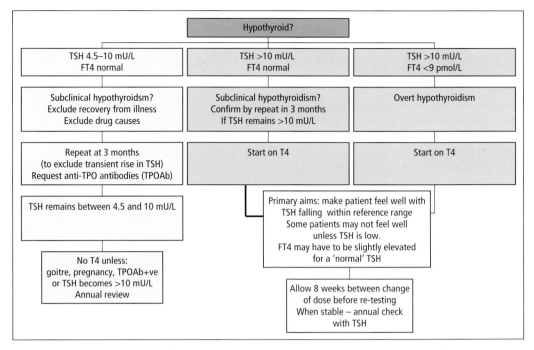

Figure 8.5 Interpretation of thyroid function tests in suspected hypothyroidism.

[FT3] are increased; this condition is known as T3 hyperthyroidism or T3 thyrotoxicosis.

Patients with a hormone profile suggestive of hyperthyroidism may get an isotope scan (technetium Tc-99m pertechnate) to identify the cause. A diffuse increased uptake of isotope is consistent with Graves disease, whilst the presence of 'hot nodules' with surrounding areas of reduced isotope uptake would be consistent with nodular hyperthyroidism. Poor uptake of isotope across the gland is consistent with thyroiditis.

Subclinical hyperthyroidism (FT4 and FT3 normal; TSH low)

Thyroid disease presents as a spectrum of clinical and biochemical features of varying severity. The clinical diagnosis of mild thyroid disorders is often difficult since the patient may have few if any clinical features and the only biochemical abnormality may be an abnormal plasma [TSH]. The combination of a persistent abnormality in [TSH], together with normal thyroid hormone concentrations, is known as 'subclinical thyroid disease'. This description is unsatisfactory, since it rests solely on the results of chemical investigations. Many clinically euthyroid patients with multinodular goitre or with exophthalmic Graves disease have 'subclinical hyperthyroidism', that is, [TSH] below 0.01 mU/L and [FT4] and [FT3] in the upper part of their respective reference ranges. Before assigning this diagnosis, however, other causes of a low TSH should be excluded, including NTI, pregnancy and drugs that suppress TSH (dopaminergic drugs, high dose glucocorticoids). The tests should be repeated 1–2 months later and if the abnormalities persist the patient should be referred to an endocrinologist to establish the diagnosis and give optimal treatment (Figure 8.4).

Management of hyperthyroidism

The therapeutic objective is to maintain [FT4] in the upper half of the reference range after treating with anti-thyroid drugs, radioiodine or subtotal thyroidectomy. Monitoring every 4–6 weeks for the first few months is required. Measurement of [TSH] is not a reliable guide of thyroid status during the first 4–6 months of treatment for hyperthyroidism, since [TSH] may still be suppressed even when plasma thyroid hormone concentrations have become abnormally low. [TSH] can be used to determine the adequacy of treatment after normal thyrotroph responsiveness has returned.

After radioactive iodine treatment, the likelihood that patients will eventually develop hypothyroidism is high. Annual follow-up of these patients is essential. Patients treated by subtotal thyroidectomy may have temporary disturbances of thyroid function tests in the early post-operative period but in the long-term are more likely to remain euthyroid than are patients treated with radioactive iodine. Annual follow-up is still required however.

Patients with subclinical hyperthyroidism who are not treated should be monitored every 6–12 months.

Hypothyroidism

Overt primary hypothyroidism (FT4 low; TSH high)

[TSH] is invariably increased, often to more than 20 mU/L, as feedback inhibition of the pituitary (Figure 8.3) is diminished. [FT4] and [total T4] are usually low. FT3 and total T3 measurements are of no value here, since normal concentrations are often observed.

Subclinical primary hypothyroidsm (FT4 normal; TSH high)

Many cases of subclinical hypothyroidism are transient. It is essential to confirm that abnormalities in TSH are persistent or progressive. Studies suggest that the average patient will not get any clinical benefit from T4 therapy until TSH rises above approximately 10 mU/L. If a profile consistent with subclinical hypothyroidism is found, the tests should be repeated at 3 months to

exclude a transient rise in TSH. Measurement of anti-thyroid peroxidase antibodies (TPOAbs) can help to determine if an autoimmune process is present and help predict risk of progression to overt hypothyroidism.

Management of overt and subclinical hypothyroidism

T4 therapy

The aim of thyroxine therapy is to make patients feel well and restore TSH and FT4 to within the reference range. In some patients FT4 may have to be above the reference range to achieve a 'normal' TSH. Some patients report they 'feel better' only when T4 is given at a dose that produces a low or undetectable TSH, but there have been some reports of decreased bone mineral density in post-menopausal women on T4 who have a TSH less than 0.1 mU/L. As a consequence many endocrinologists will attempt to fine-tune the T4 dose to allow the patient to feel well with a TSH that lies within the reference range.

The value of treating patients with subclinical hypothyroidism is controversial, but, in general, it is believed that only patients with a TSH greater than 10 mU/L will derive any benefit from therapy. If the TSH lies between 4.5 and 10 mU/L then T4 therapy is often withheld unless the patient has clear features of hypothyroidism; annual monitoring must be done and treatment initiated when TSH rises above 10 mU/L. Some endocrinologists may treat all patients with subclinical hypothyroidism who have positive anti-TPOAbs (Figure 8.5). This is because such patients have a high risk of developing overt disease and thus therapy is initiated with a view to preventing them developing debilitating symptoms.

Some over-the-counter medications can impair T4 absorption. These include calcium carbonate, soy protein, aluminium hydroxide and ferrous sulphate. Patients should be advised not to take T4 within 4 h of taking other medication.

The requirement for T4 is likely to increase in hypothyroid patients who become pregnant or who are commenced on proton pump inhibitors, H2 antagonists, anti-convulsants or oestrogen-containing oral contraceptives.

Following a change in the prescribed dose of thyroxine, it may be 6–8 weeks before the thyroid function tests again stabilise, and repeat testing within this time frame may produce misleading results. Some hypothyroid patients may not take their replacement thyroxine regularly, but may take some shortly before attending the follow-up clinic. Such poor compliance is indicated by finding that the [FT4] and [TSH] are both abnormally high.

T3 therapy is rarely required and there is no consistent evidence to recommend the use of combined therapy with T3 and T4. The aim of T3 therapy is to normalise TSH. Measurement of FT4 is of no value in assessing patients on T3. Serum T3 measurements are of limited value due to the variability of T3 concentrations in blood after a T3 dose.

Paediatrics and the neonate

Plasma TSH is widely used to screen for congenital hypothyroidism in the neonate. Marked changes in thyroid function occur in the early days of life, with an initial surge in TSH and thyroid hormone after delivery, followed by a marked decline in hormone levels over the next few days. Hormone levels then show a slow decline until adult values are reached at about the age of 10. It is essential to apply appropriate age-related reference ranges.

Pregnancy

Marked changes in thyroid hormone concentration and [TSH] occur throughout pregnancy, and it is essential to use trimester-related reference ranges. The diagnosis and management of thyroid disease in pregnancy is not straightforward, and close liaison between GP, endocrinologist, obstetrician and community midwife is essential. Thyroid disease and pregnancy is covered in Chapter 11.

Thyroid cancer

Patients with thyroid cancer (papillary and follicular) usually present with a thyroid swelling or nodule. A biopsy using a fine needle aspirate is required to make the diagnosis. Most patients are clinically euthyroid at presentation with normal [TSH], [FT4] and [FT3]. Treatment usually involves total thyroidectomy followed by an ablative dose of radioiodine to destroy any residual thyroid tissue and metastases. Lifelong therapy with sufficient thyroxine to suppress [TSH] to undetectable levels is required in order to prevent metastases from growing (see Chapter 16 p. 251).

Situations in which thyroid function test results may be misleading

Non-thyroidal illness and the sick euthyroid syndrome

Patients attending or admitted to a hospital suffering from any of a wide range of chronic or acute NTIs often have abnormalities in thyroid function tests. The abnormalities found depend on the severity of the illness (Figure 8.6). A low [T3] may often be found even though the patients are clinically euthyroid; this has been termed the *sick euthyroid syndrome*.

Several mechanisms are involved, including:
• Alterations in the hypothalamic–pituitary–thyroid axis, for example resulting from increased release of cytokines, dopamine, cortisol and somatostatin, which inhibit TSH release.

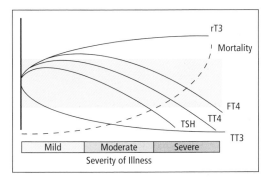

Figure 8.6 The effects of illness on the concentration of thyroid hormones and thyrotrophin. The profile for FT4 is that obtained with the reference method of equilibrium dialysis. The FT4 profile found using routine assays is method dependent. FT3 shows a similar profile to total T3. The shaded area represents the reference range.

- Changes in the affinity characteristics and in the plasma concentrations of the thyroid hormone-binding proteins. These changes give rise to alterations in the plasma concentrations of both the free and total thyroid hormones.
- Impaired uptake of thyroid hormones by the tissues.
- Decreased production of T3 in the peripheral tissues.
- Changes in the T3 occupancy and function of the T3 receptors.

The contribution of each of the above mechanisms may vary with the severity and stage of the illness, and thus the pattern of thyroid function tests may be extremely variable and may mimic the profile seen in primary or secondary thyroid disease. Interpretation of thyroid function tests is complicated further by the effects of drugs and methodological problems associated with free hormone measurements.

Although TSH is the most reliable test of the thyroid function, in hospitalised patients, it is worth remembering that in these patients:

- A low TSH is twice as likely to be due to NTI as to hyperthyroidism.
- An increased TSH is as likely to be due to recovery from illness as to hypothyroidism.
- Because of the poor predictive value of thyroid function tests in hospitalised patients, these tests should only be requested if the reason for hospital admission is considered on clinical grounds to be related to a thyroid problem.

Drug treatment

Drugs may interfere with TSH secretion or the production, secretion, transport and metabolism of thyroid hormones (Table 8.4). Some drugs modify thyroid status while others produce abnormal thyroid function test results in otherwise euthyroid subjects. Certain agents impair the absorption of thyroxine from the gut, and patients on thyroxine therapy should be advised to take their thyroxine at least 4h apart from these medications. Patients taking thyroxine are likely to require an increase in replacement dose if drugs such as phe-

Table 8.4 Examples of drugs that alter thyroid hormone synthesis, secretion and metabolism

Mechanism	Example of drug
Decrease in TSH secretion	Dopamine, glucocorticoids, octreotide, cytokines
Decrease in thyroid hormone secretion*	Lithium, amiodarone, iodide
Induce hyperthyroidism	Lithium, amiodarone, iodide
Decrease in thyroidal synthesis*	Carbimazole, methimazole, propylthiouracil, lithium
Increase in TBG	Oestrogens, tamoxifen, heroin, methadone,
Decrease in TBG	Androgens, glucocorticoids, anabolic steroids
Displacement of thyroid hormones from plasma proteins	Furosemide, fenclofenac, salicylates, NSAIDs, mefanamic acid, carbamazapine
Increased hepatic metabolism	Proton pump inhibitors, H2 antagonists, Phenytoin, carbamazepine, rifampacin, barbiturates
Impaired T4 and T3 conversion	β-Antagonists, amiodarone*, radiocontrast dyes, iopanoic acid
Impaired absorption of thyroxine[†]	Cholestyramine, aluminium hydroxide, ferrous sulphate, calcium, soya protein
Altered immunity[‡]	Interleukin-1, interferons, TNF-α
Modified thyroid hormone action	Amiodarone

* Cause a decrease in thyroid hormone synthesis or secretion and alter thyroid status.

† Interfere with absorption from the GI tract. Patients on T4 therapy should be advised to take their T4 at least 4h apart from these medications.

‡ These cytokines can cause transient hypothyroidism or thyrotoxcosis. The mechanism is unclear. Other drugs listed produce abnormal thyroid function tests but patients remain euthyroid. Amiodarone, lithium and iodine are exceptions (see text).

nytoin or carbamazepine, proton pump inhibitors or H2 antagonists are prescribed that increase hepatic metabolism of T4. Phenytoin, carbamazepine, furosemide and salicylate compete with thyroid hormone binding to serum-binding proteins and may increase [FT4]. However, it is important to note that the influence of drugs on modifying free thyroid hormone concentrations may be method specific. For example, depending on the method, [FT4] may be measured as normal, high or low in patients given heparin or taking phenytoin or carbamazepine.

Amiodarone, lithium and interferon can induce thyroid dysfunction. For example, the anti-arrhythmic drug amiodarone is an iodine-containing drug that has complex effects on thyroid metabolism. These include inhibition of T4 to T3 conversion, inhibition of thyroidal iodine uptake and inhibition of T4 entry into cells. The drug may also induce a destructive thyroiditis. Patients may have an altered thyroid hormone profile without thyroid dysfunction, but 14–18% of patients taking amiodarone may develop clinically significant hypothyroidism or amiodarone-induced thyrotoxicosis. It is important to evaluate patients before they commence therapy with amiodarone. This should include clinical examination and a basal measurement of TSH, FT4, FT3 and TPOAbs. After starting treatment, these tests should be repeated at 6 months and thereafter every 6 months including the year after the drug is stopped. Lithium can also cause hypothyroidism or less commonly hyperthyroidism. Patients taking lithium should have their thyroid function tests at 6–12-month intervals.

Secondary thyroid disorders

[TSH] is normal in about half of patients with central (pituitary) hypothyroidism, but [FT4] and [total T4] are usually low. Circulating TSH has been shown to have reduced bioactivity in hypopituitarism. It should be stressed that the most common cause of a normal [TSH] with low [FT4] and [FT3] is NTI, but it is essential to consider hypopituitarism in all patients with this combination of results. In patients with *secondary hypothyroidism*, the objective of replacement therapy is to maintain [FT4] in the upper third of the reference range.

Very rarely is hyperthyroidism due to a TSH-secreting tumour. Persistent hyperthyroid symptoms associated with elevated [FT4] and [FT3] and raised or normal TSH is consistent with this diagnosis, once the common problems of assay interference or NTI have been eliminated. The concentration of the α-subunit in the circulation is often increased in these patients.

Abnormal pituitary T3 receptor function is another rare cause of hyperthyroidism. In this disorder, the thyrotroph is resistant to the normal negative feedback regulation, so that plasma thyroid hormone levels are raised, and there are hyperthyroid symptoms and a normal or raised [TSH]. This is termed 'end-organ resistance'.

Assay interference from endogenous heterophilic antibodies

Some individuals have antibodies in their plasma that react with a range of animal immunoglobulins (heterophilic antibodies). These antibodies interfere with a wide range of immunoassays that are used to measure hormones. For example, a normal or elevated TSH result may be found in some thyrotoxic patients due to this type of assay interference.

Causes of abnormal results for thyroid hormone measurements in euthyroid subjects

1 *Abnormal plasma TBG concentrations* occur frequently, leading to parallel changes in total thyroid hormone concentrations. The affinity and binding capacity of TBG for thyroid hormones may be diminished by NTI and by drugs (e.g. salicylates), leading in turn to decreases in [total T3] and [total T4]. Thyroid hormone concentrations may be increased in pregnancy or by oestrogen-containing medication that increases [TBG]. Genetic causes of low and high [TBG] also exist.

Free hormone concentrations are unrelated to changes in the concentration of these proteins, but, in practice, some methods for free hormone measurement are unreliable and produce results that are influenced by changes in the concentration and binding capacity of albumin.

2 *Genetic variants of both albumin and pre-albumin* have been described which have a high affinity for T4. These variants give rise to increased [total T4] but other tests are usually normal and the patient is clinically euthyroid.

3 *Endogenous antibodies to thyroid hormone* may occur in a few patients with autoimmune thyroid disease. These antibodies interfere with many of the assay methods for both free and total thyroid hormones and produce apparently elevated results. Plasma TSH measurements provide the most reliable indications of thyroid status in these patients, as they are not affected by these antibodies.

Miscellaneous chemical tests and thyroid disease

TRH test

The only indication for the TRH test is in distinguishing secondary hyperthyroidism (due to a TSH-secreting tumour) from end-organ resistance to the action of thyroid hormones (due to a nuclear T3 receptor defect). Both of these conditions cause increased thyroid hormones with a slightly raised (or inappropriately normal) plasma [TSH], and the patients may appear clinically hyperthyroid.

In normal subjects, after IV TRH, serum [TSH] increases by more than 2 mU/L above the basal level at 20 min and returns towards the basal value at 60 min. Patients with T3 receptor defects also show a TSH response in a TRH test, but the TSH response is absent in patients with TSH-secreting tumours. Also, serum [α-subunit] of TSH are increased, often markedly, in patients with thyrotroph adenomas, whereas normal concentrations are present in patients with T3 receptor defects. There is no increase in the [TSH] response to TRH in patients with primary hyperthyroid-

ism, and an absent response may also occur in hypopituitarism. In hypothyroidism, the response is exaggerated.

Anti-thyroid peroxidase antibodies (TPOAbs)

These are present in the serum of patients with a wide range of immunologically mediated thyroid disorders (e.g. Hashimoto's thyroiditis, Graves' disease). They may also be found in a small proportion of apparently healthy individuals, but the appearance of TPOAbs often precedes the development of overt thyroid disorders. The measurement of TPOAbs is of clinical use (1) in the diagnosis of autoimmune thyroid disorders and (2) as a risk factor for thyroid dysfunction during treatment with interferon, interleukin-2, lithium or amiodarone.

The highest titres of these antibodies are found in the serum of patients with Hashimoto thyroiditis but are present only in 90% of these patients.

Thyrotrophin receptor antibodies (TRAbs)

'Thyroid-stimulating immunoglobulins' (TSIs) are IgG antibodies directed against the TSH receptors in the thyroid, and are involved in the pathogenesis of Graves' disease by promoting hormone synthesis and thyroid hypertrophy. TSIs can only be measured using a bioassay that monitors the release of cyclic AMP from cultured thyrocytes. For routine use, TRAbs are measured by assessing the ability of a patient's serum to inhibit the binding of labelled TSH to a dispersion of TSH receptors. It should be recognised that some TRAbs do not stimulate thyroid hormone production but rather they block the action of the TSH receptor; thus TRAb and TSI assays are not strictly comparable.

TRAb measurements are of value in:
• Predicting relapse, in patients who are to have their anti-thyroid medication withdrawn. If TRAbs are still strongly positive, then the patient has a high risk of immediate relapse.

- Predicting neonatal hyperthyroidism in babies born to mothers with high TRAbs after 20 weeks of pregnancy (TRAbs cross the placenta and stimulate the foetal thyroid).
- Distinguishing between postpartum thyroiditis and Graves disease. Undetectable TRAbs are found in thyroiditis, while TRAbs are positive in 97% of patients with Graves disease.
- Investigation of suspected euthyroid Graves ophthalmopathy.

Tests affected by thyroid dysfunction

Several other chemical tests may be affected by changes in thyroid status.

Hyperthyroidism

- GTTs may show a diabetic type of response.
- Plasma cholesterol may be low.
- Liver function tests may be abnormal.
- Plasma calcium and ALP may be increased.
- Sex hormone-binding globulin (SHBG) may be increased.

Hypothyroidism

- Hyponatraemia.
- Hypercholesterolaemia.
- Hyperprolactinaemia.
- SHBG may be decreased.
- Creatine kinase may increase.

Keypoints

- Serum [TSH] is usually the single best test for assessing thyroid status. Plasma [TSH] is elevated in primary hypothyroidism and suppressed to <0.01 mU/L in primary hyperthyroidism. A normal plasma [TSH] usually excludes a primary thyroid disorder.
- Serum [FT4] can help assess the severity of thyroid disease and distinguish subclinical (normal thyroid hormone concentrations) from overt (abnormal thyroid hormone levels) disease.
- Serum [FT3] can help determine the severity of hyperthyroidism and identify patients with T3 hyperthyroidism.
- Free thyroid hormone measurements correlate more closely with thyroid status than total hormone measurements, the latter being heavily influenced by changes in the concentration of thyroid hormone-binding proteins.
- Thyroid function tests are often abnormal in patients with NTI, and should not be requested in hospitalised patients unless the presenting complaint might be due to thyroid disease.
- In certain situations (NTI, secondary thyroid disease, early treatment of hyperthyroidism and early pregnancy), TSH results may be misleading.
- Screening for thyroid disease is warranted in the elderly, women at menopause when presenting with non-specific symptoms and in patients presenting with features of a thyroid disorder. Ideally TSH and FT4 should be measured to ensure hypopituitarism is not missed.
- Annual monitoring using serum [TSH] of patients at high risk of developing thyroid disorders is warranted (e.g. diabetes, Down's and Turner's syndrome, amiodarone, lithium and post-neck irradiation).
- Screening for thyroid disease in pregnancy (and pre-conception) is warranted in patients with features of a thyroid disorder or who have other autoimmune diseases or a family history of thyroid disease (see Chapter 11).
- TSH receptor antibodies are helpful in identifying the cause of hyperthyroidism and in predicting neonatal hyperthyroidism in babies born to mothers with Graves disease
- The aim of T4 replacement is to make the patient feel well and restore TSH to within the reference range.

Case 8.1

A 30-year-old housewife attended her GP. She had lost weight (6 kg in the previous 3 months), was irritable and felt uncomfortable in the recent spell of hot weather. She was taking an oestrogen-containing oral contraceptive. On clinical examination, her palms were sweaty, and she had a fine tremor of the fingers when her arms were outstretched. There was no thyroid enlargement or bruit, and no eye signs. The following results were reported for thyroid function tests:

Serum	Result	Reference range
TSH	<0.01	0.2–4.5 mU/L
FT4	19	9–21 pmol/L
Total T4	160	70–150 nmol/L
FT3	12.1	2.6–6.2 pmol/L
Total T3	6.5	0.9–2.4 nmol/L

What is the diagnosis in this patient, and on which results was this diagnosis based?

Comments: The patient had T3 thyrotoxicosis, and the diagnosis was based on the increased plasma [FT3] and undetectable [TSH], in the presence of a normal plasma [FT4]. The fact that the patient was taking an oestrogen-containing oral contraceptive would account for the increased plasma [total T4] and some of the increase in [total T3], since the oestrogen content in the oral contraceptive would cause an increase in plasma [TBG].

In patients with thyrotoxicosis but no goitre, it is important to perform a thyroid isotope scan to help determine the cause of the hyperthyroidism. This patient's thyroid showed a diffuse and increased uptake of TC-99m pertechnate, and TSH receptor antibodies were detected in her serum. This patient had Graves disease but no goitre; this is thought to arise when thyroid-stimulating Igs are present that stimulate the pathways required for thyroid hormone synthesis but the Igs do not stimulate thyroid growth.

Case 8.2

A 65-year-old widow had been receiving treatment for primary hypothyroidism with thyroxine (150 mg/day) for the previous 12 months. She felt well and was clinically euthyroid; her weight had been steady. Results of thyroid function tests performed at a routine follow-up out-patient attendance were:

Serum	Result	Reference range
TSH	0.2	0.2–4.5 mU/L
FT4	28	9–21 pmol/L
FT3	6.0	2.6–6.2 pmol/L

Are these results indicative of satisfactory therapeutic control, or would you want to adjust the patient's dosage of thyroxine?

Comments: The aim of thyroxine replacement treatment for primary hypothyroidism is to keep the patient clinically euthyroid and to render plasma [TSH] normal (it would have been much increased before thyroxine treatment was started). In some of these patients, it is necessary to give sufficient thyroxine to increase the plasma [FT4] to above the upper reference value in order to normalise plasma [TSH]. In this patient, although she was clinically euthyroid, the plasma [FT4] was above normal and [TSH] was below normal, but not so suppressed as to be undetectable (i.e. it was not <0.01 mU/L). It was decided not to reduce the thyroxine dosage, and to reassess the patient 3 months later. If the abnormal TSH persisted, then a lower dose of T4 (125 µg) should be tried.

Case 8.3

A 35-year-old secretary attended for follow-up review of her treatment for Graves disease. Carbimazole administration (15 mg three times/day) had been started 1 month before. The results for thyroid function tests were as follows:

Serum	Result	Reference range
TSH	<0.01	0.2–4.5 mU/L
FT4	<5	9–21 pmol/L
FT3	2.5	2.6–6.2 pmol/L

Comment on the acceptability of these results. If they are not acceptable, what would you do?

Comments: Plasma TSH measurements are not a reliable indicator of thyroid status in the early months of treating hyperthyroid patients, as the responsiveness of the thyrotrophs lags behind the fall in plasma [FT4] and [FT3] for several weeks. During these early months, plasma free thyroid hormone measurements provide the most reliable indication of thyroid status. In this patient, the results for plasma [FT4] and [FT3] clearly indicated the need to reduce the dosage of carbimazole immediately.

Case 8.4

A 38-year-old factory worker attended her GP because she was always tired and had a feeling of discomfort in her neck. She had been gaining weight. On clinical examination, she was found to have a goitre. The following results were reported for thyroid function tests:

Serum	Result	Reference range
TSH	18	0.2–4.5 mU/L
FT4	10	9–21 pmol/L
FT3	4.2	2.6–6.2 pmol/L

TPOAbs were present in the patient's serum in very high concentration.
   What is the diagnosis? Comment on whether all these tests needed to be requested in this patient.

Comments: The patient has hypothyroidism. However, she still had sufficient functioning thyroid tissue, when stimulated by the high plasma [TSH], to be able to maintain plasma [FT4] and [FT3] within their reference ranges. It should be noted that it was not appropriate to have requested the FT3 measurement, since about 50% of patients with hypothyroidism have a normal plasma [FT3].
   The very high concentration of TPOAbs in this patient's serum indicates that she had hypothyroidism due to Hashimoto thyroiditis.

Case 8.5

A 28-year-old female office worker presented to her GP complaining she had developed what she described as a persistent sore throat following a cold she had 2 weeks earlier. The throat pain was worse when she turned her head or swallowed. She also complained of feeling very tired. There was no past medical history of note.
   On examination she was pyrexial, had a fine tremor and tachycardia (90 beats/min). Her thyroid was firm but tender and appeared to be slightly enlarged.
   The GP took a blood sample and the following results were found:

(continued on p. 132)

Case 8.5 *(continued)*

Haematology

The erythrocyte sedimentation rate (ESR) was markedly increased.
Leucocytes and other haematology were normal.

Biochemistry

Serum	Result	Reference range
TSH	<0.01	0.4–4.5 mU/L
FT4	40	10–21 pmol/L
FT3	10	2.6–6.2 pmol/L

The patient was referred to an endocrinologist and seen 2 weeks later. Her thyroid gland was no longer painful and repeat blood tests were performed.
The ESR remained elevated.

Serum	Result	Reference range
TSH	<0.01	0.4–4.5 mU/L
FT4	23	10–21 pmol/L
FT3	7	2.6–6.2 pmol

Anti-thyroid peroxidase antibodies were negative. The uptake of Tc-99m pertechnate by the thyroid was found to be negligible.
What is the likely diagnosis?

Comments: The patient has viral thyroiditis (also known as de Quervain thyroiditis). This induced a transient hyperthyroidism.
The very low uptake of radioiodine is due to the low TSH (TSH is required to trap iodine) and the fact that thyroid follicular cells are damaged.
She returned to the clinic 4 weeks later for review and was found to be biochemically hypothyroid (raised TSH low FT4). No treatment with thyroxine was required as the hypothyroidism is usually transient in this disorder.

Chapter 9

Disorders of the adrenal cortex and medulla

The adrenal gland consists of two distinct tissues of different embryological origin: the outer cortex and the inner medulla. The cortex secretes glucocorticoid, mineralocorticoid and sex steroid hormones which are synthesised from cholesterol obtained from both high-density lipoprotein (HDL) and low-density lipoprotein (LDL) in plasma. The medulla secretes catecholamines, principally adrenaline. Disorders of the adrenals are uncommon, but they are easily diagnosed and can be readily treated. The need for specific and sensitive screening tests is therefore important; additional tests can then be used to confirm or refute the results of screening tests.

After a brief review of the control of steroid hormone secretion from the adrenal cortex and the action of the different steroid hormones, the investigation of adrenocortical hyperfunction and hypofunction will be discussed. Finally, the investigation of catecholamine hypersecretion from an adrenomedullary tumour (phaeochromocytoma) is discussed.

Regulation of adrenal steroid hormone synthesis and secretion

Three zones can be recognised in the adrenal cortex (Figure 9.1). The outermost zona glomerulosa is

Lecture Notes: Clinical Biochemistry, 8e. By G. Beckett, S. Walker, P. Rae & P. Ashby. Published 2010 by Blackwell Publishing.

the site of synthesis of aldosterone, the principal mineralocorticoid. The deeper layers of the cortex, the zona fasciculata and zona reticularis, synthesise glucocorticoids, of which cortisol is the most important in man. Sex steroid production also occurs in the adrenal cortex, mainly in the zona reticularis and to some extent in the zona fasciculata.

Glucocorticoid secretion

Glucocorticoids have widespread metabolic effects on carbohydrate, fat and protein metabolism. In the liver, cortisol stimulates gluconeogenesis, amino acid uptake and degradation, and ketogenesis. Lipolysis is increased in adipose tissue, and proteolysis and amino acid release promoted in muscle. Glucocorticoids are also involved to some extent in regulating sodium and water homeostasis and the inflammatory and stress responses. In the circulation, glucocorticoids are mainly protein bound (~90%), chiefly to CBG (cortisol-binding globulin or transcortin). Plasma [CBG] is increased in pregnancy and with oestrogen treatment (e.g. oral contraceptives). It is decreased in hypoproteinaemic states (e.g. nephrotic syndrome). Changes in plasma [cortisol] occur in parallel to changes in [CBG]. The biologically active fraction of cortisol in plasma is the free (unbound) component, though usually the total (i.e. bound plus free) concentration of cortisol is measured for diagnostic purposes.

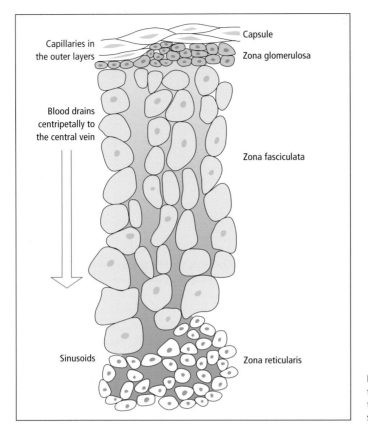

Figure 9.1 The morphological zonation of the adrenal cortex, showing the three types of cells and their particular structural arrangement.

In the figure:
- Capsule
- Capillaries in the outer layers
- Zona glomerulosa
- Blood drains centripetally to the central vein
- Zona fasciculata
- Sinusoids
- Zona reticularis

ACTH is the main stimulus to cortisol secretion. Three factors regulate ACTH (and therefore cortisol) secretion:

1 *Negative feedback control* ACTH release from the anterior pituitary is stimulated by hypothalamic secretion of CRH. Increased plasma [cortisol] or synthetic glucocorticoids suppress secretion of CRH and ACTH (Figure 9.2).

2 *Stress* (e.g. major surgery, emotional stress) leads to a sudden large increase in CRH (and ACTH) secretion; the negative feedback control mechanism is temporarily over-ridden.

3 *The diurnal rhythm of plasma [cortisol]* This control mechanism is related to the rhythm of an individual's sleeping–waking cycle (Figure 9.3). Cortisol levels are highest at the start of the working day, falling to the lowest levels in late evening with the onset of sleep.

Aldosterone secretion

The principal physiological function of aldosterone is to conserve Na^+, mainly by facilitating Na^+ reabsorption and reciprocal K^+ or H^+ secretion in the distal renal tubule and in other epithelial cells. Although its rate of production is less than 1% of the rate of cortisol production, aldosterone is a major regulator of water and electrolyte balance, as well as blood pressure.

The renin–angiotensin system is the most important system controlling aldosterone secretion (Figure 9.4). *Renin* is a proteolytic enzyme produced by the juxtaglomerular apparatus of the kidney and released into the circulation in response to a fall in circulating blood volume or renal perfusion pressure, and by loss of Na^+. Renin then acts on angiotensinogen (a 248 amino

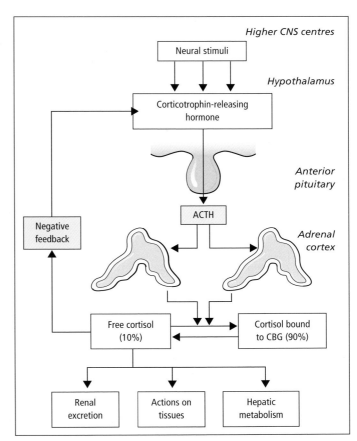

Figure 9.2 The hypothalamic–anterior pituitary–adrenal axis and the fate of cortisol following its release. CBG = cortisol-binding globulin.

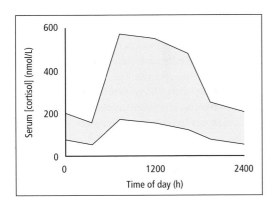

Figure 9.3 The diurnal rhythm of cortisol secretion; the shaded area represents values that lie within the reference range. There is a similar rhythm for the secretion of ACTH by the anterior pituitary. Patients with Cushing's syndrome lose this diurnal variation.

acid peptide produced by the liver) in plasma to produce angiotensin I (AI), a decapeptide which is then converted by ACE in the lung to the octapeptide angiotensin II (AII). AI and particularly AII stimulate aldosterone production in the adrenal glomerulosa. Measurements of both aldosterone and renin are often helpful to establish whether aldosterone production is autonomous. Under normal circumstances, plasma [aldosterone] varies with posture, and measurement of [aldosterone] in the supine and erect position is also helpful in elucidating the cause of hyperaldosteronism (p. 145). An increase in plasma [K⁺] also stimulates aldosterone, while ACTH is relatively unimportant, except possibly in stress conditions and in congenital adrenal hyperplasia (CAH) due to 21-hydroxylase deficiency (p. 299).

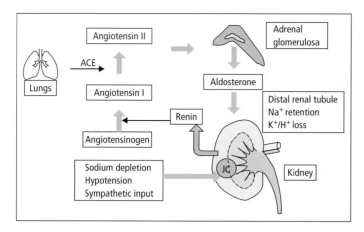

Figure 9.4 The renin–angiotensin system. Renin is released from the renal juxtaglomerular cells (JC) in response to hypotension, low blood volume or sodium depletion. Renin catalyses the conversion of angiotensinogen in plasma to angiotensin I. During passage through the lung, angiotensin-converting enzyme (ACE) catalyses the production of angiotensin II from angiotensin I. The angiotensin II stimulates release of aldosterone from the adrenal glomerulosa and the mineralocorticoid then promotes reabsorption of sodium in the distal tubules of the kidney.

No specific aldosterone-binding protein has been demonstrated.

Androgen secretion

The zona reticularis and to some extent the zona fasciculata produce the androgens androstenedione, dehydroepiandrosterone (DHEA) and dehydroepiandrosterone sulphate (DHEAS). The measurements of these androgens are important in the investigation of hirsutism, virilisation (p. 162) and CAH (p. 298).

The pathways for the production of the various adrenal steroids are shown in Figure 9.5

Investigation of suspected adrenocortical hyperfunction

Hyperfunction of the adrenal cortex can lead to overproduction of cortisol (Cushing's syndrome) or aldosterone (Conn's syndrome).

Cushing's syndrome

This can be ACTH dependent or ACTH independent (Figure 9.6; Table 9.1). If iatrogenic causes are excluded (e.g. use of hydrocortisone, prednisolone or dexamethasone), then the condition is caused by tumours that release either ACTH or cortisol. Approximately 70% of cases are due to a pituitary adenoma secreting ACTH (this is known as Cushing's disease). Ectopic ACTH secretion (often from a small-cell carcinoma of the bronchus or a carcinoid tumour) is the cause of approximately 10% of the cases. Glucocorticoid-secreting adrenal adenoma or carcinoma are each responsible for about 10% of the cases. Most ACTH-dependent forms of Cushing's syndrome lead to diffuse bilateral adrenocortical hyperplasia, but about 10–15% of patients with ACTH-driven Cushing's syndrome demonstrate a macronodular hyperplasia.

While Cushing's syndrome is uncommon, many of the clinical features of the disease such as hypertension, obesity, menstrual irregularities, depression, glucose intolerance or diabetes are commonly seen in general practice. It is therefore essential that patients with suspected Cushing's syndrome should be investigated according to a logical scheme that involves the use of simple screening tests to establish a likely diagnosis of Cushing's syndrome before the more involved investigations are carried out to establish the cause.

Some patients have 'cyclical Cushing's syndrome' in which there is intermittent and cyclical abnormal secretion of ACTH. This may be reflected by a history of variable and intermittent depression with anxiety, or variability in the severity of the symptoms and signs characteristic of Cushing's syndrome. Such patients may require tests to be performed on a number of occasions to make the diagnosis; salivary cortisol measurements

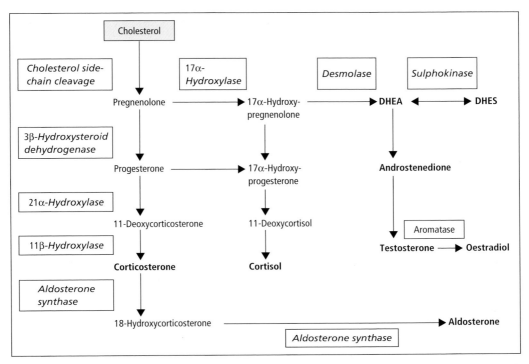

Figure 9.5 Steroid biosynthetic pathways in the adrenal cortex. Enzymes are shown in the boxes, and major steroid products are shown in bold. The conversion of corticosterone to aldosterone is restricted to the zona glomerulosa.

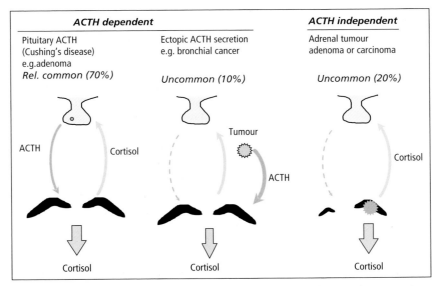

Figure 9.6 Pathological causes of Cushing's syndrome. Cushing's disease is caused by a pituitary adenoma autonomously secreting ACTH. The production of ACTH from the pituitary is suppressed (dotted arrow) when Cushing's syndrome is caused by an ectopic ACTH-secreting tumour or an adrenal adenoma autonomously secreting cortisol.

Table 9.1 Causes of adrenocortical hyperfunction

ACTH dependent
Pituitary (Cushing's disease)
Ectopic
Ectopic CRH or related peptides
ACTH therapy
ACTH independent
Adrenal adenoma
Adrenal carcinoma
Glucocorticoid therapy
Micronodular hyperplasia (partially ACTH dependent)

provide a convenient means of providing this long-term assessment.

A suggested plan of investigation is shown in Figure 9.7. Table 9.2 gives a summary of the commonly observed (but not invariable) findings in these hormonal tests.

Tests used to establish if a clinical diagnosis of Cushing's syndrome is likely

Initial screening tests

Low-dose dexamethasone suppression test

The best initial screening test for adrenocortical hyperfunction is to perform, as an outpatient, a low-dose/overnight dexamethasone suppression test. Under normal circumstances, dexamethasone suppresses the secretion of CRH (negative feedback – Figure 9.2); ACTH and cortisol levels thus fall to below 50 nmol/L.

In the *overnight suppression test*, the patient takes dexamethasone (1 mg) at 11–12 pm the night before attending the clinic. Serum [cortisol] is measured on a blood specimen taken the following morning at 8–9 am. A cortisol concentration in serum of less than 50 nmol/L in this morning sample effectively excludes Cushing's syndrome. This test performed using a 1 mg dose of dexamethasone has a false-positive rate of 12.5% with a false-negative rate of less than 2%.

The *48-h suppression test* is superior, but less convenient than the overnight test. Dexamethasone (0.5 mg) is taken every 6 h, beginning at 9 am on the first day, and serum [cortisol] is measured 48 h

later (interpretation as for the overnight test). The true-positive rate is reported to be better than 97%, with a false-negative rate of less than 1% for the 48-h test.

Drugs that induce hepatic microsomal enzymes (e.g. phenytoin, phenobarbitone) may increase dexamethasone metabolism, with premature lowering of its blood level below that required to achieve suppression of CRH secretion (false-negative result).

Urinary free cortisol (UFC)

Cortisol undergoes hepatic metabolism with the production of a number of metabolically inactive compounds that are excreted in the urine mainly as conjugated metabolites (e.g. glucuronides). A small amount of cortisol is excreted unchanged in the urine. Urinary cortisol excretion is related to the biologically active plasma [free cortisol] during the period of urine collection.

The measurement of UFC excretion in a 24-h collection is an acceptable screening test, but it suffers from the disadvantage that an incomplete collection of urine may lead to a false-negative result. Cushing's syndrome is excluded if the cortisol excretion is less than 250 nmol/24 h. Even if a complete urine collection is obtained, the test has a false-negative rate of 8–15%.

Interpretation of screening tests

The screening tests usually serve to distinguish simple non-endocrine obesity from obesity due to Cushing's syndrome. Abnormal results may, however, be obtained in depressed or extremely anxious patients, in the presence of severe intercurrent illness or in alcoholism (pseudo-Cushing syndrome). Further tests (as an inpatient) may be required to rule out pseudo-Cushing syndrome and help determine the specific cause of the adrenocortical hyperfunction (Figure 9.7).

Confirmatory tests

Diurnal rhythm of plasma cortisol

In normal subjects, plasma cortisol is highest in the morning and lowest around midnight (Figure 9.3). Patients with Cushing's syndrome lose this

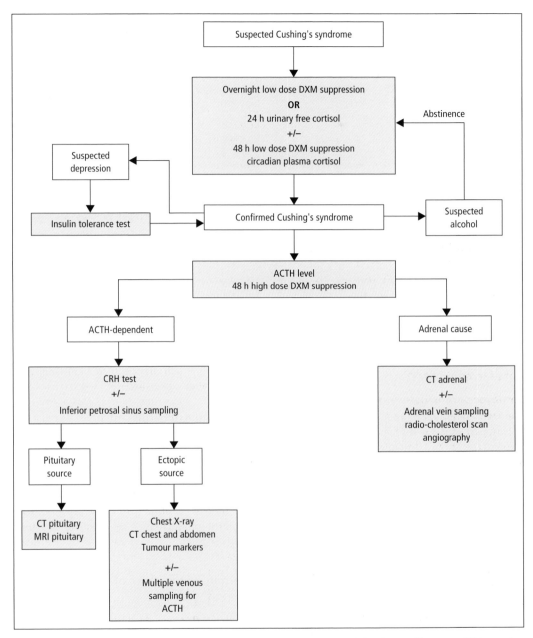

Figure 9.7 Algorithm for the investigation of suspected Cushing's syndrome and elucidation of its cause. CRH = cortico-trophin-releasing hormone; CT = computed tomography; DXM = dexamethasone; MRI = magnetic resonance imaging. Some investigators may prefer to perform the CRH test rather than the insulin tolerance test.

Table 9.2 Results of hormonal tests in patients with adrenal hyperfunction

Test	Cushing's disease	Adrenal tumour	Ectopic ACTH-secreting tumour
Tests to confirm the diagnosis			
Serum [cortisol] at 10 pm	Increased	Increased	Increased
Dexamethasone, low-dose test	Not suppressed	Not suppressed	Not suppressed
Urinary cortisol*	Increased	Increased	Increased
Diurnal rhythm	Lost	Lost	Lost
Insulin-induced hypoglycaemia	No response	No response	No response
Tests to differentiatee cause			
Plasma [ACTH]	Normal or increased	Not detectable	Increased or much increased
Dexamethasone, high-dose	Suppressed	Not suppressed	Not suppressed
CRH test	Increased response	No response	No response

* This test may be performed on a 24-h collection of urine or on an early morning specimen when the results are expressed as the urinary cortisol : creatinine ratio.

rhythm such that in most patients, the 8 am plasma [cortisol] is normal but the 10 pm plasma [cortisol] is raised. Patients need to be hospitalised for at least 48 h prior to stress-free venepuncture (e.g. in-dwelling catheter) to obtain meaningful results. It is also convenient to collect a series of 24-h urine samples for urine free cortisol measurement.

Patients with pseudo-Cushing syndrome may also show abnormal diurnal variation in cortisol; however, in response to a hypoglycaemic stimulus, the pseudo-Cushing patient will increase secretion of CRH, ACTH and cortisol; in true Cushing's syndrome, there is little or no response (see next section).

In alcoholism, other clues (e.g. raised mean cell volume (MCV), abnormal liver function tests) may be helpful; abstinence will lead to normalisation of the HPA axis.

Insulin hypoglycaemia test

This tests the integrity of the HPA axis, but is only occasionally necessary to allow true Cushing's syndrome to be distinguished from depressive illness. The test is contraindicated in patients with epilepsy or heart disease.

Insulin is administered intravenously (typically 0.15 U/kg) to lower blood glucose to 2.2 mmol/L or less while monitoring serum [cortisol]. Samples for simultaneous measurement of glucose and cortisol

are taken basally (before insulin) and at 30, 45, 60 and 90 min after IV insulin injection. The test requires close supervision, with glucose available for immediate injection if symptoms of severe hypoglycaemia develop. Failure to achieve a glucose level of 2.2 mmol/L invalidates the test, and repetition, with insulin incremented in steps of 0.05 U/kg, may be necessary.

Interpretation of results

Serum [cortisol] normally reaches its maximum at 60 or 90 min, the level reached being at least 500 nmol/L with an increment above the basal (pre-insulin) level of at least 145 nmol/L. Patients with Cushing's syndrome, whatever the cause, show little or no increase in serum [cortisol], despite the production of an adequate degree of hypoglycaemia.

Determining the cause of Cushing's syndrome

Once the diagnosis is established, other investigations may help to determine the cause (Table 9.2); difficulties sometimes arise in distinguishing between ectopic ACTH production and Cushing's disease. Biochemical results need to be considered together with the findings from other methods of investigation, particularly radiological, for example MRI and CT scanning.

Plasma [ACTH]

ACTH is unstable and samples must be collected into EDTA with the plasma being separated and frozen within 30 min of collection. Temporary, often large, increases in these hormones may be observed as a response to emotional stress. Plasma [ACTH] should be measured on blood specimens collected both in the morning and in the evening (e.g. at 8 am and 10 pm). If ACTH is undetectable, this is diagnostic of a functional adrenal tumour, and should be confirmed by an abdominal CT or MRI scan to detect an adrenal mass. Rare types of nodular adrenocortical disease (also ACTH independent) are also described.

If the patient has Cushing's disease (pituitary-dependent Cushing's syndrome), ACTH will be present in plasma in normal or increased amounts, particularly in the evening specimen. Results for plasma [ACTH] overlap considerably for patients with Cushing's disease and ectopic ACTH secretion. However, a very high plasma [ACTH] points to an ectopic ('non-endocrine') origin.

The following additional tests are used to distinguish Cushing's disease from ectopic ACTH secretion.

High-dose dexamethasone suppression test

This uses 2 mg of dexamethasone 6-hourly for 48 h in an attempt to suppress cortisol secretion. Basal (pre-dexamethasone) serum cortisol or 24-h urine free cortisol is compared with values obtained at the end of the 48-h period. Suppression is defined as a fall to less than 50% of the basal value. An overnight suppression test using a single dose of 8 mg of dexamethasone is reported to achieve similar diagnostic accuracy to the standard 48-h high-dose test.

About 90% of patients with Cushing's disease show suppression of cortisol output. In contrast, only 10% of patients with ectopic ACTH production show suppression.

CRH stimulation test

This test measures the ACTH and cortisol levels prior to and at 15, 30, 45, 60, 90 and 120 min after injection of 100 μg of CRH. Normal individuals (and depressed patients without Cushing's syndrome) show an increase in ACTH to peaks of less than 100 ng/L and an increase in cortisol with a peak of less than 600 nmol/L. Little or no response to CRF is found in patients with ectopic ACTH production or an adrenal tumour. Most patients with Cushing's disease show exaggerated ACTH and cortisol responses to human CRH (Figure 9.8). In distinguishing between Cushing's disease and ectopic ACTH production, the CRF tests have a specificity of about 95%. Together, the high-dose dexamethasone suppression test and the CRH test

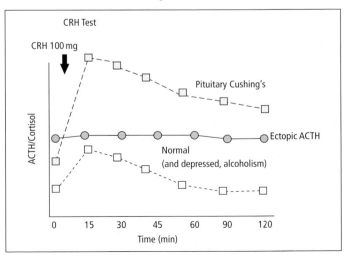

Figure 9.8 The cortisol and ACTH response in the CRH test. An exaggerated response is seen in Cushing's disease (pituitary adenoma), while a flat response is seen in ectopic ACTH production and adrenal adenoma. The test is usually not required for confirmation of adrenal adenoma as in such patients the diagnosis is made on the basis of an undetectable ACTH concentration.

provide almost 100% specificity and sensitivity in the diagnosis of Cushing's disease.

Other chemical tests

1 *Potassium* Hypokalaemic alkalosis may be a prominent feature of ectopic ACTH production, possibly due to the increased output of mineralo-corticoids or high cortisol levels (with renal loss of K^+ and H^+ in the urine). Patients with Cushing's syndrome are often treated with diuretics (for hypertension and oedema), and this treatment may itself lower the plasma $[K^+]$.

2 *Selective venous sampling* Blood specimens can be collected from selected sites for measurement of plasma [ACTH], to help identify the source of the ACTH (e.g. an inferior petrosal sinus : peripheral vein [ACTH] ratio which increases on CRH injection would support a pituitary source for the ACTH). In patients with an ectopic ACTH syndrome, there is no ACTH gradient between the inferior petrosal sinus samples and the samples drawn from peripheral veins.

3 *Pituitary function tests* (Chapter 7) may be abnormal in Cushing's syndrome due to the suppressive effect of cortisol on the hypothalamus and pituitary. LH and TSH responses to luteinising hormone-releasing hormone (LHRH) and to TRH are often impaired, and the increase in plasma [growth hormone] in response to hypoglycaemia is reduced.

4 *Tumour markers* As many as 70% of patients with ectopic ACTH secretion also secrete one or more marker peptides (e.g. carcinoembryonic antigen, gastrin, somatostatin and calcitonin), so a peptide tumour marker screen may assist in difficult cases.

5 *Glucose tolerance test* Patients with adrenocortical hyperfunction may develop steroid-induced diabetes and have a diabetic type of response to an OGTT (p. 94).

Treatment

Adrenal adenomas are treated by unilateral adrenalectomy. After surgery it may be many months or even years before the suppressed adrenal recovers, and treatment with dexamethasone may be required as a temporary measure. Pituitary-dependent Cushing's disease is treated by selective removal of the pituitary microadenoma by transphenoidal surgery. Again dexamethasone cover may be required until the HPA axis recovers from suppression. A non-suppressible serum cortisol post-operatively suggests that the patient has not been cured even if basal cortisol secretion has fallen to normal.

Treatment of ectopic ACTH syndrome involves removal of the tumour or occasionally bilateral adrenalectomy if the source of ACTH cannot be found.

Investigation of suspected adrenocortical hypofunction

Adrenocortical insufficiency may be primary (e.g. destruction of the gland itself by tuberculosis or autoimmune disease) or secondary (e.g. hypothalamic or pituitary disease leading to ACTH deficiency or after long-term steroid therapy). The causes are listed in Table 9.3.

In primary adrenal failure, patients present with lethargy, weakness, nausea and weight loss. They are typically hypotensive, with characteristic

Table 9.3 Causes of adrenocortical hypofunction

Primary adrenocortical insufficiency (Addison's disease)
1. Autoimmune adrenalitis
2. Infective (e.g. tuberculosis (TB), cytomegalovirus, histoplasmosis, meningococcal)
3. Secondary tumour deposits
4. Infiltrative lesions (e.g. amyloidosis, haemochromatosis)
5. CAH or hypoplasia
6. Drugs (e.g. etomidate)

Secondary to pituitary disease
1. Congenital deficiency (isolated or with GH deficiency)
2. Pituitary tumours (functional or non-functional)
3. Infections (e.g. TB, syphilis)
4. Secondary tumour deposits
5. Vascular lesions (e.g. postpartum haemorrhage)
6. Trauma
7. Iatrogenic (e.g. surgery or radiotherapy)
8. Secondary to hypothalamic disease
9. Others

hyperpigmentation affecting the buccal mucosa, scars and skin creases. The condition may present itself when a patient suffers from trauma or infection, or undergoes surgery. Patients with primary adrenal failure usually have deficiencies of both glucocorticoids and mineralocorticoids. Often there is hypoglycaemia with hyponatraemia, hyperkalaemia, raised serum urea levels and acid–base disturbance. The condition is life threatening, and requires urgent investigation if suspected.

The hypotension and electrolyte abnormalities are generally less severe in secondary adrenal insufficiency, with preservation of aldosterone secretion; the patient is typically pale. Where hypothalamic or pituitary disease is the cause, associated deficiency of other pituitary hormones may be found (Chapter 7). An enlarging pituitary tumour often first affects gonadotrophin secretion (with loss of libido and secondary sexual characteristics), followed by loss of growth hormone, thyrotrophin and ACTH.

The diagnosis of adrenocortical hypofunction is relatively straightforward, once the suspicion of the condition arises. Patients should be immediately referred to a hospital, and blood should be collected for basal measurements of serum urea, electrolytes, glucose, cortisol and plasma ACTH concentrations *before* the patient is given cortisol. Definitive tests for the diagnosis of this condition should be carried out later, after the crisis. A suggested plan of investigation is shown in Figure 9.9.

Diagnosis of primary adrenal hypofunction (Addison's disease)

Cortisol and ACTH measurements

A normal serum [cortisol] at 8 am (or normal 24-h UFC) does *not* exclude Addison's disease; patients may be able to maintain a normal basal output but be unable to secrete adequate amounts of cortisol in response to stress. Nevertheless, a serum [cortisol] below 50 nmol/L at 8 am is strong presumptive evidence for Addison's disease, while a value (at 8 am) of 500 nmol/L or more (in the absence of steroid therapy) makes the diagnosis extremely

unlikely. Simultaneous measurement of cortisol and ACTH improves diagnostic accuracy such that a low serum cortisol (<200 nmol/L) and a raised ACTH (>200 ng/L) are diagnostic of adrenal failure.

Short tetracosactrin (Synacthen) test

Stimulation of the adrenal cortex with synthetic ACTH (tetrocosactide, Synacthen, comprising the first 24 amino acids of ACTH) allows confirmation of the diagnosis of Addison's disease and an assessment of adrenocortical reserve. For patients with equivocal results, it allows a firm diagnosis to be made or dismissed. Basal cortisol is measured and a further measurement is taken 30 min after an IM injection of 0.25 mg tetracosactrin.

A normal response is defined as a rise in serum [cortisol] to at least 500 nmol/L. A normal response excludes primary adrenocortical insufficiency. Conversely, failure of cortisol to respond to Synacthen, together with an elevated plasma [ACTH], confirms primary adrenocortical insufficiency. Adrenocortical hypofunction secondary to hypothalamic or pituitary disease is also extremely unlikely if the response is normal, since, in the prolonged absence of ACTH, the cells of the adrenal cortex would have atrophied.

Severe emotional stress, treatment with glucocorticoids within 12 h prior to the tetracosactrin injection, and the taking of oestrogen-containing oral contraceptives may invalidate the test. Where a patient with suspected Addison's disease is receiving steroid therapy, a steroid that does not cross-react in the cortisol assay should be prescribed (e.g. dexamethasone not predisolone) unless it is possible to stop steroid therapy for 24 h prior to the tests. With this proviso, adrenal reserve in patients on steroid therapy can also be assessed using this test.

Diagnosis of secondary adrenocortical insufficiency

The finding of a low serum cortisol accompanied by a low plasma ACTH would support a diagnosis of adrenocortical insufficiency secondary to hypothalamic or pituitary disease. While the atrophied

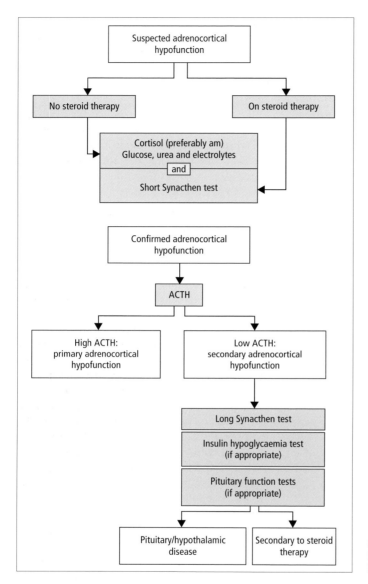

Figure 9.9 Suggested plan of investigation of adrenocortical hypofunction.

adrenocortical cells fail to respond in the short Synacthen test, the gland can become responsive over a longer period of stimulation using the so-called depot (long) Synacthen test.

Depot (long) Synacthen test

Serum [cortisol] is measured on a basal sample and on further samples taken between 5 and 8 h after IM injection of 1 mg of depot Synacthen on each of three successive days. In Addison's disease, the cortisol fails to rise above 600 nmol/L at 5–8 h after the third injection. In secondary adrenocortical insufficiency, a stepwise increase in the cortisol response after successive injections is observed. Poor responses to the long Synacthen tests may occur in patients with hypothyroidism (primary or secondary). In patients with hypothyroidism, adrenal function cannot be satisfactorily assessed until the thyroid deficiency has been corrected.

Patients who receive prolonged steroid therapy are at risk of secondary adrenal hypofunction on withdrawal of steroid treatment, and the same test can be used to assess their reserve. Occasionally, it may be necessary to test the full integrity of the HPA axis using the insulin hypoglycaemia test (reducing insulin dose to 0.1 U/kg) (p. 140).

Other pituitary function tests

Other pituitary functions will almost certainly be abnormal by the time hypopituitarism is severe enough to produce adrenocortical hypofunction. It is usual in these patients, therefore, to measure basal concentrations of FT4 and TSH, prolactin, testosterone (male), oestradiol (female), LH and FSH in plasma or serum and to investigate dynamic growth hormone responses in addition to the cortisol response (p. 109).

Adrenal antibodies A diagnosis of autoimmune Addison's disease can be made in patients who have idiopathic Addison's disease if they have adrenal antibodies in their serum.

Electrolytes Hyponatraemia is present in about 90% of cases and hyperkalaemia in 65%. Urea is also usually elevated. Acid–base disturbances are not usually observed unless complications develop (e.g. due to vomiting).

Hyperaldosteronism and hypertension

Hypertension is common and in most cases no underlying cause is apparent, that is, they have 'essential hypertension'. Hypertension may, however, be due to renal disease or adrenal disorders. Adrenal causes include Cushing's syndrome, primary aldosterone excess due to an aldosterone-secreting tumour (Conn's syndrome), ACTH-dependent aldosterone excess, congenital adrenal hyperplasia or phaeochromocytoma. Patients with hypertension who have a clinical history or features suggestive of a renal or adrenal lesion require further investigation. Unprovoked hypokalaemia

with a hypernatraemia may suggest primary mineralocorticoid excess (e.g. hyperaldosteronism), while hypokalaemia with hyponatraemia may suggest secondary aldosteronism. Young patients with hypertension and patients who are resistant to treatment with anti-hypertensive agents should also be considered for further investigation. Non-compliance with medication, excessive sodium intake and white coat hypertension should be excluded before further investigations are initiated.

Primary hyperaldosteronism (low-renin hyperaldosteronism)

Causes

• A unilateral single small (1 cm) aldosterone-producing adenoma, as originally described by Conn's (Conn's syndrome), is the cause in approximately 60% of cases. In these adenomas, aldosterone production is unresponsive to AII and thus aldosterone changes little on standing (AII increases on standing). However, the adenoma retains a diurnal rhythm and responds to changes in ACTH.
• Idiopathic aldosteronism characterised by bilateral nodular adrenal hyperplasia is the cause in 30–35% of cases. Aldosterone secretion by these nodules is exquisitely sensitive to AII but not ACTH and as such these patients show an exaggerated increase in aldosterone secretion when they move from a supine to erect posture.
• The remaining 5% of cases are due to either
  • Glucocorticoid-suppressible hyperaldosteronism (GSA), an autosomal dominant inherited disorder produced by a hybrid gene (11β-hydroxylase + aldosterone synthase), which allows aldosterone to be produced by the fasciculata under the control of ACTH. In GSA, aldosterone production can be suppressed by giving glucocorticoids.
  • Primary adrenal hyperplasia (unilateral), aldosterone-producing AII-responsive adenoma (unilateral).
  • Aldosterone-producing carcinoma (rare).
Symptoms are usually absent or non-specific, and include tiredness, muscle weakness, thirst and

polyuria. Primary hyperaldosteronism is a rare cause of hypertension (0.5–2% of cases) although some believe that the prevalence is nearer 5%. It may be suspected in a hypertensive patient with low plasma [K⁺] (<3.5 mmol/L) or in a patient where plasma [K⁺] falls below 3 nmol/L during therapy with a thiazide diuretic. However, detection of primary hyperaldosteronism is difficult since approximately 40% of such patients are normokalaemic. Common causes of hypertension with a reduced plasma [K⁺] need to be considered in the differential diagnosis (e.g. essential hypertension with diuretic therapy). If hypokalaemia is found in patients taking diuretics and primary hyperaldosteronism is suspected, then the diuretic should be withdrawn, potassium stores replenished and plasma [K⁺] measured 2 weeks later.

Investigation of suspected primary hyperaldosteronism

Screening

Some advocate that a ratio of plasma renin : plasma [aldosterone] may be used as a screening test even when patients are taking anti-hypertensive medication; however, if possible, the patient should be off medication before the test is performed. Cut-offs depend on the assay used for measurement of plasma renin and therefore local protocols and reference ranges for the investigation of suspected primary hyperaldosteronism should always be followed. Samples should be taken supine after an overnight fast. The ratio of aldosterone : renin is increased in primary hyperaldosteronism.

Further tests

Defined protocols are required and involve the patient being admitted as a day case to study responses in aldosterone when moving from the supine to erect posture. The principle of these tests is that adrenal adenomas that secrete aldosterone are sensitive to ACTH but not AII, whereas idiopathic bilateral adrenal hyperplasia is sensitive to changes in AII but not ACTH.

In normal subjects, standing decreases renal blood flow with a consequent increase in rennin, AII and aldosterone.

In order to investigate the aldosterone response to ACTH and AII, a blood sample should be taken in the early morning (8.30 am) *after the patient has been supine for at least 30 min* (ACTH is at peak diurnal concentration at this time). A further sample is taken at midday *after the patient has been standing for at least an hour* (ACTH concentrations should be lower than early morning).

It is important that local protocols are followed and that the samples are taken at the stated times since interpretation of results requires changes in ACTH to have occurred; ACTH does not have to be measured as cortisol is more convenient to measure and reflects changes in ACTH.

Interpretation

In a normal individual, supine at 8.30 am and erect at 12.30 pm, the increases in AII overcomes the effect of the fall in ACTH over this time period; this prompts [aldosterone] to increase by approximately 30%. This increase in [aldosterone] is exaggerated in bilateral nodular adrenal hyperplasia (idiopathic) and aldosterone-producing AII-responsive adenomas.

Aldosterone production in patients with an adenoma or GSA is independent of AII but becomes dependent on ACTH. In these individuals aldosterone falls between 8.30 am (supine) and midday (standing).

In GSA, aldosterone secretion and production of intermediary metabolites (e.g. 18-hydroxy metabolites of cortisol) are predominantly under the control of ACTH. Further diagnostic information can be obtained from urinary 18-hydroxycortisol measurements as these are typically less than 600 nmol/24 h in normal individuals, slightly increased or normal in patients with idiopathic adrenal hyperplasia (<1000 nmol/24 h), 1000–3000 nmol/24 h in Conn's adenoma and more than 3000 nmol/24 h in GSA.

Imaging

Imaging of the adrenals can be helpful but only after a biochemical abnormality has been identified. This is because of the high incidence of non-functional adrenal incidentalomas. Equivocal results on scanning may require adrenal venous sampling.

Treatment

Adrenal tumours are removed. Patients with bilateral adrenal hyperplasia are treated with spironolactone, a diuretic that antagonises the action of aldosterone. GSA is treated with dexamethasone.

Secondary hyperaldosteronism (high-renin hyperaldosteronism)

This is much more common, and is only sometimes associated with hypertension. It is due to conditions that stimulate the secretion of renin, often as a result of reduced renal Na^+ filtration (e.g. congestive heart failure, cirrhosis, Na^+ deprivation). Diagnosis of these conditions is usually straightforward and further investigation of the renin–angiotensin–aldosterone system is not necessary. Probably the most common cause of secondary hyperaldosteronism is diuretic therapy.

Mineralocorticoid deficiency

The most common cause of mineralocorticoid deficiency is adrenal insufficiency due to Addison's disease and some forms of CAH.

Inherited adrenocortical enzyme defects

A number of inherited enzyme deficiencies have been identified that are associated with abnormal steroid secretion or action. Many of these patients present as neonates or in childhood, but in some cases the biochemical lesion may not manifest itself clinically until adult life. CAH can be due to a deficiency in 21-hydroxylase or 11β-hydroxysteroid dehydrogenase. These deficiencies are discussed in more detail in Chapter 21.

Phaeochromocytoma

These tumours arise from chromaffin cells (90% are in the adrenal medulla; the rest can occur anywhere from the base of the brain to the testes). About 5% of tumours are bilateral and about 10% malignant. They secrete excessive amounts of noradrenaline, adrenaline and the metabolites normetadrenaline, metadrenaline and 4-hydroxy-3-methoxymandelic acid (HMMA – also known as vanillylmandelic acid or VMA). The catecholamines and their metabolites can be further metabolised in various tissues, especially the liver, to produce sulphated and glucuronide derivatives that are then excreted in urine (Figure 9.10).

Phaeochromocytoma is a rare cause of hypertension (<0.1% of cases). Characteristically, this is episodic. Even when the hypertension is present all the time, episodic attacks of symptoms (e.g. headache, pallor, palpitations, sweating, panic attacks, abdominal pain) tend to occur. Such features are important when selecting the time for collecting specimens for certain laboratory investigations.

Phaeochromocytoma sometimes occurs as a familial condition, in association with the MEN IIa and IIb syndromes (Table 16.7).

Catecholamines and their metabolites are also secreted by neuroblastomas; these are rare rapidly

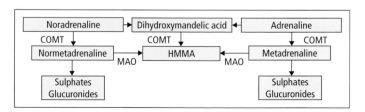

Figure 9.10 Pathways for the metabolism of catecholamines. COMT = catechol-*O*-methyltransferase; MAO = monoamine oxidase; HMMA = 4-hydroxy-3-methoxymandelic acid.

growing tumours that occur in infants and young children.

Diagnosis

The diagnosis of phaeochromocytoma depends crucially on demonstrating excessive production of catecholamines or their metabolites in plasma or urine. This is often not straightforward as a number of the tests that are commonly used to make the diagnosis produce false-negative results. The measurements of plasma-free metadrenalines or urinary fractioned metadrenalines are the most sensitive tests, having sensitivities of 99% and 97%, respectively. The measurement of plasma catecholamines (sensitivity 84%), urinary catecholamines (sensitivity 86%), urinary total metadrenalines (sensitivity 77%) or urinary HMMA (sensitivity 64%) is much less reliable for detecting phaeochromocytoma.

The measurement of plasma metadrenalines is the best diagnostic test for a number of reasons. First, the tumour produces metadrenalines continuously while the release of catecholamines is usually episodic. Secondly, stimulation of the adrenal via the sympathetic nervous system causes a large increase in the release of catecholamines but, under such circumstances, plasma free metadrenalines remain relatively unaffected. Thirdly, HMMA and metadrenalines measured in urine are produced by metabolism of catecholamines in tissues other than the tumour and are often secreted in urine as sulphated or glucuronide conjugates. Currently the measurement of plasma free metadrenalines is not a widely available test but many laboratories are able to measure urinary fractionated metadrenalines.

Urine fractionated metadrenalines

These tests use high-performance liquid chromatography (HPLC) to quantify the 24-h urinary excretion of metadrenaline and normetadrenaline (or HMMA which is less satisfactory).

Several points concerning the collection and timing of urine specimens for catecholamine investigations should be noted:

- *Drugs* can increase (e.g. vasodilators) or decrease (e.g. reserpine) the release of catecholamines. Others affect their metabolism (e.g. monoamine oxidase inhibitors), or interfere with certain analytical methods (e.g. labetalol). Investigations for phaeochromocytoma should preferably be started *before* initiation of drug treatment.
- *Diet* Interference from dietary constituents is possible (e.g. HMMA measurement requires the patient to be on a vanilla-free diet). Local laboratory requirements for any dietary restrictions should be consulted.
- *Timing of urine collections* is important in order to minimise false-negative results. When the clinical index of suspicion is high:
  - *Patients who have 'attacks'* If the patient is normotensive between attacks, a single baseline set of measurements should be made, and the patient should be instructed to start a second 24-h urine collection when the next 'attack' occurs.
  - *Patients with persistent hypertension* Determination of 24-h urinary excretion of catecholamines or metabolites needs only be performed once.

When the clinical index of suspicion is low (e.g. a middle-aged or elderly patient who is hypertensive, but without paroxysmal symptoms), there is little justification for requesting these investigations, which should be restricted to those with appropriate symptoms or young patients with hypertension.

Keypoints

- Patients with suspected adrenocortical hyperfunction should be screened by the low-dose overnight or 48-h dexamethasone suppression test, or measurement of UFC. A positive result requires confirmation (diurnal rhythm, serial 24-h urine free cortisol measurements). Pseudo-Cushing syndrome (severe depression, alcoholism, severe intercurrent illness) may need to be distinguished by the insulin hypoglycaemia test or CRH test. Plasma ACTH measurement, the high-dose dexamethasone suppression test and the CRH test and imaging help establish the cause.
- The diagnosis of primary adrenal hypofunction is best made by simultaneous measurement of cortisol and ACTH (early morning) followed by the short tetracosactrin (Synacthen) test. Secondary hypofunction is assessed by the long Synacthen test and tests of pituitary hormone reserve.
- Hyperaldosteronism is most commonly secondary (e.g. liver disease, congestive heart failure, kidney disease). Primary hyperaldosteronism (Conn's syndrome) is rare. Diagnosis is suspected in hypertensive patients with hypokalaemia (with no other explanation for low plasma K^+). Confirmation is by measurement of plama renin activity and aldosterone using strict protocols with the patient erect and supine.
- Phaeochromocytoma is a catecholamine-secreting tumour of the adrenal medulla or extra-chromaffin tissue. It is a rare cause of hypertension. Biochemical diagnosis depends on the measurement of plasma or urinary metadrenalines.

Case 9.1

A 34-year-old housewife was admitted to a hospital with a provisional diagnosis of Cushing's syndrome. As an outpatient, her serum [cortisol] had not been suppressed when an overnight dexamethasone suppression test (1 mg of dexamethasone) was performed. She was obese (weight 74 kg, height 1.7 m), hypertensive (blood pressure, 165/105 mmHg) and had wasting of the proximal limb muscles. The following results were obtained for adrenal function tests:

Test		Result		Usual response
Diurnal rhythm of serum cortisol nmol/L		400 (8 am)		Reference range 150–550 nmol/L
		380 (10 pm)		Reference range up to 200 nmol/L
Insulin hypoglycaemia test	Basal	Max response		
Plasma glucose mmol/L	4.5	1.5		Should fall below 2.2 mmol/L
Serum cortisol nmol/L	435	480		Increment of at least 145 nmol/L
Dexamethasone suppression test	Basal	After 48 h 0.5 mg qid	After 48 h 2 mg qid	
Serum cortisol nmol/L	420	410	500	Cortisol should suppress to <50 nmol/L
Plasma ACTH ng/L	<2			Reference range 7–51 ng/L

How would you interpret these results?

Comments: These results are consistent with a diagnosis of Cushing's syndrome due to an adrenal adenoma (low basal ACTH, no cortisol suppression with high dose dexamethasone). These tumours account for 5–10% of all cases of Cushing's syndrome. Ultrasound examination and imaging confirmed the presence of a tumour in the right adrenal, and the patient was treated successfully by right adrenalectomy.

Case 9.2

A 58-year-old man was admitted to a hospital with weight loss and respiratory distress. He was pigmented and his blood pressure was 140/80. Urea electrolytes, a random cortisol and an overnight (1 mg) dexamethasone test gave the following results:

Serum	Result	Reference range
Urea	8.6	2.5–6.6 mmol/L
Sodium	144	135–145 mmol/L
Potassium	2.0	3.6–5.0 mmol/L
Total CO_2	45	22–32 mmol/L
Cortisol (Random)	1650	150–550 nmol/L
Post-overnight dexamethasone	1530	<50 nmol/L

Further investigation revealed the following:

Test	Result				Usual response
Dexamethasone suppression test	Basal	After 48 h, 0.5 mg qid	After 48 h, 2.0 mg qid		
Serum cortisol nmol/L	1350	1420	1100		Suppression to <50 nmol/L
Plasma ACTH ng/L		220	180		Suppression to <2 ng/L

A CRH test showed a flat response for cortisol and ACTH.
  How would you interpret these results?

Comments: The very high [cortisol] and [ACTH] that are not suppressed by dexamethasone (overnight, low-dose and high-dose dexamethasone test) together with the marked hypokalaemic alkalosis strongly suggest that the patient has Cushing's syndrome caused by ectopic ACTH production. The flat response to the CRH test supports this diagnosis. Imaging demonstrated that the patient had carcinoma of the bronchus.

Case 9.3

A 25-year-old woman presented to her GP complaining of tiredness, loss of appetite and some weight loss. She also complained of feeling dizzy when she stood up and generally feeling very depressed. She appeared pigmented, which she attributed to sunbathing, but on closer examination her buccal mucosa were also pigmented. Her blood pressure (supine) was 110/70. A blood sample was taken and the following was found:

Serum	Result	Reference range
Urea	8.0	2.5–6.6 mmol/L
Sodium	130	135–145 mmol/L
Potassium	5.2	3.6–5.0 mmol/L
Cortisol	160	150–550 nmol/L

How would you interpret these results in light of the clinical presentation? What further tests should be performed?

Comments: Addison's disease is likely in this patient as she has hypotension, hyponatraemia, mild hyperkalaemia and hyperpigmentation affecting the buccal mucosa. Although the result for the random cortisol is within the reference range, it is rather low for someone who is likely to be somewhat stressed, and many patients who present with Addison's disease have low normal [cortisol].

(continued on p. 151)

Case 9.3 *(continued)*

The GP referred the patient to the endocrine clinic where a short Synacthen test was performed with the following results.

Serum	Result	Reference range
Basal cortisol	170	150–550 nmol/L
Basal ACTH	450	7–50 ng/L
Cortisol 30-min post-Synacthen	190	>500 nmol/L

Anti-adrenal antibodies were present in high concentration.

The high basal [ACTH], borderline low basal serum [cortisol] and lack of cortisol response to the short Synacthen test confirmed a diagnosis of primary adrenal failure. The presence of anti-adrenal antibodies suggests that she has autoimmune primary adrenal failure. She was given glucocorticoid and mineralocorticoid replacement therapy.

Case 9.4

A 68-year-old retired woman with long-standing type 2 diabetes presented with continued problems of obesity and poorly controlled hypertension. The GP noticed that she had plethoric moon facies and a blood pressure of 210/115 mmHg. An overnight dexamethasone (1 mg of dexamethasone) suppression test failed to suppress her cortisol below 530 nmol/L and ACTH below 40 ng/L. Urea, sodium, potassium and total CO_2 were all within the reference range but her glucose was 22.0 mmol/L. Further tests performed as an outpatient at the endocrine clinic gave the following results for adrenal function tests:

Test	Result		
	Basal	After 48 h, 0.5 mg qid	After 48 h, 2.0 mg qid
Dexamethasone Serum cortisol 9 am	520	230	110

Interpretation

A CRH test gave the following results:

Time (min)	Cortisol (nmol/L)	Time (min)	Cortisol (nmol/L)
0	590	60	1220
15	710	90	890
30	1300	120	735
45	1660		

What is the likely diagnosis? What further investigations should be performed?

Comments: These results are consistent with a diagnosis of Cushing's syndrome due to a pituitary adenoma secreting ACTH (Cushing's disease). Approximately 90% of patients with Cushing's disease suppress cortisol to less than half of the basal values when given high-dose dexamethasone. Most patients with Cushing's disease show an exaggerated cortisol response (>600 nmol/L) following CRH injection. In this patient MRI showed bilateral adrenocortical hyperplasia and a microadenoma (~5 mm in diameter) in the anterior pituitary. If imaging had failed to demonstrate an adenoma then petrosal sinus sampling for ACTH may have been required to detect the source of the ACTH. She was treated surgically by transphenoidal removal of the microadenoma. Cure is likely if the patient develops hypocortisolism in the first few days to weeks after surgery. During this post-operative period, they require glucocorticoid replacement therapy.

Chapter 10

Investigation of gonadal function, infertility, menstrual irregularities and hirsutism

Infertility in women and menstrual irregularities are relatively common clinical problems. They often have an endocrine cause and result from abnormal ovarian, thyroid, hypothalamic, pituitary or adrenal function. The laboratory can help with the diagnosis of these endocrine abnormalities. Biochemical tests are also useful in screening hirsute women for the presence of occult ovarian or adrenal tumours. Endocrine causes of male infertility are rare, but biochemical tests play an important role in assessing such patients.

This chapter outlines the function of the hypothalamic–pituitary–gonadal axis, and describes the biochemical tests that are required for the investigation of infertility, menstrual disorders and hirsutism. Guidance on interpretation of the test employed is also provided.

Male gonadal function

Spermatogenesis and its control

Spermatogenesis takes place in the seminiferous tubules, and requires normal functioning of both the Leydig and the Sertoli cells.

Lecture Notes: Clinical Biochemistry, 8e. By G. Beckett, S. Walker, P. Rae & P. Ashby. Published 2010 by Blackwell Publishing.

Leydig cells produce testosterone, the principal androgen, under the control of LH. Sertoli cells provide other testicular cells with nutrients, and also produce several regulatory proteins, of which inhibin, activin, Mullerian inhibitory hormone (MIH) and androgen-binding protein (ABP) are the best characterised. Sertoli cell function is regulated by FSH. Testosterone has crucial paracrine actions in the testes which are required for normal spermatogenesis and fertility.

The entire hypothalamic–pituitary–testicular axis (Figure 10.1) must function normally for spermatogenesis. GnRH from the hypothalamus stimulates the release of LH and FSH; its effect on LH release is more marked than that on FSH release. The secretion of GnRH, and thus of LH, occurs in pulses; the secretion of FSH is less markedly pulsatile. The amplitude and frequency of the pulses of LH release appear to be important in exerting effects on testosterone production.

The secretion of LH is under negative feedback control from plasma [free testosterone], and the release of FSH is inhibited by inhibin and stimulated by activin, both released by Sertoli cells. High testicular [testosterone] is ensured by the anatomical proximity of Leydig, Sertoli and spermatogenic cells, and by the local release of ABP. Inhibin is a dimeric glycopeptide comprising a 20 kDa α-subunit and a 15 kDa β-subunit. Two forms of β-subunit occur, thus two forms of inhibin (inhibin A and inhibin B) occur, although in males inhibin

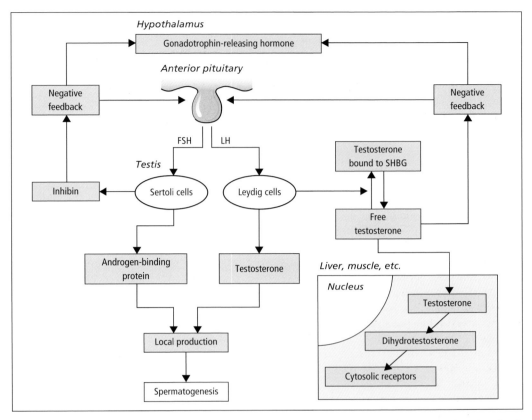

Figure 10.1 The hypothalamic–pituitary–testicular axis. SHBG = sex hormone-binding globulin. Activin from Sertoli cells stimulates FSH release.

B is the most important form in plasma. Both FSH and testosterone are necessary for inhibin production in normal men. Activin is a dimer of inhibin β-subunits and has a stimulatory action on FSH release. MIH causes regression of the Mullerian ducts, and in the absence of MIH and testosterone the ducts differentiate into female internal genitalia.

Transport, metabolism and actions of testosterone

In the circulation in males, about 60% of testosterone is strongly bound to sex hormone-binding globulin (SHBG), 38% is weakly bound to albumin while approximately 2% is unbound (free). These proportions vary somewhat and are dependent on the relative concentrations and affinities of albumin and SHBG. Since a large proportion of testosterone is bound to SHBG, the factors that alter the concentration or affinity of SHBG will have a significant effect on the circulating total testosterone concentration. Factors that modify the concentration of SHBG are shown in Table 10.1. There is continued debate concerning which components of circulating testosterone are capable of exerting bioactivity on target tissues. Classically androgens have been considered to exert their effect through interactions with a cytosolic receptor that then translocates to the nucleus and interacts with androgen-responsive genes. As such it was believed that only the small unbound 'free' fraction could enter cells and exert a biological effect. However, some consider that both the 'free'

Table 10.1 Causes of abnormal SHBG in males and females

Increased SHBG	Decreased SHBG
Anorexia nervosa	Obesity
Hyperthyroidism	Hypothyroidism
Hypogonadism (males)	Polycystic ovarian syndrome (females)
Cirrhosis	Glucocorticoids
Anti-convulstants	Androgens
Oestrogens	

Table 10.2 Causes of hypogonadism in the male

Primary hypogonadism (low testosterone, high LH, FSH)	
Klinefelter's syndrome	Testicular torsion
Androgen resistance	Trauma
Androgen synthesis defects	Iron overload
Anorchia or cryptoorchidism	Drugs including alcohol
Epididimo-orchitis (e.g. mumps)	
Secondary hypogonadism (low testosterone, LH, FSH low or normal)	
Kallman's syndrome	Opiates, cocaine, anabolic steroids
Hypothalamic–pituitary disease	Excessive exercise
Isolated GnRH deficiency	Stress
Panhypopituitarism	Weight loss
Destructive pituitary tumour	Moderate illness (acute or chronic)
Cushing's syndrome	Iron overload
Hyperprolactinaemia	Oestrogen-secreting tumours

and 'albumin-bound fraction' of testosterone may be able to enter cells and thus be the 'bioavailable testosterone' fraction. Few laboratories measure the 'free' testosterone concentration, as this is technically demanding. Some laboratories may provide a measure of 'bioavailable testosterone'. Most laboratories will offer a 'free androgen index' (FAI) which requires the measurement of [SHBG] and [total testosterone] and applying these in the formulae:

$$FAI = \frac{[\text{total testosterone}]}{[\text{SHBG}]}$$

This effectively corrects for changes in SHBG but it does not take into account changes in the albumin-bound fraction. The FAI is unreliable in males and tends to overestimate the serum [free testosterone]; its use should be confined to females. More complicated mathematical formulae based on the law of mass action have been produced that can calculate [free testosterone] and estimate [bioavailable testosterone] from measured serum [total testosterone], [albumin] and [SHBG]. These formulae do not take into account changes in the affinity of SHBG and albumin but appear to work well for male subjects.

Androgens are thought to exert their action in target tissues through high-affinity cytosolic receptors that transport the androgens into the cell nucleus. In the nucleus, the androgens then interact with androgen receptors, which in turn modify the expression of androgen-responsive genes. In many tissues, testosterone is converted to the more biologically active compound 5α-dihydrotestosterone (5α-DHT) by 5α-reductase. It

would seem that some actions of testosterone might be mediated through oestrogen receptors after local conversion of testosterone to oestrogen by the enzyme 'aromatase'. It has thus become apparent that many of the actions of testosterone may be regulated in target tissues by both 5α-reductase and aromatase. In addition, since oestradiol and testosterone bind to SHBG with differing affinities, changes in the concentration of SHBG may modify the relative clearance rates of testosterone and oestradiol and thus alter the ratio of these hormones in plasma; this may in turn have a biological consequence.

Investigation of infertility and male hypogonadism

Endocrine causes of subfertility are rare in men. Most infertile males are eugonadal, with oligospermia due to failure of the seminiferous tubules. In a eugonadal male with a normal sperm count, endocrine investigations are not required. Causes of male hypogonadism are given in Table 10.2.

If on two occasions the sperm count is less than 20×10^6/ml and/or motility is poor in more than 50% of the sperm, measurements of serum [LH], [FSH] and [testosterone] should be made to determine whether hypogonadism is caused by a primary defect in the testes or in the hypothalamic–pituitary region. Both forms lead to infertility (Figure 10.2). Azoospermia with a raised FSH suggests severe seminiferous tubular damage, while azoospermia with normal FSH and normal testicular volume indicates bilateral genital tract obstruction. Plasma [prolactin] should also be determined (p. 108), as hyperprolactinaemia can lead to diminished libido, hypogonadism and impotence.

Misleadingly high values for LH and FSH might be observed because of pulsatile release. Serum [total testosterone] results are affected by changes in serum [SHBG]. 'The calculated serum [free testosterone]' should be derived for all males who have abnormalities in serum [SHBG] or a low total testosterone. The calculation of the FAI provides an unreliable and often misleading estimate of free testosterone in males and its use should be avoided in male patients.

Hypergonadotrophic and hypogonadotrophic hypogonadism

Causes of hypogonadism are listed in Table 10.2

Primary gonadal failure: hypergonadotrophic hypogonadism

The primary abnormality is in the testes, and serum [testosterone] is reduced while gonadotro-

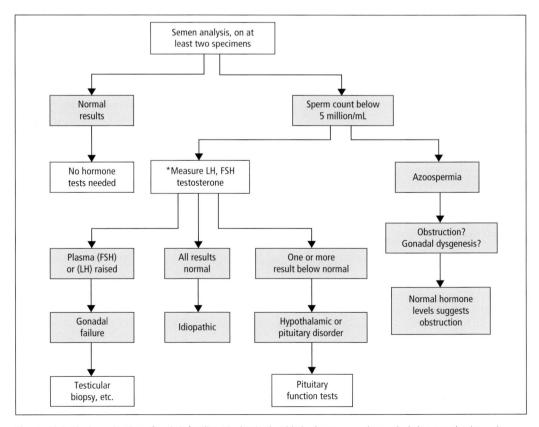

Figure 10.2 The investigation of male infertility. *Prolactin should also be measured to exclude hyperprolactinaemia.

phins are increased. This group of conditions includes congenital defects such as Klinefelter syndrome (usually 47XXY) and acquired lesions due to drugs, viruses or systemic diseases that affect testicular function. In some cases of abnormal spermatogenesis, FSH may be raised but LH and testosterone may remain normal.

Hypothalamic–pituitary disease: hypogonadotrophic hypogonadism

The primary abnormality is in the hypothalamus or the pituitary; the deficiency may be part of a generalised failure of pituitary hormone production. Serum gonadotrophins and [testosterone] are often both reduced, but in some cases gonadotrophins may remain within the reference range. Low testosterone is a common finding in those who have moderate to severe chronic or acute illnesses.

hCG, injected daily for several days, can be used to help differentiate between hypergonadotrophic (primary) and hypogonadotrophic (secondary) hypogonadism. A failure to show a rise in serum [testosterone] suggests inadequate Leydig cell function whilst an exaggerated response suggests secondary hypogonadism.

Disorders of male sex differentiation

Many conditions have been described, all rare. In some, the gonads degenerate; in others, there is an enzyme defect affecting steroid synthesis. In a third group, there is androgen resistance at the end organ, and a fourth group consists of the true hermaphrodites.

The testicular feminisation syndrome is inherited as an X-linked recessive, caused by a mutation in a gene coding for the androgen (testosterone) receptor, in which genetic (XY) males develop female secondary sexual characters; serum [testosterone] is abnormally high. In many of the other conditions, plasma [testosterone] is low, both in childhood and in adult life.

Erectile dysfunction (impotence)

This is most commonly caused by diabetes, neurological disorders, cardiovascular disease medication

such as β-blockers, alcohol abuse, thyroid disease, liver and renal disease and psychological problems. Testosterone deficiency and hyperprolactinaemia are uncommon causes of erectile dysfunction; such patients often complain of loss of libido. Patients with this condition should have glucose, lipids, thyroid function tests and renal function assessed in addition to testosterone and prolactin.

A common clinical problem is the patient with erectile dysfunction who has a slightly low testosterone and calculated free testosterone yet a 'normal' LH and FSH. A repeat blood sample should be taken between 8.30 and 11 am (since testosterone falls during the day) and if a low testosterone is confirmed an assessment of basal pituitary function should be carried out (Chapter 7). If no evidence of pituitary dysfunction is found some endocrinologists may still advocate a trial of testosterone replacement therapy; others argue that a fall in testosterone represents the normal pattern of ageing and would not give such therapy.

Andropause

In men, total and free testosterone concentrations tend to decline from about the age of 40. Whether this decline in testosterone is responsible for some of the functional changes that occur with age such as decreased muscle strength and decline in libido remains controversial. The long-term benefits and potential risks (e.g. prostate cancer) of testosterone treatment in older men are at present still being debated.

Gynaecomastia in males

Breast development occurring in males other than in the neonate or during puberty usually has a pathological cause. About 25% of cases of gynaecomastia are idiopathic but the principal endocrine causes are conditions that lead to an imbalance of oestrogen and androgens (Table 10.3). These include decreased androgen activity in hypogonadism and increased oestrogen production resulting from a variety of endocrine tumours; these tumours may synthesise oestrogens or secrete hCG, which then acts as a stimulus of oestrogen production. Thyrotoxicosis, hyperprolactinaemia, renal failure, liver failure and androgen resistance are other pathological causes that lead to an imbalance of oestrogens and androgens. Drugs account for about 20% of cases of gynaecomastia, and over 300 drugs have been reported as having the potential for producing the condition. Most drugs cause gynaecomastia by modifying the androgen/oestrogen ratio by direct or indirect mechanisms. In the elderly, mild gynaecomastia may commonly occur as a result of a decline in testosterone production.

Table 10.3 Some causes of gynaecomastia

Hypogonadism (primary or secondary)	Haemachromotosis
Drugs – including cannabis, methadone, cimetidine, phenothiazines, oestrogens	Tumours – including testicular, adrenal, bronchus, liver, haematological, etc.
Thyrotoxicosis	Chronic renal failure
Cushing's syndrome	Liver disease
Congenital adrenal hyperplasia	Hyperprolactinaemia

Over 300 drugs have been reported to cause gynaecomastia, and in many, the mechanism is uncertain.

Patients require full endocrine investigation, including measurement of serum oestrogens, androgens, gonadotrophins, prolactin, hCG and SHBG. Tests of liver, renal and thyroid function should also be performed and a full drug history taken.

Female gonadal function

Menstrual disorders and infertility

The changes that occur in normal menstrual cycles depend on cyclical variations in the output of FSH and LH, influenced by the output of GnRH (Figure 10.3). The effects of GnRH on LH and FSH release, in terms of the amounts secreted at different stages of the menstrual cycle, are strongly influenced by negative feedback control effects exerted by oestradiol-17β and progesterone.

The developing Graafian follicles in the ovaries respond to the cyclical stimulus of gonadotrophins by secreting two oestrogens, oestradiol and oestrone; these are metabolised to a third oestrogen, oestriol. After ovulation, the corpus luteum secretes progesterone as well as oestrogens. The changes in the uterus are determined by the

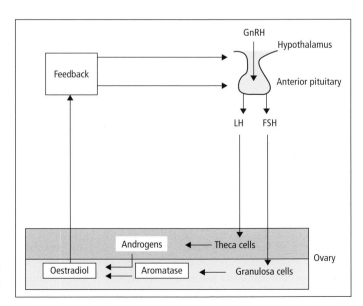

Figure 10.3 The hypothalamic–pituitary–ovarian axis. Activins, inhibins and progesterone also have a role in regulating the cycle.

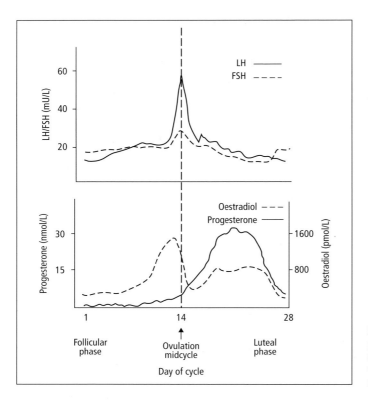

Figure 10.4 Cyclical changes in the plasma concentrations of the pituitary gonadotrophins and the principal ovarian steroid sex hormones in a normal 28-day menstrual cycle.

Table 10.4 Reference ranges in men and women for the plasma concentrations of the pituitary gonadotrophins and of the principal sex hormones

Hormone	Males	Menstruating female			
		Early follicular	**Mid-cycle**	**Luteal**	**Post-menopausal**
FSH (IU/L)	1.5–9.0	3.0–15.0	<20	3.0–15.0	30–115
LH (IU/L)	1.5–9.0	2.5–9.0	<90	2.5–9.0	30–115
Oestradiol (pmol/L)	<200	110–180	550–1650	370–700	<100
Testosterone (nmol/L)	10–30	0.4–3.0			

These values may vary between laboratories depending on the methods used.

ovarian steroid output at each stage. These changes are modified if pregnancy occurs.

Changes in plasma concentrations of FSH, LH and the principal gonadal steroids in the normal menstrual cycle (i.e. a cycle unmodified by oral contraceptives) are shown diagrammatically in Figure 10.4. Reference ranges for these hormones are given in Table 10.4, but these may vary slightly between laboratories.

Oestrogens act on several target tissues, including the uterus, vagina and breast; progesterone mainly acts on the uterus, and is essential for the maintenance of early pregnancy. Both oestrogens and progesterone are important in the control of the hypothalamic–pituitary–ovarian axis. Oestradiol may stimulate or inhibit the secretion of gonadotrophins, depending on its concentration in plasma; the stimulating effect of oestradiol can be prevented by high plasma [progesterone]. Inhibins and activins also play a role in regulating ovarian function and they change during the cycle; however, their measurement is not performed as part of routine investigation. Inhibin B originates from developing follicles while inhibin A is derived from the dominant follicle and corpus luteum.

Ovarian dysfunction and its investigation

The complex relationships between the hypothalamus, pituitary, ovary and uterus in controlling gonadal function mean that abnormality in any of these organs may cause abnormal menstruation and infertility. Other endocrine diseases (e.g. Cushing's syndrome, thyroid disease) and general ill-health or stress can also have these effects. The patient history may provide important clues as to the cause of the problem. The regularity of the cycle is an important determinant of the rate of conception. Oligomenorrhoea, defined as an interval between periods of more than 6 weeks but less than 6 months, is often due to polycystic ovarian syndrome (PCOS; see below). Amenorrhoea (no periods for >6 months) has many causes (Table 10.5). Details of general health and weight fluctuations are also important since weight loss is a common cause of amenorrhoea, while a large increase in body weight may precipitate PCOS. Presentation of amenorrhoea with galactorrhoea may suggest hyperprolactinaemia, although hyperprolactinaemia can occur without galactorrhoea. Menstrual disturbance with features of hyperandrogenism (hirsutism, acne, etc.) are often due to PCOS.

Oligomenorrhoea and amenorrhoea

Women with oligomenorrhoea or amenorrhoea may present because of concerns they have regarding their bleeding pattern, infertility, hirsutism, virilism or a combination of these.

Physiological causes of amenorrhoea (pregnancy, lactation) and anatomical abnormalities should first be excluded as the possible cause. Amenorrhoea may be primary, that is, the patient

Table 10.5 Endocrine causes of amenorrhoea and infertility

Site of lesion	Examples
Hypothalamus	Anorexia nervosa Severe weight loss Stress (psychological and/or physical) GnRH deficiency (Kallmann's syndrome) Tumours (e.g. craniopharyngioma, acromegaly)
Anterior pituitary	Hyperprolactinaemia Hypopituitarism Functional tumours (e.g. Cushing's disease) Isolated deficiency of FSH or of LH
Ovaries	PCOS Ovarian failure* Ovarian dysgenesis – Turner's syndrome Ovarian tumours
Receptor defect	Testicular feminisation syndrome
Other endocrine diseases	Diabetes mellitus Thyrotoxicosis Adrenal dysfunction (e.g. late-onset CAH)

* Ovarian failure may be autoimmune, chromosomal, iatrogenic (e.g. after cancer therapy) or idiopathic.

has never menstruated, in which case abnormal development is a likely cause, or secondary to various causes (Table 10.5). Investigation of primary amenorrhoea is required if the patient has reached the age of 16 and has undergone normal secondary sexual development or at the age of 14 if the patient has no breast development.

Measurements of plasma concentrations of prolactin, FSH, LH, oestradiol, TSH and FT4 are required. In addition, plasma testosterone should be measured if PCOS is suspected and other androgens such as androstenedione and DHEAS concentrations may need to be measured if there is hirsutism or virilisation. Figure 10.5 summarises one scheme for interpreting the investigations commonly performed in patients with menstrual abnormalities or who are infertile.

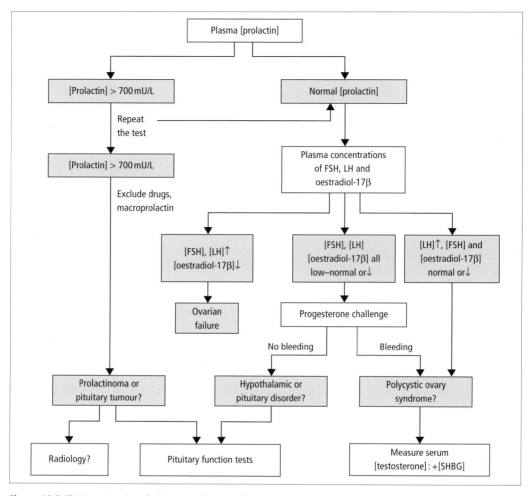

Figure 10.5 The investigation of oligomenorrhoea and amenorrhoea. It is assumed that other endocrine causes of these conditions (e.g. pregnancy, thyroid disease) have been excluded.

Plasma [prolactin] high This finding needs to be confirmed by repeating the investigation, and macroprolactinaemia should be excluded (p. 109). Even then, it must be interpreted with caution, since stress, certain drugs, hypothyroidism and chronic renal failure can all lead to marked elevations in plasma [prolactin] (see Table 7.2). About 20% of women with secondary amenorrhoea and ovulatory failure have *hyperprolactinaemia*; some of these patients have galactorrhoea. These patients may respond to treatment with dopamine agonists.

Plasma [prolactin] normal As indicated in Figure 10.5, the results from the measurement of plasma concentrations of FSH, LH and oestradiol-17β should then be interpreted.

1 *Plasma [FSH] and [LH] high, [oestradiol-β] low.* There is primary ovarian failure, due to a chromosomal abnormality, chemotherapy or autoimmune disease, or it may be due to a premature menopause.

2 *Plasma [LH] high, [FSH] and [oestradiol] normal or low.* The patient may have PCOS; a testosterone and FAI should be measured (discussed below).

3 *Plasma [FSH], [LH] and [oestradio] all low,* or at the lower limits of their reference ranges. Low BMI, stress, excessive exercise or the use of oral contraceptives should be first excluded as a cause. The patient may have hypothalamic, pituitary or other endocrine disease but, before this possibility is investigated, a progesterone challenge test should be performed.

In this test, the patient takes 5 mg of medroxyprogesterone daily for 5 days. Menstrual bleeding in the week following progesterone withdrawal indicates that there has been adequate priming of the endometrium by oestrogens; in these patients, PCOS may be the diagnosis.

4 *Plasma [LH], [FSH] low, [oestradiol] high.* This may be due either to sampling in the luteal phase or to pregnancy. A pregnancy test should be performed.

Infertility

Table 10.5 summarises the endocrine causes of infertility that may have to be considered, especially if there are also menstrual abnormalities. Once it has been established that the patient is not taking oral contraceptives, and that other endocrine diseases (e.g. diabetes mellitus, hypothyroidism) are not the cause of the infertility, investigation should proceed according to the schemes outlined in Figures 10.5 and 10.6, depending on whether or not the patient has normal menstruation.

In patients who menstruate normally (Figure 10.6), it is important to establish whether the cycles are ovulatory or anovulatory. In patients with a regular 28-day cycle, serum [progesterone] should be measured on one occasion between days 19 and 23 of the cycle, and the response in three separate cycles should be monitored. Patients who have long or short cycles should have serum [progesterone] measured in a sample collected 7 days prior to the expected onset of menses. If the serum [progesterone] is greater than 30 nmol/L, this indicates an ovulatory cycle, whereas levels less than 10 nmol/L strongly suggest anovulatory cycles. In patients who have a serum [progesterone] between 10 and 30 nmol/L and in whom the sample has been collected 7 days prior to onset of menses, it is thought that the cycles are ovulatory, but that there may be a defect in the luteal phase leading to decreased fertility. PCOS is the most common cause of anovulatory infertility.

The [FSH] measured in the early follicular phase (days 1–5 of the cycle) is often carried out in patients undergoing assisted conception, since an elevated [FSH] even in the presence of normal menstruation indicates diminished fertility.

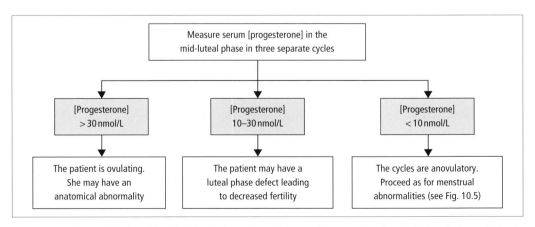

Figure 10.6 The investigation of female infertility in patients with normal menstrual cycles. In the luteal phase of a fertile ovulatory menstrual cycle, serum [progesterone] is normally >30 nmol/L. Note that samples must be taken 7 days prior to the expected onset of next menses.

Hirsutism and virilism

Hirsutism is a fairly common complaint among women. Most hirsute women have normal menstruation and no evidence of virilism. By itself, hirsutism rarely signifies an important disease, but it still requires investigation, because patients with ovarian or adrenal tumours have been described with normal menstrual cycles. Patients who have menstrual disorders in addition to hirsutism are more likely to have endocrine dysfunction.

Figure 10.7 outlines a scheme for the investigation of female hirsutism. Serum [testosterone] and [DHEAS] should be measured; in females, DHEAS is a specific adrenal product. Serum [androstenedione], an androgen originating from both the ovaries and adrenals, may also be measured. Most hirsute women have *idiopathic hirsutism* with normal levels of these steroids. Detailed investigation, however, may reveal evidence of androgen excess due, for instance, to low plasma [SHBG] accompanied by increased serum [free androgens], or to increased conversion of testosterone to 5α-DHT in the skin. Some laboratories will only measure [SHBG] when requested to do so, while others adopt a policy of reporting [SHBG] and an FAI with all total testosterone results.

A second group of hirsute women (Figure 10.7) have moderately increased serum [testosterone], 2.8–7.0 nmol/L, secondary to increased production by the ovaries or the adrenals, and often associated with menstrual irregularity. If the underlying cause is *late-onset CAH*, due to partial deficiency of 21-hydroxylase (p. 299), this can be confirmed by injecting tetracosactide (Synacthen, 250 mg IM) and measuring serum [17α-hydroxyprogesterone] 1 h later. In a patient with CAH, there will be an increase in serum [17α-hydroxyprogesterone] to

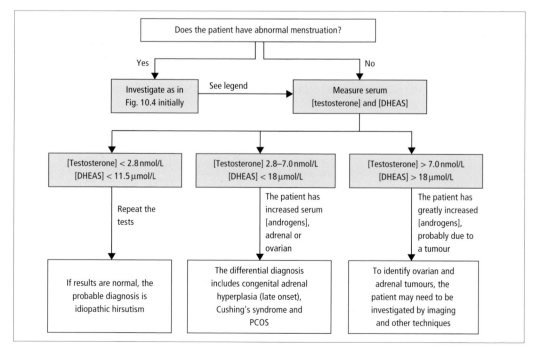

Figure 10.7 The investigation of hirsutism in females. Continue from Figure 10.5 if the results there indicate the need to measure serum [testosterone]. Reference ranges for testosterone and for DHEAS in females are, respectively, 0.8–2.8 nmol/L and 1.5–11.5 μmol/L.

more than twice the upper reference value. About 5% of hirsute women have late-onset CAH. *PCOS* (Stein–Leventhal syndrome) is a more common cause of hirsutism, with patients often having irregular menses, moderately increased serum [testosterone] and serum [DHEAS] with increased serum [LH] (see below).

A third group of hirsute women (Figure 10.7) have considerably increased serum [testosterone] and [DHEAS], and may show signs of virilism. Late-onset CAH should be excluded, as should rare causes of these abnormalities, for example ovarian or adrenal tumours.

If drug treatment is required for hirsutism, then Dianette is often given, which is effective in approximately 60% of cases. This is a formulation of cyproterone acetate (an anti-androgen) and ethinyloestradiol that suppresses secretion of gonadotrophins, reduces the secretion of ovarian androgens and also acts peripherally with anti-androgen actions. Other treatments include fluta-mide, finasteride and ketoconizole.

Polycystic ovarian syndrome (PCOS)

PCOS is very common, affecting approximately 20% of Caucasian women and more common in UK Asians. It is thought to arise during puberty, and 40% of cases are associated with obesity. The common features of PCOS are menstrual irregularities, infertility, signs of androgen excess and obesity. Although the classical profile of PCOS is that of hypersecretion of LH and androgens with normal concentrations of FSH, a wide spectrum of findings are seen and abnormalities in LH and androgens are not always present. In addition to establishing the diagnosis, it is also important to exclude disorders with similar presenting features such as CAH, Cushing's syndrome and androgen-secreting tumours. Most patients with PCOS have evidence of androgen excess but the measurement of total testosterone may not be as sensitive at detecting an abnormality as a measure of [free testosterone] such as the FAI. This is because in PCOS, the concentration of the SHBG often decreases, which in turn tends to decrease [total testosterone] and increase [free testosterone]. Androstenedione

and DHEAS may also be increased in some patients with PCOS. The absolute concentration of LH is increased in about 60% of women with PCOS while the LH/FSH ratio may also be elevated in over 90% of patients. Ultrasound often, but not always, shows the presence of cysts of 2–6 mm in the central stroma.

The cause of PCOS is unclear, but abnormalities in the adrenal, ovary, pituitary and in insulin resistance have all been suggested. Indeed the high prevalence of PCOS suggests that it may not be a single disease. Approximately 50% of women with PCOS have insulin resistance, and the ensuing hyperinsulinaemia can give rise to increased ovarian synthesis of testosterone and androstenedione. The high insulin also gives rise to reduced synthesis of SHBG and thus an increase in [free testosterone]. Impaired conversion of androgens to oestrogens in the ovary also leads to increased release of ovarian androgens. These androgens are then converted in adipose tissue by aromatase to oestrone that in turn inhibits the release of FSH and stimulates secretion of LH. These effects on the gonadotrophins tend to produce persistent anovulation and the excess LH also tends to stimulate androgen production from the theca cells, thus perpetuating the abnormalities. Figure 10.8 summarises how a cycle may be set up that tends to perpetuate the clinical problems. Clearly obesity is a risk factor since it may produce insulin resistance, and excess adipose tissue will increase oestrone production from androgens. Treatment of PCOS is directed towards interrupting the cycle by lowering LH levels with oral contraceptives, weight reduction in obese patients or enhancement of FSH production with clomiphene, etc.

The perimenopause, menopause and premature ovarian failure

Perimenopause and menopause

The perimenopause is defined as the time from the start of irregular menstrual cycles until at least 1 year after periods have ceased. This menopausal transition takes 2–8 years, with the menopause

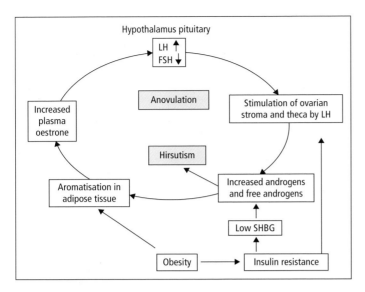

Hypothalamus pituitary

LH ↑
FSH ↓

Anovulation

Stimulation of ovarian stroma and theca by LH

Increased plasma oestrone

Hirsutism

Aromatisation in adipose tissue

Increased androgens and free androgens

Low SHBG

Obesity → Insulin resistance

Figure 10.8 Biochemical, metabolic and endocrine changes in PCOS. Treatment is aimed at breaking the cycle (see text).

occurring at an average age of about 51 years. The menopause can only be defined retrospectively when 12 months have elapsed since the last period. During the perimenopause, hormone levels in serum fluctuate erratically such that a single blood sample may not show biochemical evidence of the perimenopause. A raised serum [FSH] (>30 U/L) is the most consistent finding in the perimenopause but FSH is not invariably raised. Also women with raised FSH may continue to have further ovulatory cycles. Samples for FSH measurement should be collected if possible during the early follicular stage of the cycle. It is only later in the menopausal transition that oestradiol levels may become low. In most women, the perimenopause can be diagnosed clinically. In women over the age of 45 years with oligomenorrhoea or amenorrhoea, biochemical investigations will add little to the diagnosis of the perimenopause. Younger women with menstrual disturbances should be investigated as described earlier in this chapter. In summary (also see Figure 10.9):

- Consider whether an FSH result will actually help with clinical management.
- Provide the laboratory with the dates of the last menstrual period and if the woman is having periods take sample on days 1–5 of the cycle.

- FSH > 15 U/L on days 1–5 of the cycle is suggestive of ovarian failure or perimenopause.
- Random FSH > 30 U/L is highly suggestive of ovarian failure or perimenopause but could represent mid-cycle peak especially if the LH concentration is greater than that of FSH.
- Ovarian failure and perimenopause cannot be excluded by normal FSH levels as hormone levels fluctuate markedly in perimenopause.

Premature ovarian failure or 'premature menopause'

This refers to the occurrence of menopause before the age of 40 and may manifest itself in 1–3% of women. It may be due to genetic factors, autoimmune disorders, viral agents, chemotherapy, radiation therapy, surgery or exposure to toxic substances, or it may be idiopathic. While a normal menopause is an irreversible condition, about 50% of women with premature ovarian failure may have intermittent ovarian function and sometimes ovulate despite the presence of high gonadotrophin levels. The diagnosis of premature ovarian failure is made by finding persistently elevated serum [FSH] (>30 mU/L) on two or three occasions with samples taken 3–4 weeks apart. If premature

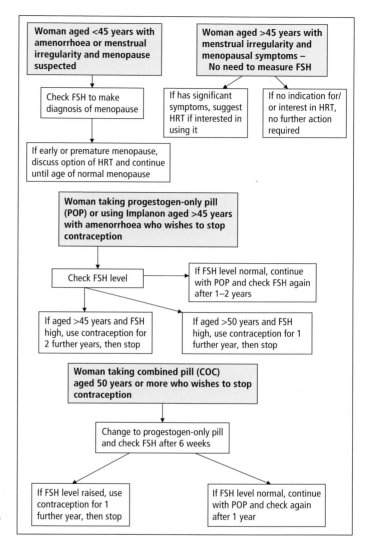

Figure 10.9 Diagnosis and management of the menopause.

ovarian failure occurs at a young age, a karyotype is often performed to identify chromosome abnormalities. There is a high prevalence of autoimmune disorders in premature ovarian failure, and additional tests may be advisable to rule out autoimmune disorders of the adrenal, parathyroid, thyroid, pancreas and GI tract. Annual follow-up to exclude these autoimmune disorders is also desirable. Risks associated with early menopause include osteoporosis and cardiovascular disease.

Some also advocate that androgen replacement should also be considered in women who are receiving hormone-replacement therapy (HRT) but who continue to experience fatigue and low libido.

Hysterectomy

Post-hysterectomy women are at risk of undergoing early menopause. Such patients should have

FSH measured annually or earlier if symptoms develop.

Hormone replacement therapy

In HRT, natural oestrogens are often used in combination with a progestogen. There is little place for the measurement of reproductive hormones in patients taking HRT because often such therapy does not suppress gonadotrophins to pre-menopausal levels and many of the natural oestrogens used are not detected by the specific assay used in the laboratory to measure oestradiol. The exception is perhaps the use of oestradiol measurements to check whether an implant containing oestradiol needs replacing; a serum [oestradiol] above 400 pmol/L suggests that the implant is still functioning. Oestradiol implants are more potent than natural oestrogens at decreasing gonadotrophin levels and may suppress LH and FSH into the pre-menopausal ranges. The effect on plasma lipids and other biochemistry and risk to the patient will depend on the particular preparation used and also on whether the hormones are given orally or as a dermal patch.

Steroid contraceptives

Combined oral contraceptives (COCs)

Ethinyl oestradiol in COCs can suppress LH and FSH to less than 15 U/L; thus primary ovarian failure cannot be excluded by the usual method of FSH testing. Patients aged 50 years or more who wish to stop contraception should be advised to change to a progestogen-only pill (POP) and check [FSH] after 6 weeks (Figure 10.9).

Progestogen-only pill (POP)

Women taking the POP or using implanon aged over 45 years with amenorrhea who wish to stop contraception should have their [FSH] measured. If [FSH] is less than 30 mU/L, the POP should be con-

tinued for a further 2 years and FSH re-checked. If FSH is more than 30 mU/L contraception should be continued for a further 2 years in women aged 45–50 years and a further 1 year in women aged over 50 years (Figure 10.9).

Young women who remain amenorrhoeic when they stop taking oral contraceptives may have premature menopause and should be investigated accordingly. Progesterone-only medications do not suppress FSH and LH to pre-menopausal levels; thus an FSH of less than 15 U/L makes primary ovarian failure unlikely in women who become amenorrhoeic when taking these medications.

Steroid contraceptives, principally those containing synthetic oestrogens, may cause diverse metabolic effects. For example, increases in plasma hormone-binding proteins and lipids may occur. Contraceptives that only contain progestogens are largely free from these effects. Progestogens largely oppose the effects of oestrogens; thus, in preparations containing combinations of oestrogen and progestogens, the net effect on the lipid profile and hormone-binding proteins, etc. will depend on the balance of these hormones in the individual preparations.

Keypoints

- Endocrine causes of infertility in the male are rare.
- Abnormal menstruation and infertility in women can arise from disease of the hypothalamus, pituitary, ovary, adrenal or thyroid.
- Pituitary and hypothalamic causes of abnormal menstruation and infertility in the female include stress, low BMI, hyperprolactinaemia and hypopituitarism.
- Ovarian causes of abnormal menstruation include polycystic ovary disease, ovarian failure and tumours.
- Hirsutism is common, and is usually idiopathic unless accompanied by menstrual disorder or virilism.
- In women over 45 years, biochemical investigations will add little to the diagnosis of the perimenopause.
- A single raised FSH should not be used as a guide to stopping contraception. Some women may continue to ovulate after a raised FSH level.

Case 10.1

A 17-year-old boy was investigated for delayed onset of puberty. There was nothing of note in his medical history, and he had not been receiving any drugs; his 14-year-old brother was already more advanced developmentally. The patient was on the twenty-fifth centile for height, and had poorly developed secondary sexual characteristics. There were no signs of endocrine disturbances. However, it was noticed that the patient had a poor sense of smell. Hormone investigations on blood samples gave the following results:

Serum	Result	Reference range
LH	1.2	1.5–9.0 U/L
FSH	<0.5	1.5–9.0 U/L
TSH	1.3	0.2–4.5 mU/L
FT4	17	9–21 pmol/L
Prolactin	200	<500 mU/L
Testosterone	2	10–30 nmol/L
Cortisol (8 am)	500	160–565 nmol/L

How would you interpret these results in light of the patient's history and clinical findings?

Comments: The findings suggest that the patient had hypogonadotrophic hypogonadism as the sole endocrine abnormality, but a combined test of pituitary functional reserve (p. 110) would be worth considering; it would provide information about growth hormone. The lack of a sense of smell is typical of Kallmann's syndrome, in which there is an isolated deficiency of GnRH. Stimulation with exogenous GnRH can be used both diagnostically and as treatment, but usually puberty is induced in these patients with sex steroids.

Case 10.2

A 17-year-old girl consulted her doctor because she was embarrassed about the amount of dark hair that was growing on her face. She told the doctor that her menstrual periods had never been regular (menarche age 13) and that she had not had a period for over 4 months. She was not pregnant. On examination, the doctor found that the patient was slightly overweight and had an extensive growth of dark hair on her lower abdomen (an escutcheon), as well as much dark hair on her upper lip, arms and legs. The patient was referred to an endocrinologist. After it was confirmed that the patient was not pregnant, the following hormones were measured in blood (reference ranges are for the early follicular phase, where relevant):

Serum	Result	Reference range
Prolactin	550	<500 mU/L
LH	23	2.5–9.0 U/L
FSH	2.0	3–15 U/L
Oestradiol	160	110–180 pmol/L
Testosterone	3.7	0.8–2.8 nmol/L
SHBG	27	30–120 nmol/L
Free androgen index	14	<7
Androstenedione	13	0.6–8.8 nmol/L
DHEAS	11	1.8–11.7 µmol/L
TSH	0.4	0.2– 4.5 mU/L
FT4	18	9–21 pmol/L

What do you think is the most likely diagnosis? What is your differential diagnosis?

(continued on p. 168)

Case 10.2 *(continued)*

Comments: This girl had the clinical and biochemical features of PCOS. The gonadotrophin pattern excludes hypogo-nadotrophic hypogonadism and ovarian failure as the cause of amenorrhoea (pregnancy had already been excluded). The testosterone concentration was high and the patient had a low SHBG giving a significantly elevated free androgen index. The androgens were not sufficiently high, however, to indicate that the patient had an androgen-secreting tumour. Late-onset CAH can present with all the features of PCOS, and could be excluded by measuring the 17-hydroxy-progesterone response to Synacthen stimulation.

Case 10.3

A 22-year-old secretary presented to her doctor complaining of a white, milk-like discharge from the nipple of each breast. She had had these symptoms intermittently for the previous month. On questioning, it was found that she had also been experiencing menstrual irregularities over the previous year, and had not had a period for at least 6 months. She was a non-smoker, and was not taking any medication.

Plasma [prolactin] was found to be markedly elevated at 1846 mU/L (reference range 60–390), and a second sample taken 2 weeks later showed a similar elevation at 1240 mU/L. Macroprolactin was not detected.

She was referred to an endocrinologist. The patient was clinically euthyroid, not pigmented and had normal secondary sexual characteristics. Visual fields were normal.

The following hormones were measured in blood:

Serum	Result	Reference range
Prolactin	1400	<500 mU/L
LH	1.6	2.5–9.0 U/L
FSH	3.5	3.0–15 U/L
TSH	2.2	0.2–4.5 mU/L
FT4	15	9–21 pmol/L

How would you interpret these results in light of the history and clinical findings? What further investigations should be performed?

Comments: The very high prolactin levels, accompanied by galactorrhoea and amenorrhoea, suggest the presence of a prolactinoma. In patients with a prolactin level >700 mU/L, stress, hypothyroidism and pharmacological causes of a raised prolactin level should be excluded, and the test should be repeated to confirm an elevated level. A CT or MRI scan of the pituitary should be performed in patients with unexplained hyperprolactinaemia. In this patient, a CT scan showed a possible low-density lesion in the anterior pituitary, which on an MRI scan was found to be a microadenoma. The patient was treated successfully with dopamine agonists.

Case 10.4

During investigations for infertility, a 27-year-old man was found to have azoospermia. On examination he he had bilateral gynaecomastia and firm but small testes. He also complained of fatigue and low libido. Results of blood tests were as follows:

Serum	Result	Reference range
Prolactin	300	<500 mU/L
LH	36	2.5–9.0 U/L
FSH	21	3.0–15 U/L
Testosterone	5	10–30 nmol/L
Oestradiol	280	<200 pmol/L
FT4	15	9–21 pmol/L
TSH	2.0	0.2–4.5 mU/L
Cortisol	400	nmol/L

What do these result suggest as regards the cause of the patient's infertility

Comments: The low testosterone with markedly raised LH and FSH suggest that the patient has primary gonadal failure (hypergonadotrophic hypogonadism). The most common cause is Kleinfelter syndrome. Chromosomal analysis in this patient showed he had karyotype 47XXY, confirming the diagnosis of Klinefelter syndrome. The disorder affects 1 in 500 men across all ethnic groups, but the diagnosis is often delayed because of substantial variation in clinical presentation. This patient was treated with regular injections of testosterone (200 mg of testosterone enanthate IM) which gave improvements in fatigue and libido. The couple were referred to an infertility clinic for artificial insemination with donor sperm.

Case 10.5

A 45-year-old shop assistant presented to her GP complaining of fatigue, weight gain, trouble sleeping, anxiety and hot flushes. Her periods were regular.

Her hormone profile was as follows, with the sample being taken at day 3 of her menstrual cycle.

Serum	Result	Reference range
Prolactin	500	<500 mU/L
LH	9.0	2.5–9.0 U/L
FSH	25	3.0–15 U/L
Oestradiol	120	110–180 pmol/L
TSH	6.5	0.2–4.5 mU/L
FT4	12	9–21 pmol/L

How would you interpret these results in light of the history and clinical findings?

Comments: The high FSH would be consistent with the perimenopause, which would also explain her symptoms. The thyroid function tests are consistent with subclinical hypothyroidism, but with such a modest elevation in TSH it is unlikely that this mild thyroid disorder is contributing to her clinical problems. The thyroid function tests should be repeated in 3 months time to exclude transient elevation of TSH. If the raised TSH were confirmed, the patient should have T4 therapy commenced if TSH became greater than 10 mU/L. For management of the menopause see Figure 10.9.

Chapter 11

Pregnancy and antenatal screening

Pregnancy is associated with many hormonal, physiological and metabolic changes. This chapter considers how the results of biochemical tests may be affected, how they may help in the diagnosis and management of some complications of pregnancy, and how biochemical tests are applied in antenatal screening programmes for the identification of pregnancies at risk of foetal neural tube defects (NTDs) and trisomy 21.

The foetoplacental unit

The placenta produces several proteins, including hCG and (human) placental lactogen. It also produces large amounts of steroid hormones and is the main source of progesterone during pregnancy.

Human chorionic gonadotrophin

There are several pregnancy-specific proteins, all of which normally originate in the trophoblast. The most commonly measured is hCG. Following synthesis, hCG is secreted into the maternal circulation. There is a surge in maternal [hCG] in early pregnancy, peak blood levels being reached at 12 weeks; thereafter, production of hCG rapidly

Lecture Notes: Clinical Biochemistry, 8e. By G. Beckett, S. Walker, P. Rae & P. Ashby. Published 2010 by Blackwell Publishing.

declines. hCG becomes detectable in urine about 10 days after conception, and this forms the basis of readily available pregnancy tests.

Trophoblastic tumours secrete hCG. These tumours can occur in males and females, and they include hydatidiform mole and choriocarcinoma, both of which may secrete hCG in very large amounts. A female who is found to be excreting hCG, and who is not pregnant, most frequently has a tumour of the trophoblast; in males, testicular teratoma is the most common source (p. 250).

Steroids in pregnancy

Oestrogens and progesterone are secreted by the corpus luteum during the first 6 weeks of pregnancy, but after this the placenta is the most important source of these steroids. Oestriol is the oestrogen produced in the greatest amounts, but oestradiol-17β and oestrone are also produced in large amounts. The placenta cannot synthesise oestriol *de novo*, but it can produce oestriol from C-19 adrenal steroids that are supplied by the foetal adrenal in the form of DHEAS. The oestriol produced in this way is secreted into the maternal and foetal circulation. Oestriol production thus requires the involvement of both the placenta and the foetus, and recognition of this interdependence led to the concept of the foetoplacental unit.

Effect of pregnancy on biochemical tests

Reproductive hormones

Serum [prolactin], [oestrogens] and [testosterone] show a steady increase in pregnancy, as does the concentration of SHBG. The concentrations of growth hormone and the pituitary gonadotrophins are decreased. However, some less specific methods for the measurement of LH may show cross-reaction with hCG, leading to apparent high LH levels.

Cortisol

There are large increases in serum [cortisol] due to increased serum [CBG], but the diurnal rhythm is retained. However, increased free and total cortisol levels in pregnancy may also be related to resetting of the sensitivity of the HPA axis and not merely to raised levels of CBG, progesterone or CRH. There is also an increase in serum [free cortisol] and in the 24-h urinary excretion of cortisol. This may be related to a resetting of the HPA axis and also the production of an ACTH-like substance by the placenta that is not completely suppressible by low- or high-dose glucocorticoids such as dexamethasone. This may help to explain why pregnant women often show intolerance of glucose and occasionally develop Cushingoid

features. These changes make the diagnosis of Cushing's syndrome difficult in pregnancy, and several variations in the work-up, when compared with non-pregnant women, may be required. An absence of diurnal variation is a useful clue to the diagnosis.

Thyroid function tests

During pregnancy, oestrogen production increases and TBG concentrations rise, leading to an increase in total T4 and total T3. There is also a large increase in the concentration of hCG, a hormone that has a mild stimulatory effect on thyroid hormone production. As a consequence, [FT4] and [FT3] may increase slightly during the early part of the first trimester, which, through the normal negative feedback loop, leads to a fall in serum TSH sometimes to undetectable concentrations. In the second and third trimesters, the serum [FT4] and [FT3] decrease and may fall below the reference range derived from non-pregnant women (Figure 11.1). The magnitude of this fall in free thyroid hormones is method dependent. After delivery, levels of thyroid hormones and TSH normally return to the pre-pregnant state. Trimester-related reference ranges should be applied for TSH and thyroid hormones if these are available; for free hormones, these reference ranges are also method dependent.

Figure 11.1 Changes in TSH, thyroid hormones, hCG and TBG in normal pregnancy. For TSH and thyroid hormones it is important to use gestational or trimester-related reference ranges. In some pregnancies TSH may fall to <0.1 mU/L in the first trimester. Total T3 and FT3 follow the same pattern as total T4 and FT4, respectively.

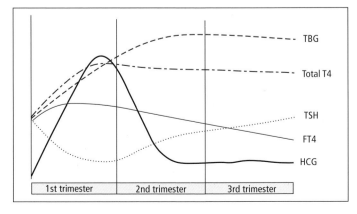

Plasma volume and renal function

During pregnancy, the plasma volume and GFR increase, sometimes by as much as 50%. This is accompanied by decreases in, for example, serum [sodium], [urea] and [creatinine].

Serum lipids and proteins

Serum [triglyceride] may increase as much as 3-fold in pregnancy; serum [cholesterol], LDL and HDL increase to a lesser extent. Serum [albumin] and [pre-albumin] fall because of the increase in plasma volume. Plasma [fibrinogen] and [ceruloplasmin] increase.

Liver function tests

In pregnancy, the placental isoenzyme of ALP is released, and total ALP activity in serum may rise to as much as three times non-pregnant levels. In contrast, the expansion of the extracellular fluid leads to a fall (~20%) in the activities of the transaminases and GGT and in the concentration of bilirubin.

Iron and ferritin

During pregnancy, increased maternal red cell synthesis and transfer of iron to the developing foetus cause a greater demand for iron. Unless iron supplements are given, iron stores generally fall, with accompanying falls in serum [ferritin] and plasma [iron], and rises in serum [transferrin] and total iron binding capacity (TIBC).

Complications in pregnancy

Ectopic pregnancy

In ectopic pregnancy, serum [hCG] fails to rise at the normal rate (approximately doubling every 2–3 days). If levels have failed to rise by 66% in 2 days, there is a 90% chance of an abnormal pregnancy. In practice, the diagnosis is made on a high index of clinical suspicion, qualitative pregnancy tests, ultrasound and, if indicated, laparoscopy.

Diabetes mellitus

Women with type 1 diabetes are at greater risk from both diabetic and obstetric complications during pregnancy. Rates of foetal and neonatal complications including late intrauterine death, foetal distress, congenital malformation, hypoglycaemia, respiratory distress syndrome and jaundice are also increased. To minimise these risks, it is essential that maternal glucose control and HbA_{1c} are optimised prior to conception and that tight control is maintained throughout pregnancy. Particular emphasis is placed on the need for careful home glucose monitoring (4–6 times a day) and intensive insulin regimens. Women should aim to maintain blood glucose and HbA_{1c} concentrations as near to the non-diabetic range as possible without excessive risk of hypoglycaemia. Type 2 diabetes is less common during the reproductive years, but its management during pregnancy should follow the same intensive pattern.

'Gestational diabetes mellitus' is the term used to describe the abnormal glucose tolerance or diabetes mellitus that may develop during pregnancy. It is particularly important to identify women with undiagnosed type 1 or type 2 diabetes mellitus as urgent action is required to normalise metabolism. The diagnosis of gestational diabetes mellitus is made on the basis of an OGTT. Glucosuria detected at routine antenatal testing may suggest the need for an OGTT, but may have no significance, since the renal threshold for glucose tends to be lowered in pregnancy. One approach is to screen women with appropriate risk factors, such as a family history of diabetes mellitus, or a previous large baby. Also, glucosuria is more significant if detected on the second specimen of urine passed after an overnight fast (i.e. the first specimen passed is discarded). Mild abnormalities should be reassessed not less than 6 weeks after delivery. In the majority of cases of gestational diabetes, the response to a GTT reverts to normal after the pregnancy, but about 50% of patients go on to develop diabetes mellitus within the next 7 years.

Thyroid disorders

Screening for thyroid disorders in pregnancy

The following categories of patient should have TSH **and** FT4 measured preferably prior to conception or, if not, at booking:

- Current thyroid disease
- Previous history of thyroid disease
- Family history of thyroid disease
- Goitre or other features of thyroid disease
- Type 1 and type 2 diabetes.

Management of thyroid disease requires close liaison between the GP, endocrinologist, obstetrician and community midwife.

Hypothyroidism

The developing foetal brain requires optimal thyroxine levels from early in the first trimester of pregnancy. The foetus relies on maternal thyroxine until 12 weeks gestation, when its own thyroid gland develops. Overt untreated hypothyroidism is associated with foetal loss, gestational hypertension, placental abruption, poor perinatal outcome and severe neurodevelopmental delay. The offspring of women with subclinical hypothyroidism, whose FT4 levels are in the lowest 10% of the reference range in the first trimester of pregnancy, have significant neurodevelopmental delays at the age of 2 years.

There is an increased requirement for T4 in pregnancy, and mothers with hypothyroidism are required to have the dose of T4 increased by 25–50 mg/day when pregnancy occurs. It is thus very important to ensure adequate thyroxine replacement from as early as 5 weeks gestation.

Assessing hypothyroidism in pregnancy

Ideally women with established hypothyroidism should be seen pre-pregnancy to ensure that they are euthyroid. They should also be encour-

aged to present as soon as they become pregnant in order that their thyroxine dose may be increased and TSH and FT4 are monitored regularly. The ideal monitoring regimen is to assess [TSH] and [FT4]:

- Before conception (if possible)
- At diagnosis of pregnancy or at antenatal booking
- Every 6–10 weeks with a minimum of at least once in each trimester
- 2–6 weeks postpartum.

Patients with previous Graves disease who have been rendered euthyroid or hypothyroid through radioiodine treatment or surgery must also have [TRAbs] measured early in pregnancy irrespective of the thyroid function test profile. *If TRAbs are undetectable* they do not need to be repeated. *If TRAbs are positive* the consultant obstetrician and consultant endocrinologist should be informed as a scan and possibly anti-thyroid medication may need to be given if the [TRAbs] is very high.

T4 replacement and pregnancy

T4 requirements increase by up to 50% by 20 weeks and then plateau. Thus:

- When pregnancy is confirmed the daily T4 dose should be increased by 25 µg and rechecked after approximately 2 weeks. Further dose increases may be required to achieve a satisfactory [FT4] (ideally [FT4] in the upper third of the reference range) and a TSH of 0.4–2 mU/L.
- Patients newly diagnosed with hypothyroidism whilst pregnant should have T4 treatment commenced immediately and be closely monitored to ensure an optimal [FT4] and [TSH] is achieved.
- TSH and FT4 should be monitored approximately every 6–8 weeks for the first 20 weeks. If the thyroid function tests are unstable, the patient should be seen by a consultant obstetrician and consultant endocrinologist as early as possible as growth scans may need to be performed in the third trimester.
- The T4 dose should be reduced to pre-pregnancy at 2–6 weeks postpartum and TSH and FT4 rechecked 6–8 weeks later.

Hyperthyroidism

All women with hyperthyroidism in pregnancy need to be seen by a consultant endocrinologist and a consultant obstetrician to ensure appropriate management.

Patients being treated with anti-thyoid drugs require careful monitoring during pregnancy as these drugs cross the placenta and can induce foetal hypothyroidism. Similarly, TRAbs in maternal blood also cross the placenta and may give rise to intrauterine and neonatal thyrotoxicosis if present in high concentration. For these reasons it is essential to identify new cases of Graves disease in pregnancy and also to assess [TRAbs] status preconception or at booking in patients with previous Graves disease irrespective of their current thyroid status.

Managing hyperthyroidism in pregnancy

The aim is for good control of hyperthyroidism on the minimum dose of carbimazole/propylthiouracil possible.

If TRAbs are positive the endocrinologists and obstetricians should be informed. Such women should be advised to deliver in hospital and be scanned at 32 weeks to assess foetal goitre. Paediatricians should be informed on the woman's admission to the labour ward and FT4 and TSH measured in cord blood taken to assess the thyroid status of the baby.

Hyperemesis gravidarum – undetectable TSH

Patients with hyperemesis gravidarum and some 'normal' pregnancies are associated with a mild transient 'physiological' hyperthyroidism during the first trimester due to the stimulatory action of high [hCG] on the thyroid. In approximately 3% of pregnancies the TSH in the first trimester will be suppressed to <0.01 mU/L and [FT4/FT3] may be slightly elevated. It is essential to exclude Graves disease in such pregnancies, and [TRAbs] should be measured and an endocrine and obstetric opinion sought if these are positive.

Postpartum thyroiditis

This occurs in 5% of women within 2–6 months of delivery or miscarriage. It presents with non-specific symptoms such as tiredness, anxiety and depression. Typically the patient will initially have a hyperthyroid hormone profile, which will resolve or be followed by a transient hypothyroidism neither of which usually require treatment. Occasionally, thyroid function may not return to normal after postpartum thyroiditis, and persistent hypothyroidism may require treatment with T4.

Postpartum patients should have thyroid function tests checked at 8–12 weeks if they have, symptoms of thyroid disease, goitre, previous history of postpartum thyroiditis or other autoimmune disorder.

If a hyperthyroid profile is found (i.e. TSH <0.01 mU/L; FT4/FT3 raised) an endocrine opinion is warranted to differentiate postpartum thyroiditis from other causes of hyperthyroidism such as Graves disease; a [TRAbs] measurement will be helpful for this.

Pre-eclampsia

Pre-eclampsia is a major cause of maternal and foetal morbidity and mortality, affecting approximately 3% of primagravidae. It usually develops during the third trimester, often after 32 weeks. The biochemical abnormalities that are most commonly of value in the diagnosis of pre-eclampsia are proteinuria, raised serum creatinine, abnormal liver function tests and a raised serum urate. These are usually found in association with hypertension.

At the antenatal clinic, urine specimens should also be routinely tested for protein. Proteinuria, if detected, may be the first evidence of pre-eclampsia and, as the condition worsens, proteinuria in excess of 1 g/24 h may occur. Patients with pre-eclampsia may develop impaired renal function with increasing serum [creatinine] and [urea] as the renal impairment worsens, or as a result of vomiting and dehydration. A serum [urea] of 7.0 mmol/L should be regarded as definitely abnormal, since plasma [urea] is normally reduced in pregnancy due to the increase in plasma volume.

Impaired renal function causes reduced tubular clearance of urate. Serum [urate] may be measured to assess the severity of pre-eclampsia and to provide an index of prognosis. A serum [urate] greater than 0.35 mmol/L before 32 weeks' gestation, or greater than 0.40 mmol/L after 32 weeks, is significantly raised.

Intravascular coagulation and hepatic ischaemia can result in the HELLP (Haemolysis, Elevated Liver enzymes and Low Platelets) syndrome which is seen in 4–12% of women with pre-eclampsia. Serum [LDH] may also increase as a result of haemolysis, and renal function tests may be abnormal.

Obstetric cholestasis

Obstetric cholestasis usually occurs in the third trimester of pregnancy and affects approximately 0.5% of all pregnancies in the UK. The prevalence varies between populations and it is thought to relate to a genetic predisposition resulting in increased susceptibility to environmental and hormonal factors, especially oestrogens. The foetus is at risk from intrauterine/perinatal death, foetal distress and spontaneous pre-term delivery.

While a prominent clinical feature is generalised pruritus, itching is common in pregnancy and it is important to distinguish obstetric cholestasis from other forms of liver disease. The most sensitive and important biochemical test is the measurement of serum bile acids which may be elevated by up to 100 times normal. However, there is no correlation between serum bile acid concentrations and foetal outcome. Most affected women will also have increased levels in at least one other liver function test. While bilirubin is raised only infrequently, modest elevations in transaminase levels (2- to 3-fold) or GGT may also be observed. Because of the presence of the placental isoenzyme, the reference range for ALP is so wide in the third trimester of pregnancy that its measurement contributes little to the diagnosis.

Pre-natal diagnosis of foetal abnormalities

Neural tube defects

The foetal liver begins to produce α-fetoprotein (AFP) from the sixth week of gestation, and the highest concentration of AFP in foetal serum occurs in the mid-trimester, after which it falls progressively until term. Amniotic fluid [AFP] increases steadily during early pregnancy, reaching maximum levels at 13–14 weeks and declining thereafter. In contrast, maternal serum [AFP] (MSAFP) continues to rise and peaks in the third trimester.

If the foetus has an open NTD, abnormal amounts of AFP are present in both amniotic fluid and maternal serum. [MSAFP] is measured as a screening test for NTDs, with a view to identifying those women who should be further investigated by detailed ultrasound examination. If the diagnosis of open NTD is confirmed, termination of pregnancy can be offered. Other causes of high [MSAFP] include multiple pregnancy and some rare, non-neurological foetal abnormalities (e.g. oesophageal or duodenal atresia, abdominal wall defects, renal anomalies).

The optimum timing for screening is 15–18 weeks of gestation when approximately 80% of NTD-affected pregnancies can be identified. False-negative results may be obtained with closed NTDs where the lesion is covered by a membrane. Because [MSAFP] varies throughout pregnancy, it is normally expressed as multiples of the median (MOM) for the relevant gestation age. Therefore, reliable dating of the pregnancy is essential for the correct interpretation of results.

Screening for trisomy 21

The overall incidence of trisomy 21 is approximately 1 in 800 pregnancies, and affected pregnancies can be identified by chromosome analysis of cells obtained at amniocentesis in the mid-trimester. The incidence of trisomy 21 varies greatly with maternal age; a 37-year-old woman has a chance of

1 in 250 of carrying an affected foetus at term, whereas for a woman aged 25 years, this is reduced to approximately 1 in 1100. However, since women aged over 35 years represent only 5–7% of total pregnancies, only 30% of Down's syndrome pregnancies can be detected by performing amniocentesis in this older group.

Abnormalities in a number of maternal serum analytes are associated with Down's syndrome pregnancies. These include decreased [MSAFP], [pregnancy-associated plasma protein A (PAPP-A)] and [unconjugated oestriol], and increased serum total [hCG], [free βhCG] and [inhibin A]. Each of these parameters shows overlap between trisomy 21 pregnancies and the normal population. However, if the distributions of the concentrations of these analytes for affected and normal pregnancies are known, a likelihood ratio for the chance of a foetus with trisomy 21 can be calculated. This is combined with the maternal age-related risk of trisomy 21 in order to calculate the overall probability that the pregnancy may be affected. Women with a high risk of carrying an affected child may then be offered amniocentesis.

Second trimester screening

Second trimester screening for trisomy 21 has now become an established part of obstetric practice. Protocols vary between centres but generally involve the measurement of [MSAFP] and either serum total [hCG] or [free βhCG]. These programmes usually achieve detection rates of approximately 60% for a false-positive rate of about 5%. The inclusion of serum [unconjugated oestriol] and [inhibin A] as additional markers improves screening performance by enhancing sensitivity and, importantly, reducing the number of false positives for a given detection rate.

First trimester screening

Screening may also be performed in the first trimester when risks are calculated using a combination of maternal age, biochemical measurements (maternal serum [free βhCG] and [PAPP-A]) and the ultrasonographic measurement of foetal nuchal translucency thickness, which is increased in trisomy 21 pregnancies. First trimester screening can yield detection rates of better than 80% for a false-positive rate of approximately 5%, and is likely to become firmly established as nuchal translucency measurements become more widely available.

Keypoints

- The impact of physiological changes must be taken into account when interpreting biochemical data in pregnancy.
- To minimise maternal and foetal risks in pregnant patients with diabetes, it is essential that maternal glucose control is optimised prior to conception and that tight control is maintained throughout pregnancy.
- It is important to recognise hypothyroidism early in pregnancy and institute immediate therapy with thyroxine. The dose of thyroxine required for adequate control in pregnancy is usually 25–50 µg/L higher than that required to control non-pregnant patients adequately.
- Hyperthyroid patients will also require careful monitoring and management during pregnancy. The measurement of TRAbs may be helpful in identifying situations where there may be a risk of intrauterine or neonatal thyrotoxicosis and also in differentiating Graves disease from hyperemesis gravidarum.
- The biochemical abnormalities that are most commonly of value in the diagnosis and monitoring of pre-eclampsia are proteinuria, raised serum creatinine, abnormal liver function tests and a raised serum urate.
- The most sensitive biochemical test for the diagnosis of obstetric cholestasis is the measurement of serum bile acids, which may be elevated by up to 100 times the normal value.
- Maternal serum AFP is used to screen for foetal NTDs, usually between 15 and 18 weeks gestation. If elevated concentrations are found, a detailed ultrasound scan is indicated.
- Second trimester screening for trisomy 21 is performed using maternal serum AFP, hCG and sometimes unconjugated oestriol and/or inhibin A.
- First trimester screening for trisomy 21 involves the measurement of free βhCG and PAPP-A with the ultrasonographic measurement of foetal nuchal translucency thickness.

Case 11.1

A 24-year-old housewife was 4 months pregnant when she consulted her doctor because she felt extremely uncomfortable in the current warm weather. She was concerned because, 20 years before, her mother had had similar symptoms and had been found to have Graves disease. Furthermore, she had read an article in a medical column in a magazine concerning the potential hazards to the foetus if the mother had Graves disease.

The patient showed no signs or symptoms of thyroid disease. However, the doctor decided to request the following thyroid function tests (reference ranges for TSH and free thyroid hormones relate to the second trimester of pregnancy):

Hormone	Result	Reference range
TSH	<0.01	0.06–3.4 mU/L
FT4	14	9–16 pmol/L
Total T4	190	70–150 nmol/L
FT3	4.5	3.2–6.2 pmol/L
Total T3	3.0	0.9–2.4 nmol/L
TRAbs	<1	<2.5 U/L

How would you interpret these results?

Comments: Serum [TSH] was below the limits of sensitivity of the assay. Undetectable TSH could be due to hyperthyroidism, but it could also be due to the mild thyrotrophic action of the high plasma [hCG] that is found in pregnancy.

Serum [TBG] increases in pregnancy. This causes increases in plasma [total T4] and [total T3] without, at the same time, causing raised levels of the free thyroid hormones. When interpreting results for serum [FT4] and [FT3] in pregnant women, it is important to use the appropriate trimester-related reference ranges. In this patient, the results for these analyses were both normal, and the TRAbs were not detectable in the patient's serum; thus Graves disease was not the cause of the low serum [TSH].

It was concluded that the undetectable TSH was due to the effects of hCG and the patient was reassured that she had a normal pregnancy. A repeat blood test 1 month later showed that TSH had become detectable as the hCG levels fell.

Case 11.2

Antenatal screening tests for NTDs and trisomy 21 were performed on a 34-year-old schoolteacher who was seen by the community midwives. The results were as follows:

Maternal age	33.9 years
Age-related chance of trisomy 21	1 in 533
Gestational age	17 weeks 4 days
Weight-adjusted maternal serum AFP MOM*	0.74
Weight-adjusted maternal serum hCG MOM*	2.09
Calculated chance of trisomy 21	1 in 189

* Result expressed as multiples of the median (MOM).

How would you interpret these results?

Comments: Serum [AFP] and [hCG] are expressed as MOMs for the appropriate gestational age. The relatively low AFP MOM indicates that the foetus is unlikely to be affected by an NTD (the normal action limit that triggers further detailed ultrasound investigation is 2 MOM).

(continued on p. 178)

Case 11.2 *(continued)*

In pregnancies affected by trisomy 21, the AFP MOM tends to be reduced and the hCG MOM increased. This pattern was observed in the current pregnancy. However, because there are no clearly defined cut-offs between unaffected and affected pregnancies, the overall chance that the pregnancy may be affected is calculated by modifying the maternal age-related risk using the likelihood ratios derived from the overlapping AFP and hCG distributions. If the combined chance is >1 in 250, amniocentesis and chromosomal analysis are offered.

In this woman, the chance that the foetus may be affected by trisomy 21 was increased to 1 in 189 when the biochemical markers were taken into account. She underwent amniocentesis, and chromosomal analysis indicated that the pregnancy was affected by trisomy 21.

Case 11.3

A 32-year-old woman, in her second pregnancy, was seen during the 29th week of gestation. She complained of pruritus which had increased in severity over the past 2 weeks, particularly affecting her palms and the soles of her feet. She had experienced intermittent epigastric pain and complained of nausea and vomiting. Her blood pressure was 135/78. The following biochemistry results were obtained:

Serum	Result	Reference range*
Urea	2.0	1.0–3.8 mmol/L
Creatinine	62	40–80 µmol/L
Bilirubin	10	3–14 µmol/L
ALT	131	10–40 U/L
GGT	79	5–44 U/L
Bile acids	178	<14 µmol/L

* Pregnancy-specific ranges

Comments: A provisional diagnosis of obstetric cholestasis was made in view of the elevations in serum bile acids and liver enzymes. This was confirmed following a negative liver ultrasound examination and after obtaining negative viral screens for hepatitis A, B and C, Epstein–Barr and cytomegalovirus, and negative liver autoimmune screens for chronic active hepatitis and primary biliary cirrhosis. The patient was treated with ursodeoxycholic acid and the pruritus and abnormal liver function tests resolved within 3 weeks. A healthy girl was born vaginally after induction at 38 weeks 2 days.

Chapter 12

Cardiovascular disorders

In this chapter we discuss biochemical tests in the diagnosis of acute coronary syndromes, and also in disorders of skeletal muscle. The use of a biochemical marker of heart failure is described. Cardiovascular risk factors, with a particular emphasis on lipids, are discussed, and the use of these risk factors to calculate an estimate of overall cardiovascular risk is described.

The diagnosis of myocardial infarction

The diagnosis of myocardial infarction has for the past two decades been based on WHO criteria which comprise a typical history of chest pain, the presence of diagnostic ECG abnormalities and a rise in biochemical markers. The presence of two or more of these three has defined the diagnosis. In recent years, this long-established definition has been overtaken by the advent of the troponins, which are more sensitive biochemical markers. Many studies have shown that troponins are released in some patients without conventional ECG changes of infarction, in particular elevation of the ST segment and T wave inversion. These patients are found to be at increased risk of subsequent cardiac events. This has given rise to the

Lecture Notes: Clinical Biochemistry, 8e. By G. Beckett, S. Walker, P. Rae & P. Ashby. Published 2010 by Blackwell Publishing.

concept of 'acute coronary syndromes', which comprise unstable angina with or without a rise in troponin, non-ST segment elevation myocardial infarction and ST segment elevation myocardial infarction. The use of troponin measurement thus potentially reveals biochemical changes that would not previously have been detected in patients with chest pain. This has major implications in the definition of myocardial infarction, and of course for the patients who may now be given this diagnosis, but who would formerly have been reassured that they had not had an infarct.

A task force drawn from a number of expert bodies has published a consensus 'Universal Definition of Myocardial Infarction' (see Further reading, p. 193). This places biomarkers central to the definition, requiring the detection of a rise and/or fall of a biomarker (preferably troponin). At least one troponin value should be above the 99th centile of a 'normal' population, and the assay should have an analytical performance at this level defined by a coefficient of variation of less than 10%. This is a challenging analytical standard that not all currently available assays meet. In addition there should be at least one of:
- symptoms of ischaemia
- ECG changes indicative of new ischaemia
- development of pathological Q waves in the ECG
- imaging evidence of new loss of viable myocardium or new regional wall motion abnormality.

This new definition is not yet universally adopted. There are implications for the laboratory in potential increases in testing and the analytical requirements, for cardiology services in the increase in patients receiving a diagnosis of myocardial infarction, and of course for patients (and their families, employers and insurers) receiving this diagnosis who would not previously have done so.

Biochemical tests in myocardial infarction and ischaemia

After myocardial infarction, a number of intracellular proteins are released from the damaged cells. The proteins of major diagnostic interest include:
• Troponin I and troponin T
• Enzymes, such as creatine kinase (CK), CK-MB, aspartate aminotransferase (AST) and lactate dehydrogenase (LDH)
• Myoglobin
• Ischaemia-modified albumin.
The troponins and CK will be considered in detail below, since they are the most widely established biochemical indices of myocardial damage, with the troponins largely taking the place of the enzymes in recent years. CK is, however, still widely used in some countries, and retains a use in the investigation of muscle disorders. Myoglobin is also a sensitive index of myocardial damage, and it

rises very rapidly after the event. However, it is non-specific, since it is raised following any form of muscle damage. It is not in wide laboratory use, but has a role in point of care analysers in the emergency setting. A negative result on an appropriately timed sample can be used to rule out myocardial damage and thereby determine early patient management. A positive result requires further investigation. Ischaemia-modified albumin is a new early and sensitive biochemical marker of myocardial ischaemia, but is non-specific and not widely available. Its role in patient management is yet to be determined.

Time-course of changes

After a myocardial infarction, the time-course of plasma biochemical markers always follows the same general pattern (Figure 12.1). After an initial 'lag' phase of at least 3h, during which levels remain normal, they rise rapidly to a peak between 18 and 36h, and then return to normal at rates that depend on the half-life of each marker in plasma. The biphasic response of troponins with a rapid rise and prolonged elevation, and the rapid rise and fall of CK and CK-MB activity should be particularly noted. In patients treated with thrombolytic agents, the general pattern of plasma marker changes shown in Figure 12.1 is slightly modified. Following successful thrombolytic therapy (e.g.

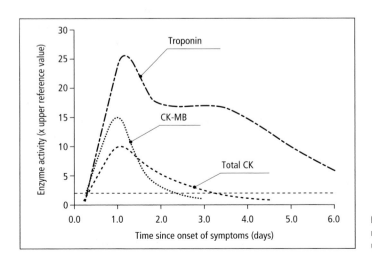

Figure 12.1 Patterns of biochemical markers in the first few days after an uncomplicated myocardial infarction.

Table 12.1 Time-course of plasma biochemical marker elevation after myocardial infarction

Enzyme	Abnormal activity detectable (h)	Peak value of abnormality (h)	Duration of abnormality (days)
Troponin T or I	4–6	12–24	3–10
CK-MB isoenzyme	3–10	12–24	1.5–3
Total CK	5–12	18–30	2–5
'Heart-specific' LDH	8–16	30–48	5–14

with streptokinase), there is a 'washout' of markers from the infarcted area, and levels rise rapidly to reach an early peak, at 10–18 h.

Optimal times for blood sampling

A sample taken on admission, if elevated, will make the required diagnosis, but if not elevated will not rule out the diagnosis if insufficient time has elapsed for a significant CK or troponin rise to have occurred. A sample taken between 6 and 12 h after the onset of symptoms will give more reliable results (Table 12.1).

Except for the occasional patient seen for the first time 2 days or more after the episode, in whom troponin measurements might still be useful, it is very rarely of any value to take samples for plasma markers after 48 h from the onset of symptoms that suggest a diagnosis of myocardial infarction.

Troponin

The troponin complex is exclusively present in striated muscle fibres and regulates the calcium-mediated interactions of actin and myosin. It comprises equimolar quantities of the structurally unrelated proteins troponin T, troponin I and troponin C. Troponin T binds tropomyosin; troponin I is an inhibitory protein and troponin C is responsible for binding calcium. Three distinct isoforms of troponin T and I exist, one each in slow twitch and fast twitch fibres of skeletal muscle, and one in cardiac muscle. These cardiac-specific forms of troponin can be recognised and measured in the plasma. There are two isoforms of troponin C, one found in slow twitch and cardiac muscle, and one in fast twitch muscle, so

there is not a troponin C species unique to myocardium.

In human heart the cardiac-specific troponin T and troponin I are largely insoluble, but 3–5% exists as a soluble cytoplasmic pool. Following cardiac myocyte necrosis, this soluble fraction probably accounts for the early rapid release of troponin into the circulation, and the slower release of the insoluble fraction accounts for the prolonged plateau of troponin release. The existence of the cardiac-specific isoforms of these troponins makes them the most specific of all the biochemical markers for cardiac damage. Under normal circumstances there is no cardiac troponin T or I detectable in the circulation by currently available assays, so any detectable rise is of significance, contributing to the high sensitivity of these tests. However, troponin may also sometimes be elevated in renal failure, severe heart failure and acute pulmonary embolism.

In general, although the initial rise in cardiac troponins after myocardial infarction occurs at about the same time as CK and CK-MB, this rise continues for longer than for most of the enzymes because of continuing release of 'insoluble' protein from the infarcted muscle. Cardiac troponin measurements are particularly useful in excluding the diagnosis of myocardial damage, particularly after 12 h following chest pain or other symptoms, and in patients who are likely to have concurrent cardiac and skeletal muscle damage.

Creatine kinase

There are three principal CK isoenzymes, each comprising two polypeptide chains, either B or M; these give the dimers BB, MB and MM.

- Skeletal muscle has a very high total CK content; over 98% normally comprises CK-MM and less than 2% CK-MB. CK-MB may rise to 5–15% in some patients with muscle disease, and also in athletes in training.
- Cardiac muscle also has a high CK content. It comprises 70–80% CK-MM and 20–30% CK-MB. As a general rule, cardiac muscle is the only tissue with more than 5% CK-MB. Before troponin analyses were widely available, CK-MB measurement was useful in confirming the cardiac origin of a raised CK.
- Other organs, such as brain, contain less CK, often CK-BB. However, CK-BB rarely appears in plasma and is not of diagnostic importance. Plasma normally contains more than 95% of its CK as CK-MM.

CK is used in the diagnosis of myocardial infarction and some muscle diseases (see below). Increases, sometimes large, may occur after trauma or surgical operations, IM injections, in comatose patients, in diabetic ketoacidosis, acute renal failure and hypothyroidism, and after prolonged muscular exercise, especially in unfit individuals.

Creatine kinase and muscle disease

Plasma CK, AST, LDH and ALT activities may be increased in muscle disease. However, plasma total CK is usually the measurement of choice, irrespective of the aetiology of the disorder, since it is increased in the greatest number of cases and shows the largest changes.

- *Muscular dystrophy* In Duchenne-type dystrophy, high plasma CK activity is present from birth, before the onset of clinical signs. During the early clinical stages of the disease, very high activities are usually present, but these tend to fall as the terminal stages of the disease are reached. Smaller CK increases are present in other forms of muscular dystrophy. About 75% of female carriers of the Duchenne dystrophy gene have small increases in plasma CK activity.
- *Malignant hyperpyrexia* This is a rare but serious disorder, characterised by raised body temperature, convulsions and shock following general anaesthesia. Many of the patients show evidence of

myopathy. Extremely high plasma CK activities are seen in the acute, post-anaesthetic stage, but smaller increases often persist and can also be detected in the relatives of affected patients. Pre-operative screening of plasma CK is not a reliable way of detecting patients liable to develop malignant hyperpyrexia, and should be limited to those patients with a family history of anaesthetic deaths or of malignant hyperpyrexia.

- *Miscellaneous muscle diseases* CK is variably increased in various myopathies, including that due to a side effect of treatment with β-hydroxy-β-methylglutaryl-coenzyme A (HMG-CoA) reductase inhibitor ('statin') cholesterol-lowering drugs. It is also raised in polymyositis.
- *Neurogenic muscle disease* Plasma CK activity is usually normal in peripheral neuritis, poliomyelitis and motor neuron disease.

CK-MB isoenzyme

CK-MB is a more sensitive and specific test for myocardial damage than total CK. Its use has been largely overtaken by the widespread availability of troponin measurement. If troponin measurement is not readily available, plasma CK-MB measurements (preferably by a mass measurement method) are the best alternative. Measurement of CK alone is no longer recommended because of its lack of specifity.

CK-MB is available on some point of care analysers.

The diagnosis of heart failure

Heart failure is a complex clinical condition in which the heart's ability to pump is compromised by one or more of a number of underlying conditions, commonly ischaemic heart disease, but also heart valve abnormalities. The prognosis is poor if untreated, with a 2-year survival rate of under 50%.

The diagnosis of heart failure can be difficult, especially since the usual presenting symptoms such as breathlessness or ankle swelling are common and can be due to many different conditions. Physical examination is neither sensitive nor specific for heart failure, even in expert hands,

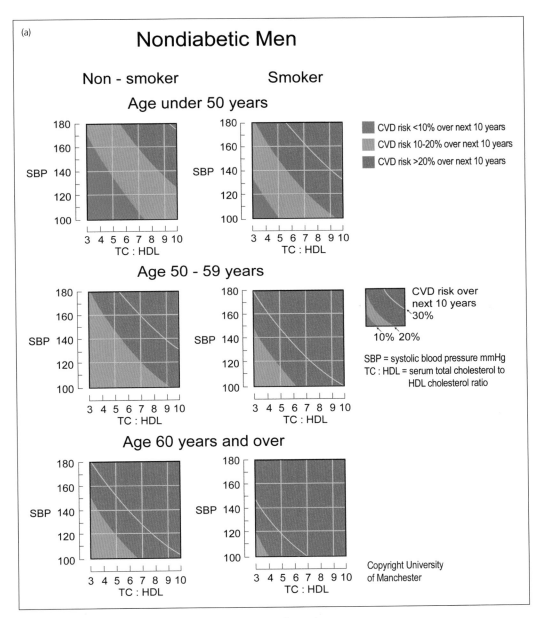

Figure 12.3 Cardiovascular risk prediction charts (Williams et al. 2004).

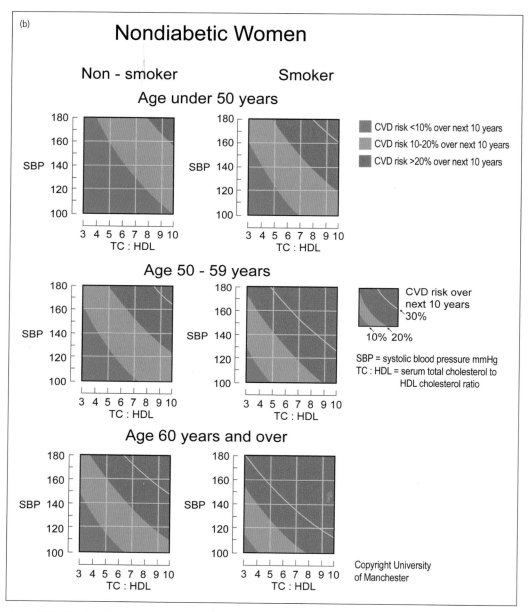

Figure 12.3 (Continued)

with incorrect diagnoses in up to 50% of patients. The definitive diagnosis is best made by echocardiography, but access to this may be limited or delayed. BNP is a neurohormone secreted by cardiac myocytes in response to volume expansion and pressure overload, and plays a role in circulatory homeostasis. In heart failure the level of BNP increases, enabling differentiation of cardiac and pulmonary causes of breathlessness. It has an evolving role in the diagnosis of heart failure in both primary care and the emergency setting, since it costs considerably less than echocardiography, and the result can be available much more rapidly.

Laboratory and point of care assays for BNP and for the inactive peptide N-terminal-proBNP (NT-proBNP) are available, and provide qualitatively similar information. Their accuracy is greatest in patients with more severe disease and poorest in those already receiving treatment. Levels rise with age, so age-related cut-offs should be used.

A number of other conditions can cause elevated BNP levels but, in a patient who is not on heart failure treatment, if levels are below the cut-off level then heart failure is highly unlikely, and the patient should be investigated for other conditions. If the level is elevated the patient should proceed to further assessment, including echocardiography. The introduction of this strategy has the potential to speed up accurate diagnosis of heart failure, and to save money by restricting the use of echocardiography to those patients most likely to benefit from its use.

The diagnosis of thromboembolic disease

Laboratory investigations have a part to play in the investigation of possible thromboembolic disease. As the fibrinolytic system breaks down clots formed of cross-linked fibrin, degradation products are produced, including D-dimers. Under normal circumstances these are not detectable in the circulation, but are present in thromboembolic disease and in disseminated intravascular coagulation. Measurement of D-dimer levels is used in the diagnosis (or, more accurately, exclusion) of thromboembolic disease such as deep venous thrombosis

(DVT) and pulmonary embolism (PE). In carefully selected patients at relatively low risk of DVT or PE, a normal result can effectively rule out these conditions, avoiding the need for more expensive and time-consuming imaging techniques. Careful clinical assessment is needed, since false-positive results are possible in non-thrombotic pathologies such as neoplasia, recent surgery, myocardial infarction and trauma.

Both laboratory and point of care tests are available for D-dimers and can help in the immediate management of patients presenting with symptoms or signs suggestive of DVT or PE, since a negative result offers reassurance. A positive result will require further investigation.

Cardiovascular risk factors

Many factors are associated with or cause increased cardiovascular risk. These can pragmatically be divided into those which cannot be influenced and those which can be influenced and reduction of which has been demonstrated to reduce risk. Those that cannot be influenced include a family history of premature vascular disease, age and pre-existing vascular disease. Those whose modification has an established role include cigarette smoking and hypertension (not considered further here), diabetes (see Chapter 6) and the hyperlipidaemias, especially hypercholesterolaemia. Lipid metabolism and the hyperlipidaemias are covered in some detail below, followed by a description of how cardiovascular risk is assessed and treated. Other novel biochemical markers of vascular risk are briefly described.

Lipids

Lipids act as energy stores (triglycerides) and as important structural components of cells (cholesterol and phospholipids). They also have specialised functions (e.g. as adrenal and sex hormones). The main lipids, being insoluble in water, are transported in plasma as particulate complexes with proteins, the lipoproteins.

From the clinical viewpoint, it is the strong relationship between plasma lipid levels and the incidence of ischaemic vascular disease, particularly of the coronary arteries, that is of major importance. In the following section, we outline:

- The biochemistry of the main body lipids.
- The mechanisms for lipid transport in plasma.
- The importance of lipids, and other factors, in the pathogenesis of arterial disease.
- The role of plasma lipid measurements in the management of hyperlipidaemia and in cardiovascular risk reduction.

Cholesterol

This is a steroid that is present in the diet, but it is mainly synthesised in the liver and small intestine, the rate-limiting step being catalysed by HMG-CoA reductase. Cholesterol is a major component of cell membranes, and acts as the substrate for steroid hormone formation in the adrenals and the gonads. It is present in plasma mainly esterified with fatty acids. The body cannot break down the sterol nucleus, so cholesterol is either excreted unchanged in bile or converted to bile acids and then excreted. Cholesterol and bile acids both undergo an enterohepatic circulation.

Triglycerides

These are fatty acid esters of glycerol, and are the main lipids in the diet. They are broken down in the small intestine to a mixture of monoglycerides, fatty acids and glycerol. These products are absorbed, and triglycerides are resynthesised from them in the mucosal cell. Most of these exogenous triglycerides pass into plasma as chylomicrons (see below).

Endogenous triglyceride synthesis occurs in the liver from fatty acids and glycerol. The triglycerides synthesised in this way are transported as VLDL (see below).

Fatty acids

These are mostly straight-chain monocarboxylic acids. They are mainly derived from dietary or tissue triglyceride, but the body can also synthesise most of them, apart from certain polyunsaturated

(essential) fatty acids. Fatty acids act as an alternative or additional energy source to glucose.

Phospholipids

These have a structure similar to triglycerides, but a polar group (e.g. phosphorylcholine) replaces one of the three fatty acid components. The presence of both polar and non-polar (fatty acid) groups gives the phospholipids their characteristic detergent properties. Phospholipids are mainly synthesised in the liver and small intestine; they are important constituents of cells, and are often present in cell membranes.

Lipoproteins

Cholesterol and its esters, triglycerides and phospholipids are all transported in plasma as lipoprotein (Table 12.2) particles. Fatty acids are transported bound to albumin.

Lipoprotein particles comprise a peripheral envelope, consisting mainly of phospholipids and free cholesterol (which each have both water-soluble polar and lipid-soluble non-polar groups) with some apolipoproteins, and a central non-polar core (mostly triglyceride and esterified cholesterol). The molecules in the envelope are distributed in a single layer in such a way that the polar groups face out towards the surrounding plasma, while the non-polar groups face inwards towards the lipid core in which the insoluble lipids are carried. Most lipoproteins are assembled in the liver or small intestine. Five main types of lipoprotein particle can be recognised:

1 Chylomicrons are the principal form in which dietary triglycerides are carried to the tissues.

2 VLDLs are triglyceride-rich particles that form the major route whereby endogenous triglycerides are carried to the tissues from the liver and, to a lesser extent, from the small intestine.

3 Intermediate-density lipoproteins (IDLs or 'VLDL remnants') are particles formed by the removal of triglycerides from VLDLs during the transition from VLDLs to LDLs.

4 LDLs are cholesterol-rich particles, formed from IDLs by the removal of more triglyceride and apoli-

Table 12.2 Properties of the five main classes of lipoproteins

Property	Chylomicrons	VLDL	IDL	LDL	HDL
Physical properties					
Diameter (nm)	100–500	30–80	25–30	20–35	5–10
Density (kg/L)	<0.95	<1.006	1.006–1.019	1.019–1.063	>1.063
Electrophoresis	Stay at origin	Pre-β	β	β	α_1
Lipoprotein composition (approximate percentages)					
Triglyceride	90	65	35	10	5
Cholesterol	5	20	40	50	35
Phospholipid	5	10	15	20	35
Protein	1	5	10	20	25
Apolipoprotein composition*	C, B, E, (A)	C, B, E, (A)	B, (C, E, A)	B	A, C, E, (B)

* The main apolipoprotein components are listed in descending order of amount (trace components in parentheses).

poprotein. Increased plasma [LDL cholesterol], and hence plasma [total cholesterol], is positively correlated with the incidence of ischaemic heart disease.

5 HDLs act as a means whereby cholesterol can be transported from peripheral cells to the liver, prior to excretion. Increased plasma [HDL cholesterol] is negatively correlated with the incidence of ischaemic heart disease, presumably explained by its role in transporting cholesterol from the periphery.

6 A sixth type of lipoprotein particle, Lp(a), is synthesised in the liver and has about the same lipid composition as LDL (see below). The physiological role of Lp(a) is not known. Plasma [Lp(a)] is positively associated with the incidence of ischaemic heart disease, independently of other lipoprotein fractions. The effect may be due to competition between Lp(a) and plasminogen for endothelial cell receptors, thereby inhibiting thrombolysis.

The apolipoproteins

The protein components of the lipoproteins, the apolipoproteins, are a complex family of polypeptides that promote and control lipid transport through the circulation and lipid uptake into tissues. They are separable into four main groups (apoA, B, C and E), some of which may be subdivided, and apo(a).

- *ApoA* is synthesised in the liver and intestine. This is initially present in chylomicrons in lymph, but rapidly transfer to HDL.
- *ApoB* is present in plasma in two forms, $apoB_{100}$ and $apoB_{48}$. $ApoB_{100}$ is the protein component of LDL, and is also present in chylomicrons, VLDL and IDL. $ApoB_{48}$ (the N-terminal half of $apoB_{100}$) is only found in chylomicrons. $ApoB_{100}$ is recognised by specific receptors in peripheral tissues (see below).
- *ApoC*. This family of three proteins (apoC-I, apoC-II and apoC-III) is synthesised in the liver and incorporated into HDL.
- *ApoE* is synthesised in the liver, incorporated into HDL and transferred in the circulation to chylomicrons and VLDL. There are three major isoforms (apoE2, apoE3 and apoE4) at a single genetic locus, giving rise to several genotypes (E3/3, E2/3, E2/4, etc.). ApoE is probably mainly involved in the hepatic uptake of chylomicron remnants and IDL; it binds to apoB receptors in the tissues.
- *Apo(a)* is present in equimolar amounts to $apoB_{100}$ in Lp(a). It has a high carbohydrate content and has a similar amino acid sequence to plasminogen.

Enzymes involved in lipid transport

Four enzymes of relevance to clinical disorders need to be described:

185

• Lecithin cholesterol acyltransferase (LCAT) transfers an acyl group (fatty acid residue) from lecithin to cholesterol, forming a cholesterol ester. In plasma, this reaction probably takes place exclusively on HDL, and may be stimulated by apoA-I.

• Lipoprotein lipase is attached to tissue capillary endothelium and splits triglycerides (present in chylomicrons and VLDLs) into glycerol and free fatty acids. Its activity increases after a meal, partly as a result of activation by apoC-II, which is present on the surface of triglyceride-bearing lipoproteins.

• Hepatic lipase has an action similar to that of lipoprotein lipase.

• Mobilising lipase, present in adipose tissue cells, controls the release of fatty acids from adipose tissue into plasma. It is activated by catecholamines, GH and glucocorticoids (e.g. cortisol), and inhibited by glucose and by insulin.

Metabolism of plasma lipoproteins

The above description of the lipoproteins and apolipoproteins is an oversimplification, and the following points should be emphasised:

• Plasma lipids and apolipoproteins exist in a dynamic state. There is interchange of lipids both between different lipoprotein particles and with tissues.

• There is considerable variation in the size and composition of individual lipoprotein particles within each lipoprotein class.

Chylomicron metabolism

Chylomicrons (Figure 12.2) are formed in the intestinal mucosa after a fat-containing meal, and reach the systemic circulation via the thoracic duct. They then transfer apoA to HDL and acquire apoC and apoE from HDL. The apoC-II activates lipoprotein lipase in the tissues, and triglycerides are progressively removed from the hydrophobic core of the chylomicrons. As the size of the particles decreases, the more hydrophilic surface components (apoC, unesterified cholesterol and phospholipid) transfer to HDL. The triglyceride-poor chylomicron remnants are taken up by the liver, where they are catabolised.

VLDL and IDL metabolism

Most VLDL is secreted into plasma by the hepatocytes ('endogenous' VLDL), but some originates from the intestinal mucosa ('exogenous' VLDL) (Figure 12.2). Hepatic VLDL synthesis is increased whenever there is increased hepatic triglyceride synthesis, for example when there is increased transport of fatty acids to the liver, or after a large carbohydrate-containing meal.

When first produced, VLDL consists mainly of triglycerides and some unesterified cholesterol, with $apoB_{100}$ and lesser amounts of apoE. ApoC-II is then acquired, mainly from HDL, and triglycerides are removed from the VLDL 'core' in a manner analogous to that for chylomicrons. The residual particles are known as 'VLDL remnants', or IDLs, which are either rapidly converted to LDL or removed from the circulation to the liver.

LDL metabolism

LDL probably all arises from VLDL metabolism in man. The LDL particles are rich in cholesterol esters, probably derived from HDL; $apoB_{100}$ is the only apolipoprotein. LDL is removed from the circulation by two processes; one regulated, the other unregulated.

• The *regulated mechanism* involves the binding of LDL to specific $apoB_{100}$ receptors present on the 'surface pits' of hepatocytes and other peripheral tissue cells. The entire LDL particle is incorporated into the cell by invagination of the cell membrane. Inside the cell, the particle fuses with lysosomes; apoB is then broken down and the cholesterol esters are hydrolysed, thereby making unesterified cholesterol available to the cell. The size of the intracellular cholesterol pool regulates:

  • The rate of cholesterol synthesis in the cell, through the effect of cholesterol on HMG-CoA reductase.

  • The number of LDL-apoB receptors on the cell surface.

• The *unregulated mechanism* involves receptor-independent mechanisms of cholesterol uptake by cells; these are present particularly in macrophages.

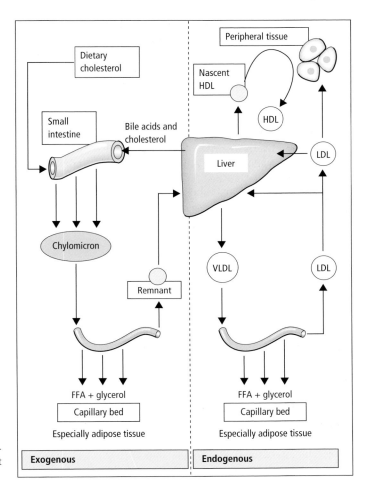

Figure 12.2 Endogenous and exogenous triglyceride metabolism (see text for details).

These mechanisms are brought into operation especially when plasma [cholesterol] is increased.

HDL metabolism

This heterogeneous group of particles is formed in the liver and intestinal mucosa. The HDL particles then undergo fairly complex exchanges of lipid and protein with other plasma lipoproteins. However, the main point to note is that free cholesterol in tissues transfers to HDL in plasma. The cholesterol is then esterified by LCAT and transferred to LDL, which, in turn, is mainly taken up by the liver (see above). Thus,

HDL forms the principal route whereby cholesterol can return from peripheral tissues to the liver.

Investigation of plasma lipid abnormalities

Most laboratories measure plasma [total cholesterol], [HDL cholesterol] and [triglycerides]. Further tests to characterise the lipoprotein abnormalities may be indicated in a few patients. The investigations are mainly of value in the investigation and management of ischaemic vascular disease.

Plasma total cholesterol

Diet, for example recent meals, does not affect plasma [cholesterol] much in the short term. This means that random [cholesterol] can be measured to assess cardiovascular risk. Plasma [cholesterol] is affected by both within-individual and between-individual factors. However, these tend to be long-term effects, as follows:

- *Diet* The amount and the composition of dietary fat affect plasma [cholesterol]. In particular, those fats containing mainly polyunsaturated fatty acids, such as those in fish and vegetable oils, tend to lower plasma [cholesterol], whereas those fats containing mainly saturated fatty acids, such as animal fat and butter, tend to raise plasma [cholesterol]. Dietary fibre may have a small effect in lowering plasma [cholesterol]. The consumption of 1–3 units of alcohol per day causes a significant rise in plasma [HDL cholesterol]. Dietary cholesterol intake has relatively little effect on plasma [cholesterol].
- *Exercise* Regular exercise tends to cause a rise in plasma [HDL cholesterol] and a small fall in plasma [total cholesterol].
- *Age* In developed countries, plasma [cholesterol] rises with age. This is probably related to diet.
- *Sex* In pre-menopausal women, plasma [total cholesterol] is lower than in men, and plasma [HDL cholesterol] is higher. These differences disappear after the menopause.
- *Race* It is likely that the marked racial differences, with particularly high plasma [cholesterol] in north Europeans, are mainly due to dietary and environmental factors rather than genetic differences.

Numerous studies have shown that the incidence of ischaemic heart disease is directly correlated with plasma [cholesterol], even within the 'reference range'. There is no clear cut-off between values for normal risk and increased risk, although risk rises particularly rapidly above about 6.5 mmol/L. Because of this association, it is inappropriate to employ reference ranges for plasma [cholesterol] in the usual way, as these imply health without increased risk of disease. Instead, it seems more appropriate to define a desirable concentration (e.g. <5 mmol/L).

Plasma [total cholesterol] is a rather unsatisfactory measurement, since it represents the sum of the various ways in which cholesterol is transported in plasma. In fact, although raised plasma [LDL-cholesterol] is associated with an increased risk of ischaemic heart disease, raised plasma [HDL-cholesterol] is associated with a decreased risk of ischaemic heart disease and seems to have a protective effect.

Plasma triglycerides

Plasma [triglycerides] also show variations with age and sex, but more especially with diet. There is, in addition, a very considerable within-individual variation, which makes interpretation of a single result difficult.

Plasma LDL

Plasma [LDL] can be measured by ultracentrifugation, but this is not a practical technique for routine clinical laboratory use. The following formula can be used to calculate [LDL] if the measurements were made on a fasting sample:

[LDL cholesterol] = [total cholesterol] – [HDL cholesterol] – [triglyceride]/2.2

where all measurements are in mmol/L. This formula assumes the absence of chylomicrons since the sample was taken in the fasting state, and therefore the total cholesterol is distributed between LDL, HDL and VLDL. The molar ratio of triglyceride to cholesterol in VDL is 2.2, as long as the [triglyceride] is less than 4.5 mmol/L. The formula is therefore not valid if [triglyceride] is greater than 4.5 mmol/L.

LDL exists in a range of sizes and densities. There is evidence that the small dense subfractions of LDL are particularly atherogenic. There are no readily available routine laboratory methods for examining LDL subfractions, but surrogate markers for the presence of these small dense LDL species are low or low-normal [HDL] and high or high-normal [triglyceride]. This combination is sometimes referred to as an 'atherogenic lipid profile'. Measurement of apoB levels may provide similar information.

Specimen collection

It is important to collect specimens for plasma lipid and lipoprotein studies under the appropriate conditions:
• The patient should have been leading a normal life in terms of diet (including alcohol consumption) and exercise for at least the previous fortnight.
• Blood specimens should be collected after an overnight fast of 10–14h, if triglyceride measurements are to be performed.
• Venous stasis should be minimal.
Results of plasma lipid and lipoprotein investigations can be misleading in specimens collected during or within a few weeks after a serious illness (e.g. a myocardial infarction or a major operation). They often then show reduced plasma [cholesterol] and sometimes hypertriglyceridaemia. However, specimens collected within 24h of a myocardial infarction will still be representative of [cholesterol] before the infarction.

Routine investigations

One or more of the following investigations should be requested in patients suspected to be at increased risk of ischaemic heart disease or of a lipid disorder:
• Plasma [cholesterol]. This may be sufficient, if decisions about secondary prevention of cardiovascular disease are to be made (see below).
• Plasma [HDL-cholesterol], if plasma [cholesterol] is raised or if additional risk factors are present. This can be used to calculate the [cholesterol] : [HDL cholesterol] ratio, which correlates well with cardiovascular risk and which is used in a number of methods developed to calculate overall cardiovascular risk in making decisions about primary prevention of cardiovascular risk (see below). It is also needed for the diagnosis of hyper-a-lipoproteinaemia (see below).
• Plasma [fasting triglycerides]. This is a weak independent risk factor for cardiovascular disease, a risk factor for acute pancreatitis if greater than 10mmol/L, and is used in the calculation of [LDL].

Specialised investigations

A large number of specialised investigations, including ultracentrifugation, apolipoprotein and enzyme studies and molecular genetic studies, may occasionally be helpful.

The primary hyperlipoproteinaemias

The causes of hyperlipoproteinaemia (Table 12.3) are complex, and different disease mechanisms can give rise to similar lipid patterns. The approach

Table 12.3 The primary hyperlipoproteinaemias (genetic classification)

Hyperlipoproteinaemia	Concentrations in plasma		Lipoproteins mainly affected
	Cholesterol	Triglycerides (fasting)	
Familial hypercholesterolaemia	↑↑	N (or ↑)	LDL
Familial hypertriglyceridaemia	↑ or N	↑↑	VLDL (and chylomicrons)
Familial combined hyperlipidaemia	↑ or N	↑ or N	LDL and/or VLDL
Remnant hyperlipoproteinaemia	↑	↑	IDL and chylomicron remnants
Lipoprotein lipase deficiency (or apoC-II deficiency)	↑ or N	↑↑	Chylomicrons and VLDL

adopted here will be primarily descriptive, based on the observed lipid abnormalities.

Increased plasma lipid concentrations may be due to:

1 Genetic factors.
2 Environmental factors.
3 A combination of the above.
4 Other diseases (secondary).

Primary hypercholesterolaemia

In about 95% of patients with primary hypercholesterolaemia, the abnormality is due to a combination of dietary factors and a number of yet to be identified genetic abnormalities in handling cholesterol.

In the minority of patients who have familial hypercholesterolaemia, there is a specific genetic defect in the production or nature of high-affinity tissue $apoB_{100}$ receptors (or in the structure of the $apoB_{100}$ itself, so that it is not recognised by the normal receptor). Heterozygotes have about 50% of normal receptor activity, and homozygotes have no receptor activity. Many heterozygotes have tendon xanthomas, and over 50% will have symptoms of coronary artery disease by the fourth or fifth decade. In homozygotes, heart disease often presents in the second decade. Plasma [cholesterol] is usually raised to 8–15 mmol/L in heterozygotes, and is even higher in homozygotes.

Familial hypertriglyceridaemia

This group of conditions is associated with defects either in the production or in the catabolism of VLDL. Plasma [triglycerides] and [VLDL] are increased but, whereas plasma [cholesterol] is often also moderately increased, plasma [HDL] is often reduced. Patients have an increased risk of ischaemic heart disease.

In some patients, there is chylomicronaemia in addition to increased plasma [VLDL]. This pattern may be brought on by alcohol excess, and is also seen in diabetics. These patients may have eruptive xanthomas and attacks of acute pancreatitis.

Familial combined hyperlipidaemia

This disorder is difficult to classify, and the method of inheritance is unclear. Even in the same family, the gene does not always express itself in the same way, as there may be increased plasma [LDL] only, increased plasma [VLDL] only, or increases in both. The incidence of ischaemic heart disease is 3–4 times greater than in the general population.

Remnant hyperlipoproteinaemia

This is an uncommon disorder characterised clinically by cutaneous xanthomas and a high risk of premature ischaemic heart disease. In the plasma, there is an increase in cholesterol-rich but otherwise VLDL-like particles; these are probably IDLs (i.e. 'VLDL remnants'). Both plasma [cholesterol] and [triglycerides] are increased; plasma [LDL] is decreased.

This disorder is probably due to a combination of factors. There is abnormal conversion of VLDL to LDL. This is usually associated with the apoE2/2 genotype. However, since as many as 1% of normal individuals have this genotype, whereas the incidence of remnant hyperlipoproteinaemia is only about 1 in 5000, the genotype is insufficient in itself to cause remnant hyperlipoproteinaemia.

Remnant hyperlipoproteinaemia responds well to treatment with fibric acid derivatives (e.g. fenofibrate), so its recognition is important. Ultracentrifuge studies provide the definitive means of confirming the diagnosis.

Lipoprotein lipase deficiency

This is a rare autosomal recessive disorder causing hypertriglyceridaemia and chylomicronaemia. The incidence of ischaemic heart disease and acute pancreatitis is increased; eruptive xanthomas often occur. The primary defect is deficiency of either lipoprotein lipase or its activator, apoC-II.

Treatment involves restriction of normal dietary fat and replacement by means of triglycerides containing fatty acids of medium chain length (C8–C11); these are less prone to lead to chylomicron formation.

Other inherited defects

Hyper-α-lipoproteinaemia is an inherited abnormality, giving rise to increased plasma [HDL] and mildly increased plasma [cholesterol]. Patients have a *reduced* incidence of ischaemic heart disease. The only importance of hyper-a-lipoproteinaemia is that no treatment is required for the raised plasma [cholesterol].

Secondary hyperlipidaemia

Probably less than 20% of cases of hyperlipidaemia are secondary to other disease. Patterns of abnormality tend to vary, even within a single disease; plasma [cholesterol] or [triglycerides], or both, may be affected.

- *Hypercholesterolaemia* is often a marked feature of hypothyroidism and of the nephrotic syndrome; in these two disorders, there is increased plasma [LDL]. It also occurs in cholestatic jaundice, but in this condition there is an accumulation of abnormal discoid particles rich in phospholipid and unesterified cholesterol, and an additional abnormal lipoprotein – lipoprotein X – is detectable. Coronary artery disease tends to develop in those patients with long-standing secondary hyperlipidaemia. The immunosuppressive drugs ciclosporin and tacrolimus also cause hypercholesterolaemia.
- *Hypertriglyceridaemia*, secondary to other disease, is most commonly due to diabetes mellitus or to excessive alcohol intake. It may also occur in chronic renal disease and in patients on oestrogen therapy, protease inhibitors or retinoids.

The effects of alcohol on plasma lipids are complex. Regular drinking of small amounts increases plasma [HDL] without affecting other lipoprotein particles. Some heavy drinkers develop hypertriglyceridaemia due to increased plasma [VLDL], possibly as a result of increased direction of fatty acid metabolism into triglyceride synthesis in the liver.

The hyperlipidaemia secondary to diabetes mellitus is also complex. Increased plasma [VLDL] is the usual finding, but often plasma [LDL] is also increased, whereas plasma [HDL] is reduced.

The primary hypolipoproteinaemias

Three rare familial diseases require brief mention. Their recognition has helped with the understanding of normal lipoprotein metabolism.

- *Tangier disease* is due to an increased rate of apoA-I catabolism. Only traces of HDL are detectable in plasma, and plasma [LDL cholesterol] is also reduced. Cholesterol esters accumulate in the lymphoreticular system, probably due to excessive phagocytosis of the abnormal chylomicrons and VLDL remnants that result from the apoA-I deficiency.
- *Abetalipoproteinaemia* is associated with a complete absence of apoB. The lipoproteins that normally contain apoB in significant amounts (i.e. chylomicrons, VLDL, IDL and LDL) are *absent* from plasma. Plasma [cholesterol] and [triglycerides] are very low.
- *Hypobetalipoproteinaemia* is due to decreased synthesis of apoB. Plasma [VLDL] and [LDL], although reduced, are not absent.

Secondary hypolipidaemia

Greatly reduced plasma [cholesterol] occurs whenever hepatic protein synthesis is depressed, as in protein-energy malnutrition (PEM; e.g. kwashiorkor in children), severe malabsorption or some forms of chronic liver disease.

Other biochemical cardiovascular risk factors or markers

Very high levels of homocysteine, up to 50-fold normal, are seen in homocystinuria, an inborn error of metabolism due to deficiency of the enzyme cystathionine β-synthase. Patients develop ocular, skeletal and vascular problems, with increased arterial and venous thrombotic events at an early age, and a markedly increased mortality. Lowering homocysteine in this group of patients has been demonstrated to lower the risk of cardiovascular disease.

Much lesser elevations in homocysteine levels are associated with an increased risk of cardiovascular disease, with patients in the upper quartile having twice the risk of patients in the lowest quartile, possibly through mechanisms involving endothelial damage and the promotion of thrombosis. However, the precise relationship remains unclear, and raised [homocysteine] may yet prove to be simply a marker of increased vascular risk rather than a causative risk factor. Homocysteine levels are strongly influenced both by genetic factors and by diet. Folic acid and vitamins B_6 and B_{12} are involved in the catabolic pathways of homocysteine, and deficiencies of these vitamins can cause elevation of [homocysteine] and supplementation can cause its reduction. So far, controlled trials of the effect of supplementation of these vitamins on the development or recurrence of cardiovascular disease have had equivocal or negative results. Because of this the precise role of [homocysteine] measurement remains unclear. However, it may be measured in individuals with a personal or family history of cardiovascular disease in the absence of the conventional well-established risk factors such as hypercholesterolaemia or hypertension. Finding a high [homocysteine] under these circumstances provides a possible explanation, and can reinforce advice to ensure that the diet contains adequate amounts of folic acid and vitamins B_6 and B_{12}.

Patients with CRP, an inflammatory marker (see p. 242), at the high end of the normal range (measured with a highly sensitive assay, hsCRP) have 1.5–4 times the cardiovascular risk of those with CRP at the low end of the normal range. This has been demonstrated both in apparently healthy individuals and in patients with established vascular disease. The origin of this increased CRP can be speculated to be endothelial inflammation in association with atherosclerotic plaques. Treatment of patients with statins results in a reduction of hsCRP. The role of hsCRP measurement is not yet established, and it is not yet recommended for widespread use. It may, however, complement use of conventional major risk factors, especially in patients at moderate risk of vascular disease, in whom the finding

of an elevated hsCRP might reinforce the need for treatment.

Calculation of cardiovascular risk and its treatment by lipid lowering

It is possible to lower plasma [LDL cholesterol] by dietary and other lifestyle means, but the most effective therapy, usually leading to reductions of up to 30% or more, is achieved by HMG-CoA reductase inhibitors ('statins'). It is this class of drug that has mainly been used in the clinical trials mentioned below.

It is conventional to consider cardiovascular risk reduction under the subdivisions of 'secondary prevention' (where the patient has established vascular disease, and the goal is to prevent recurrence); and 'primary prevention' (where the patient has no overt vascular disease, and the goal is to prevent its development). Multiple sets of guidelines have been published, differing to a greater or lesser extent in detail. These all essentially agree on the division into primary and secondary prevention; on the risk factors that should be treated; the concentration of primary prevention on those at greatest overall vascular risk; and the therapeutic options available. However, the precise thresholds and targets for treatment continue to evolve. The most recent British guidelines are those published by the 'Joint British Societies' (2005) and by the National Institute for Health and Clinical Excellence (NICE) (2008) (see Further reading).

In patients with previous myocardial infarction or with angina, trial results are conclusive. Pre-existing vascular disease is the most potent risk factor for the development of further vascular disease, and the size of the population requiring treatment is relatively limited. Cholesterol reduction by about 25% reduces all-cause mortality by 30% and cardiac events by over 40%. Lifestyle interventions to discontinue smoking, adopt a healthy diet and to take exercise are important, but should not delay lipid-lowering therapy. Guidelines suggest that virtually all patients with established vascular disease should be treated with lipid-lowering drugs, irrespective of baseline cholesterol levels. The goal is to achieve a cholesterol less than 4 mmol/L or an LDL-cholesterol less than 2 mmol/L and if this is not achieved more potent statins or higher dioses should be used.

In primary prevention, large-scale clinical trials have shown that cholesterol lowering (by an average 20%) in hyperlipidaemic men can reduce cardiovascular death and non-fatal myocardial infarction by about 30%. The available evidence strongly supports the concept that those who will benefit most from treatment are those at greatest overall absolute risk. Someone with multiple modestly elevated risk factors may be at a greater risk than someone with a single markedly elevated risk factor. This means that there is a need for a means of calculating overall risk. The guidelines achieve this by the use of computer-based risk calculators or charts which stratify risk on the basis of sex, age, smoking, blood pressure and the cholesterol : HDL-cholesterol ratio (Figure 12.3, see plate section). An important caution is that these calculations do not apply to patients with inherited dyslipidaemias. An absolute risk derived from these charts of 20% or more for the development of cardiovascular disease over the next 10 years is sufficient to justify treatment. Guidelines disagree on whether there is a cholesterol target in primary prevention similar to that in secondary prevention, or whether the aim is simply to ensure that all eligible patients are treated, with simvastatin 40 mg being recommended by NICE.

Further reading

British Cardiac Society; British Hypertension Society; Diabetes UK; HEART UK; Primary Care Cardiovascular Society; Stroke Association (2005) JBS2: Joint British Societies' guidelines on prevention of cardiovascular disease in clinical practice. *Heart*, **91**, 1–52.

National Institute for Health and Clinical Excellence (2008) *NICE clinical guideline 67: Lipid modification: Cardiovascular risk assessment and the modification of blood lipids for the primary and secondary prevention of cardiovascular disease*. NICE.

Thygesen, K., Alpert, J.S. and White, H.D. (2007) Universal definition of myocardial infarction. *Journal of the American College of Cardiologists*, **50**, 2173–95.

Keypoints

- The diagnosis of acute myocardial infarction is made on the basis of a rise and/or fall in troponin above a defined level plus one of symptoms of ischaemia, ECG evidence of new ischaemia, development of pathological Q waves on the ECG or myocardial imaging information.
- In myocardial infarction, biochemical markers usually become raised after a lag period of 4–6 h after the onset of symptoms, reach a peak at 18–30 h and have returned to normal within 3–7 days.
- Measurement of [BNP] can assist in the diagnosis of heart failure.
- The main lipids of clinical importance in plasma are cholesterol and triglyceride. These are insoluble in water and are transported in plasma as protein–lipid complexes known as lipoproteins. The principal lipoproteins in plasma are chylomicrons, VLDLs, LDLs and HDLs.
- Increased plasma [cholesterol] and [triglyceride], whether primary or secondary to other diseases such as diabetes, are associated with an increased risk of arterial disease, particularly coronary atheroma leading to myocardial infarction.
- Reduction of raised plasma [cholesterol] leads to a reduced incidence of heart disease in those treated, but treatment is best targeted at those at highest overall risk.

Case 12.1

A 66-year-old man had experienced central chest pain on exertion for some months, but in the afternoon of the day prior to admission he had had a particularly severe episode of the pain, which came on without any exertion and lasted for about an hour. On admission there were no abnormalities on examination and the ECG was normal. The troponin was clearly detectable.

Comment on these results. Has he suffered a myocardial infarction?

Comments: He has an elevated troponin plus a typical history. This is sufficient to diagnose a myocardial infarction by the most recent definition, even in the absence of ECG changes.

Case 12.2

A well-trained marathon runner collapsed as he was approaching the finishing line. An ECG was normal, but CK was elevated at 9500 U/L (reference range 30–200 U/L), and the CK-MB was 14% of the total CK (normally <6%). Troponin was undetectable. Comment on these results.

Comments: The total CK is substantially elevated, and CK-MB >6% can usually be taken to mean that it is of myocardial origin. However, the normal ECG and troponin are both reassuring. In trained endurance athletes, the proportion of CK-MB in muscle increases from the normal low levels and may be as high as 10–15%. An elevated CK-MB in such individuals can no longer be taken to imply a cardiac origin for the raised CK. Extreme exercise, especially in unfit individuals, causes an elevated CK, potentially to very high levels.

Case 12.3

A 28-year-old man requested cholesterol testing because his father had died of a myocardial infarction in his thirties, his paternal grandfather had developed angina in his early forties and died suddenly in his late forties, presumably of an infarction, and there was a further history of ischaemic heart disease at a young age in his more extended family. The GP noted that he had tendon xanthomas on his knuckles and on his Achilles tendons. He took plenty of exercise, followed a healthy diet and was not overweight, did not smoke and was normotensive.
  Comment on the history and the following results:

Serum	Result	Reference range
Cholesterol	10.6	mmol/L
Triglyceride	1.4	0.6–1.7 mmol/L
HDL	1.9	0.5–1.6 mmol/L
Cholesterol : HDL	5.6	
LDL cholesterol	8.1	mmol/L

Comments: The family history and lipid results make familial hypercholesterolaemia the likely diagnosis here, and this is confirmed by the finding of tendon xanthomas. These are accumulations of cholesterol on the tendons, which are virtually pathognomonic of familial hypercholesterolaemia. The exercise he took probably accounted for the slightly high HDL, giving him an apparently quite favourable cholesterol:HDL ratio. This, with his relatively young age, the fact he did not smoke and his normal blood pressure, would give him a relatively satisfactory calculated cardiovascular risk. However, these calculations do not apply in patients with familial hypercholesterolaemia, who are at a considerably higher than calculated risk. He merits treatment with lipid-lowering drugs.

Case 12.4

A 33-year-old man was referred to the lipid clinic with a cholesterol of 10.2 mmol/L. He had a vague memory of having his cholesterol checked at a medical examination at work in his early twenties, and thought it had been normal at that time. He had been dieting for the last few months and had succeeded in losing ~3 kg, but his cholesterol had not changed. Over the preceding 2 years he had felt tired, and stressed by his work. His GP felt that he was depressed, and had been treating him with anti-depressants with little benefit. He had stopped playing football, and his muscles ached on exertion. He had put on 20 kg over this period.
  Comment on the following results:

(continued on p. 195)

Case 12.4 *(continued)*

Serum	Result	Reference range
Cholesterol	10.2	mmol/L
Triglyceride	1.1	0.6–1.7 mmol/L
HDL	1.0	0.5–1.6 mmol/L
TSH	256	0.2–4.5 U/L
FT4	<6	9–21 pmol/L
CK	12,330	30–200 U/L
Na	129	132–144 mmol/L

Comments: He has an extremely high [cholesterol] which has not improved with diet, and if his recollections were accurate had previously had a normal [cholesterol]. This raises the question of a secondary hypercholesterolaemia. He has certainly put on weight, which may increase lipids, but not usually to this extent. His symptoms of weight gain, tiredness and depression raised the possibility of hypothyroidism, and this was confirmed by his profoundly hypothyroid thyroid function tests. Hypothyroidism can also cause a myopathy, with aching muscles and very high CK, and a dilutional hyponatraemia. He thus had a full range of the biochemical abnormalities that may be seen in hypothyroidism! Treatment with thyroxine resulted in a dramatic improvement in all his symptoms apart from the muscle aching, which still persisted 6 months later. [Cholesterol] came down to a satisfactory 4.6 mmol/L without the need for any lipid-lowering medication. CK and sodium returned to normal.

Chapter 13

Liver disease

The liver plays a key role in intermediary metabolism, including the synthesis of carbohydrates, lipids and many proteins. It exchanges substances with the plasma, adding some for distribution in the body and removing others, often with subsequent metabolism. The liver is the organ mainly responsible for the detoxification of many drugs and carcinogens; it also secretes bile salts.

Liver disease is relatively common, and the measurements of serum levels of bilirubin, hepatic enzymes and albumin, as well as the prothrombin time (PT), provide simple tests to determine whether disease is present and give some guidance as to its nature.

This chapter outlines the principles governing the use and interpretation of the common liver function tests.

Structure of the liver

Only about 80% of the cells in the liver are hepatocytes (Figure 13.1); the remainder are endothelial (Kupffer) cells lining the hepatic sinusoids and vascular and supporting tissue cells. The *functional unit* of each liver acinus consists of the portal tract, surrounded by radiating cords of hepatocytes. Blood enters the acinus via the portal tract and

Lecture Notes: Clinical Biochemistry, 8e. By G. Beckett, S. Walker, P. Rae & P. Ashby. Published 2010 by Blackwell Publishing.

passes along the sinusoids towards the central vein. Hepatocytes in the periportal area, zone 1, receive relatively well-oxygenated blood, whereas the hepatocytes surrounding the central vein, zone 3, receive blood that has lost much of its oxygen and exchanged other substances with the cells of zones 1 and 2. Cells in zone 3 are the most susceptible to anoxia and injury by a wide range of toxic substances.

Cells in zone 1 have relatively high concentrations of the enzymes usually measured in blood for diagnostic purposes (e.g. ALP and the aminotransferases ALT and AST), while cells in zone 3 are relatively deficient in these enzymes. This may help to explain why some patients with centrilobular liver damage may have normal serum enzyme activities.

Liver function tests

Most laboratories perform a standard group of tests (Table 13.1), which do not assess genuine liver function but are useful for:

1 Detecting the presence of liver disease.

2 Placing the liver disease in the appropriate broad diagnostic category. This then allows the selection of further, more expensive and time-consuming investigations such as ultrasound, CT scanning, magnetic resonance spectroscopy, endoscopy and liver biopsy,

3 Following the progress of liver disease.

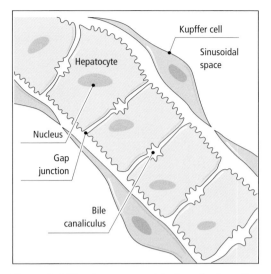

Figure 13.1 The ultrastructure of the liver. The liver ultrastructure mainly consists of hepatocytes and Kupffer cells (part of the reticuloendothelial system). The bile canaliculus is formed by the plasma membrane of two hepatocytes.

Table 13.1 Routine liver function tests (examples of widely performed groups of serum measurements)

Standard group of tests	Property being assessed
Serum albumin, PT	Protein synthesis
Serum bilirubin (total)	Hepatic anion transport
Serum enzyme activities	
ALT, AST	Hepatocellular integrity
ALP, GGT	Presence of cholestasis

Hepatic anion transport: bilirubin

Measurements of bilirubin in blood and urine are usually used to assess hepatic anion transport, although many other anions, including bile salts, are also transported by the liver. Understanding the mechanisms by which bilirubin is formed and removed is essential for the diagnosis of patients with jaundice or liver disease, since abnormal levels of bilirubin in blood can occur in patients in whom there is no liver disease.

Bilirubin production and metabolism

The pathway of bilirubin production and excretion is shown in Figure 13.2.

Production

The body usually produces about 300 mg of bilirubin per day as a breakdown product of haem. About 80% arises from red cells, with the remainder coming from red cell precursors destroyed in the bone marrow ('ineffective erythropoiesis'), and from other haem proteins such as myoglobin and the cytochromes. Iron is removed from the haem molecule, and the porphyrin ring is opened to form bilirubin.

Transport in plasma and hepatic uptake

Bilirubin is insoluble in water and is carried in plasma bound to albumin, and is thus not filtered at the glomerulus unless there is glomerular proteinuria. On reaching the liver, the bilirubin is taken into the hepatocyte by a specific carrier mechanism.

Conjugation of bilirubin and secretion into bile

In the endoplasmic reticulum of the hepatocyte, the enzyme *bilirubin UDP-glucuronyltransferase* conjugates bilirubin with glucuronic acid to produce bilirubin glucuronides which are water soluble and readily transported into bile. Secretion of bilirubin glucuronides into bile occurs against a high concentration gradient and is the rate-limiting step in removing bilirubin from the body. Secretion is a carrier-mediated energy-dependent process.

Further metabolism of bilirubin in the gut

Bilirubin glucuronides cannot be reabsorbed from the gut and are degraded by bacterial action, mainly in the colon, to a mixture of colourless,

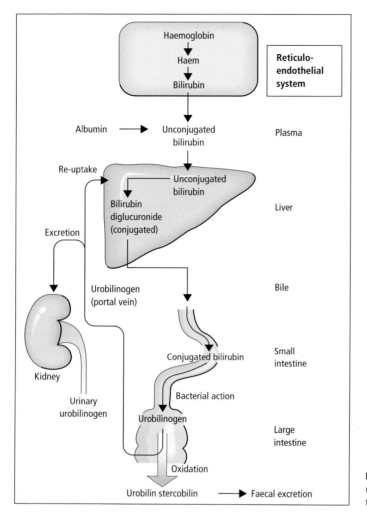

Figure 13.2 The formation and metabolism of bilirubin and its excretion into the intestine.

water-soluble compounds collectively termed urobilinogen. These compounds oxidise to brown compounds known as urobilins and stercobilins and are excreted in the faeces. A small percentage of urobilinogen is absorbed and carried to the liver in the portal blood supply, that is, it undergoes an *enterohepatic circulation*. Most of this urobilinogen is cleared by the liver, but a proportion escapes clearance and is filtered at the kidney and appears in the urine, where it can be detected using point of care urine dipsticks.

Measurements of serum bilirubin

Normally, more than 95% of bilirubin in serum is unconjugated, but in liver disease the conjugated form may predominate. For most purposes, the measurement of serum [total bilirubin] (i.e. the sum of unconjugated and conjugated forms) is sufficient, especially when results are interpreted in relation to the patient's history, findings on clinical examination and the results of urine urobilinogen and bilirubin measurements. Occasionally, it may be helpful to measure serum [conjugated bilirubin] and serum [unconjugated bilirubin] separately especially in neonates (p. 292).

Hepatocellular damage: aminotransferase measurements

Soluble cytoplasmic enzymes and, to a lesser extent, mitochondrial enzymes are released into plasma in hepatocellular damage. The measurement of the activity of ALT or AST in serum provides a sensitive index of hepatocellular damage. Serum ALT measurements are more liver specific than those of AST. Cytoplasmic and mitochondrial isoenzymes of AST exist and, in chronic hepatocellular disease (e.g. cirrhosis), serum AST tends to be increased to a greater extent than ALT. The aminotransferases are mainly located in the periportal hepatocytes, and they do not give a reliable indication of centrilobular liver damage. As with all tests based on the release of enzymes from damaged tissue, there is a lag period of some 24 h from the initiation of tissue damage to the first appearance of increased enzyme levels in the plasma.

Cholestasis: alkaline phosphatase and γ-glutamyltransferase

Some enzymes, such as ALP and GGT, are normally attached, or 'anchored', to the biliary canalicular and sinusoidal membranes of the hepatocyte. For this reason, ALP and GGT tend to be released into plasma in only small amounts following hepatocellular damage. However, they are released in much greater amounts when there is cholestasis, since their synthesis is induced and they are rendered soluble – due, at least in part, to the presence of high hepatic concentrations of bile acids.

Changes in the activities of GGT and ALP often parallel each other in cholestatic liver disease. Serum GGT has the advantage of being more liver specific, as serum ALP may also be increased due to release from bone in bone disease. However, alcohol and many drugs such as anti-convulsants may induce the expression of GGT without causing cholestasis. An isolated increase in GGT should thus be interpreted with caution.

Hepatic protein synthesis

The measurement of certain plasma proteins provides an index of the liver's ability to synthesise protein.

Albumin

In chronic hepatocellular damage, there is impaired albumin synthesis with an accompanying fall in serum [albumin]. Albumin measurements provide a fairly good index of the progress of chronic liver disease. In acute liver disease, however, there may be little or no reduction in serum [albumin], as the biological half-life of albumin is about 20 days and the fractional clearance rate is therefore low. Factors other than impaired hepatic synthesis may lead to a decreased serum [albumin]. These include loss of albumin into the extravascular compartment, ascites, increased degradation, poor nutritional status and a fall as part of the acute-phase response.

Ascites

Increased portal venous pressure, a low plasma colloid oncotic pressure and Na^+ retention due to secondary hyperaldosteronism combine to cause ascites in cirrhotic patients. This often develops when serum [albumin] falls below 30 g/L.

Coagulation factors

In liver disease, the synthesis of prothrombin and other clotting factors is diminished, leading to an increased *PT*. This may be one of the earliest abnormalities seen in patients with hepatocellular damage, since prothrombin has a short half-life (~6 h). The PT is often expressed as a ratio to a control value (the INR).

Deficiency of *fat-soluble vitamin K*, due to failure of absorption of lipids, may also cause a prolonged PT. In vitamin K deficiency, the coagulation defect can often be corrected by parenteral administration of vitamin K, but this has no effect in patients with hepatocellular damage.

Immunoglobulins

Serum Ig measurements are of little value in liver disease because the changes are of low specificity. In most types of cirrhosis, serum [IgA] is often increased, while in primary biliary cirrhosis, serum [IgM] increases greatly. In chronic active hepatitis, serum [IgG] tends to be most increased.

Serological tests

Anti-mitochondrial antibodies are present in over 95% of patients with primary biliary cirrhosis, and anti-smooth muscle and anti-nuclear factor antibodies are found in about 50% of patients with chronic active hepatitis. Viral antigens and antibody measurements are also important in detecting infective causes of liver disease.

Marker of fibrosis

A variety of markers have been described that may be of help in the assessment of hepatic fibrosis. Procollagen type III terminal peptide and hyaluronic acid (hyluronin) are the most commonly used tests.

Other liver function tests

A number of liver function tests have been described that give an indication of the functional liver mass. These tests are not often used but include the aminopyrine breath tests, the galactose elimination test and the monoethylglycinexylidide (MEGX) test. The measurement of bile acids is useful in investigating hepatic dysfunction associated with pregnancy (p. 175) and in the investigation of Gilbert's syndrome (p. 203).

Disordered metabolism

Patients with severe liver disease may have:
1 Significant *decreases in serum [urea]*, due to failure of the liver to convert amino acids and NH_3

to urea. These changes occur late in the disease. Note that there are other causes of a low serum [urea] (Table 4.2).
2 *Hypoglycaemia* due to impaired gluconeogenesis or glycogen breakdown, or both.
3 Raised concentrations of all the *serum lipid fractions*, if cholestasis is present. An abnormal lipoprotein that contains high concentrations of phospholipid, *lipoprotein X*, is present in serum in nearly all the cases of cholestasis.

The place of chemical tests in the diagnosis of liver disease

The jaundiced patient

Jaundice is due to hyperbilirubinaemia and becomes clinically apparent when the serum [bilirubin] exceeds about 50 μmol/L, although smaller degrees of hyperbilirubinaemia may be of diagnostic significance.

Measurements of serum [bilirubin] give a quantitative index of the severity of the jaundice, while serum enzyme activity measurements and point of care tests on fresh urine specimens, for bilirubin and urobilinogen, usually allow the cause of jaundice to be defined as pre-hepatic, hepatocellular or cholestatic (Figure 13.3). Further appropriate tests can then be requested (Table 13.2).

Investigations of the jaundiced patient often use the strategy shown in Figure 13.4. Increased serum [bilirubin] can arise as a consequence of increased production, impaired metabolism or decreased biliary excretion.

Pre-hepatic hyperbilirubinaemia

This is due to overproduction of bilirubin causing increased serum [unconjugated bilirubin]. It occurs in
- haemolytic anaemia
- haemolytic disease of the newborn, due to rhesus incompatibility
- ineffective erythropoiesis (e.g. pernicious anaemia)
- rhabdomyolysis.

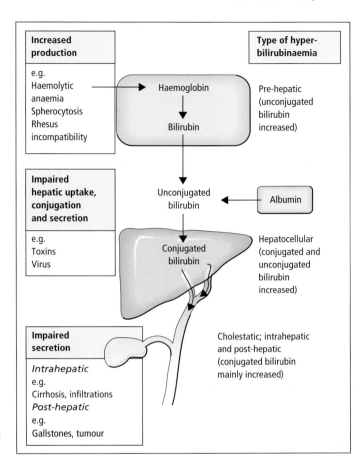

Figure 13.3 Types and causes of hyperbilirubinaemia.

Table 13.2 Bilirubin and urobilinogen measurements (examples of results in various conditions)

| Condition | Urine tests (side room) | | Serum [bilirubin] | |
	Urobilinogen	Bilirubin	Total* (μmol/L)	Conjugated
Healthy individuals	Trace	**Nil**	2–17	About 5%
Gilbert's syndrome	Trace	Nil	<50	Below 5%
Haemolytic diseases	Increased	Nil	<60	Below 5%
Hepatitis				
Prodromal	Increased	Detectable	<35	Raised
Icteric stage	Undetectable	Present	<250	Much raised
Recovery stage	Detectable	Falling	Falling	Falling
Biliary obstruction	Undetectable	Present	<400	Much raised

* Values for serum [total bilirubin] are included so as to give indications of the order of severity of the hyperbilirubinaemia that may be observed in the various conditions listed.

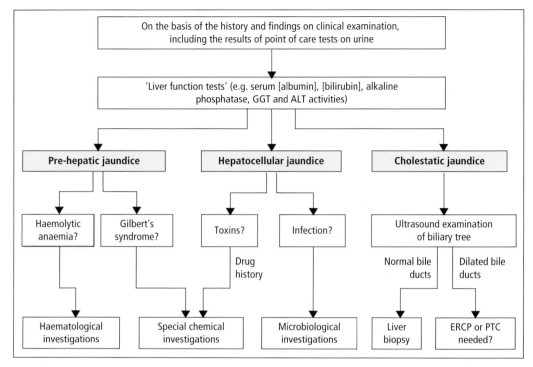

Figure 13.4 The investigation of jaundice. Endoscopic retrograde cholangiopancreatography (ERCP) or percutaneous transhepatic cholangiography (PTC) may be needed whenever the cause of dilated bile ducts is uncertain.

Hepatocellular hyperbilirubinaemia

This can arise from

1 *hepatocellular damage* caused by infective agents, drugs and toxins
2 *cirrhosis* – usually as a relatively late complication
3 *low activity of bilirubin UDP-glucuronyltransferase* in congenital deficiency (Gilbert's syndrome and Crigler–Najjar syndrome; see below), premature infants (the enzyme normally develops at about full term), or competitive inhibition of the enzyme by drugs (e.g. due to novobiocin). This leads to increased serum [unconjugated bilirubin].

Cholestatic hyperbilirubinaemia

Cholestasis may be intrahepatic or extrahepatic. In both, there is conjugated hyperbilirubinaemia and bilirubinuria.

Cholestasis commonly occurs in
- acute hepatocellular damage (e.g. due to infectious hepatitis)
- cirrhosis
- intrahepatic carcinoma (most commonly secondary)
- primary biliary cirrhosis
- drugs (e.g. methyltestosterone, phenothiazines).

Extrahepatic cholestasis is most often due to
- gallstones
- carcinoma of the head of the pancreas
- carcinoma of the biliary tree
- bile duct compression from other causes.

The congenital hyperbilirubinaemias

These are all due to inherited defects in the mechanism of bilirubin transport and metabolism.

Gilbert's syndrome

This familial autosomal dominant trait is probably present in 2–3% of men; it is 2–7 times more common in men than women. The unconjugated hyperbilirubinaemia is usually asymptomatic, and serum [bilirubin] fluctuates, higher levels tending to occur during intercurrent illness. Most patients have a serum [bilirubin] less than 50 μmol/L, but higher levels are not uncommon. Other commonly performed tests of 'liver function' are normal, and there is no bilirubinuria.

Gilbert's syndrome is caused by decreased expression of bilirubin UDP-glucuronyltransferase 1A1, due to a mutation in the promoter portion of the gene.

Gilbert's syndrome can most easily be differentiated from the mild degree of hyperbilirubinaemia in haemolytic anaemia by haematological investigations. Confirmatory tests for Gilbert's syndrome include monitoring the effects on serum [bilirubin] of a *reduced energy intake* (1.67 MJ/day; 400 kcal/day), particularly a reduction in the intake of lipids, for 72 h. This results in at least a doubling of serum [unconjugated bilirubin] in patients with Gilbert's syndrome, whereas in normal individuals it does not rise above 25 μmol/L. In simpler terms, a difference between fasted (higher) and postprandial (lower) bilirubin levels which are generally less than three times the upper limit of the reference range and where more than 70% bilirubin is unconjugated is typical of Gilbert's syndrome. The diagnosis also requires otherwise normal liver function tests. Diagnosis by genotyping is also now possible, but is not widely performed.

Crigler–Najjar syndrome

This rare condition, due to low activity of bilirubin UDP-glucuronyltransferase, gives rise to severe hyperbilirubinaemia in neonates, leading to kernicterus and often to early death.

Dubin–Johnson syndrome and Rotor syndrome

These rare disorders are characterised by a benign conjugated hyperbilirubinaemia, accompanied by bilirubinuria. In both, there is a defect in the transfer of conjugated bilirubin into the biliary canaliculus. Urinary coproporphyrins are normal in patients with Dubin–Johnson syndrome, but increased in Rotor syndrome.

Acute hepatitis

This is usually caused by viruses (hepatitis A, B, C, D and E, cytomegalovirus or Epstein–Barr). Toxins such as ethanol and paracetamol can also damage the liver. There is often a pre-icteric phase when increases in ALT and AST activities and in urobilinogen in urine occur. By the time clinical jaundice appears, serum ALT and AST activities are usually more than six times, and occasionally more than 100 times, the upper reference value. The stools may be very pale, due to impaired biliary excretion of bilirubin, and urobilinogen then disappears more or less completely from the urine. ALP activity is usually only slightly increased, up to about twice the upper reference value, but it may be considerably raised in cases (relatively uncommon) in which there is a marked cholestatic element, as occurs in acute alcoholic hepatitis.

Acute viral hepatitis usually resolves quickly, and chemical indices of abnormality revert to normal within a few weeks.

Poisoning and drugs

Findings similar to those in acute viral hepatitis are observed in patients with hepatocellular toxicity due to drugs (e.g. paracetamol overdose (p. 285), halothane jaundice, carbon tetrachloride poisoning). Drugs such as chlorpromazine and other antipsychotics may produce cholestasis, with increased serum ALP and GGT, while phenytoin, barbiturates and ethanol induce GGT synthesis without necessarily causing liver damage. Certain herbal remedies and recreational drugs such as ecstasy may also induce liver damage.

Acute liver failure

This rare condition is usually caused by paracetamol poisoning or hepatitis virus and the prognosis is often poor. It is accompanied by major metabolic disturbances including hyponatraemia, hypocalcaemia, hypoglycaemia and lactic acidosis often masked by respiratory alkalosis. The levels of the aminotransferases do not correlate well with the severity of the disease.

Chronic hepatitis

Hepatic inflammation that persists for more than 6 months is regarded as 'chronic hepatitis'. It may be due to chronic infection with hepatitis virus, alcohol abuse or be autoimmune in origin. Usually such patients have an isolated elevation in serum aminotransferase unless the disease has progressed to cirrhosis. Autoimmune hepatitis is frequently treated with azathioprine. The therapeutic action of azathioprine depends on the production of active metabolites. Toxicity can occur in patients who have low activities of the enzyme thiopurine methyl transferase (TPMT). There is a genetic polymorphism in the TPMT gene, and genotyping or phenotyping for TPMT is advisable before initiating therapy with azathioprine (p. 282).

Cholestatic liver disease

Both extrahepatic (e.g. gallstones) and intrahepatic (e.g. tumours, certain drugs) causes of obstruction cause cholestasis. The distinction between the two is often clinically important from the point of view of further investigation and treatment, but it can rarely be made by chemical tests.

Serum [bilirubin] is often greatly increased, and there is marked bilirubinuria; urobilinogen often becomes undetectable in urine. Serum ALP and GGT activities are considerably increased, often to more than three times the upper reference values, but serum ALT and AST activities are usually only moderately raised. In long-standing cholestatic jaundice, hepatic protein synthesis may be impaired and serum ALP activity may start to fall as a result, and even return to normal; this emphasises the importance of performing a baseline set of investigations as early as possible in patients with liver disease.

Serum ALP and GGT activities may be markedly increased in patients with partial biliary obstruction, due to local obstruction in one of the smaller biliary ducts, such as often occurs in both primary and secondary carcinoma of the liver. Partial biliary obstruction may have little or no effect on the capacity of the liver to excrete bilirubin, so there may be no evidence of jaundice in these patients, at least initially; bilirubin excretion in the other parts of the liver may be capable of fully compensating for the sector affected by the local biliary obstruction.

Chemical features that may help to distinguish cholestasis from hepatocellular damage are summarised in Table 13.3. These are 'typical' findings, and many cases do not follow these patterns exactly. The distinction between intrahepatic and extrahepatic cholestasis is usually made by radiological investigations, for example endoscopic retrograde cholangiopancreatography (ERCP), ultrasound or CT scanning, or by liver biopsy.

Infiltrations of the liver

The liver parenchyma may be progressively disorganised and destroyed in patients with primary or secondary carcinoma, lymphoma, amyloidosis, reticuloses, tuberculosis, sarcoidosis and abscesses. These diseases often lead to partial biliary obstruction, with the associated chemical changes described above. Serum [α_1-fetoprotein] (AFP) is often greatly increased in hepatoma (p. 250) but it can be moderately increased in chronic hepatitis and cirrhosis. Serum AFP measurements are also useful for monitoring patients who are at increased risk of developing hepatoma. Patients with liver tumours may often have elevated ALP and GGT as the only abnormality due to localised obstruction.

Cirrhosis of the liver

Alcoholism, viral hepatitis, autoimmune disease and prolonged cholestasis are the most frequent known causes of cirrhosis in Britain, although in half the cases no obvious cause is found. Less often, cirrhosis is associated with metabolic disorders such as Wilson's disease (see below), cystic

Table 13.3 Hepatocellular damage and cholestasis (serum measurements that may help to differentiate between these conditions)

Investigation	Hepatocellular damage		Cholestasis	Cirrhosis	Tumours
	Acute	Chronic			
Albumin	N or ↓	N to ↓↓	N or ↓	N or ↓	N or ↓
Bilirubin (total)	N to ↑↑	N or ↑	N to ↑↑	N or ↑	N
Aminotransferases	↑↑ or ↑↑↑	N or ↑	N or ↑	N or ↑	N or ↑
ALP	N or ↑	N or ↑	↑↑	N to ↑↑	↑
GGT	N or ↑	N or ↑	↑↑	N or ↑	↑
Igs	N or ↑	↑‡	↑†	N or ↑*	N
PT	N or ↑	N or ↑	N or ↑	N or ↑	N
Effect of parenteral vitamin K on PT	None	May correct	May correct	None	

N = normal; ↑ = increased; ↑↑ = much increased; ↑↑↑ = very much increased; ↓ = decreased; ↓↓ = much decreased.
N indicates that serum [bilirubin] is often normal when cholestasis is localised, as it often is with secondary deposits in the liver.
* Serum [IgA] is particularly increased in cirrhosis.
† Serum [IgM] is increased in primary biliary cirrhosis.
‡ Serum [IgG] is increased in chronic active hepatitis.

fibrosis (p. 300), α_1-protease inhibitor (API) deficiency (p. 243), haemochromatosis (p. 259) or galactosaemia (p. 297).

Mild cirrhosis In mild cases, no clinical abnormalities may be apparent, due to the reserve functional capacity of the liver. Serum GGT measurements provide a sensitive means of detecting mild cirrhosis, but most heavy drinkers (many of whom do *not* have cirrhosis of the liver) have raised serum GGT activities; these usually fall within 2 months of stopping drinking. Marked abnormalities in liver function tests are rarely present.

Severe cirrhosis The following clinical features may occur, either alone or in combination: haematemesis, ascites and acute hepatic decompensation, often fatal. Jaundice may develop, serum [albumin] falls and the PT becomes abnormal. Clinical deterioration accompanied by prolonged PT, a generalised amino aciduria, increased plasma [NH₃] and reduced serum [urea] may herald the development of acute hepatic failure.

Hyaluronan (also known as hyaluronic acid) is a glucosaminoglycan synthesised by the mesenchymal cells and degraded by hepatic sinusoidal endothelial cells by a specific receptor-mediated process.

Elevated levels are associated with sinusoidal capilliarisation that is seen in cirrhosis. Hyaluronan levels are significantly higher in patients with liver cirrhosis compared with hepatic fibrosis, chronic hepatitis and fatty liver. Measurement of fasting serum hyaluronan can reliably differentiate cirrhotic from non-cirrhotic liver disease and can be regarded as a useful test in the diagnosis of liver cirrhosis, particularly when a liver biopsy is contraindicated. There appears to be no significant difference in hyaluronan levels between cirrhosis caused by different aetiologies, but hyaluronan levels are increased proportionally to the severity of cirrhosis.

Copper in liver disease

The liver is the principal organ involved in copper metabolism. The amount it contains is maintained at normal levels by excretion of copper in bile and by incorporation into ceruloplasmin (see Table 16.1). The liver's copper content is increased in Wilson's disease, primary biliary cirrhosis, prolonged extrahepatic cholestasis and intrahepatic bile duct atresia in the neonate.

Wilson's disease (hepatolenticular degeneration) is a rare, hereditary, autosomal recessive disorder with a prevalence of about 1 in 30 000. The defective gene encodes a protein involved in the hepatobiliary excretion and renal reabsorption of copper. Copper is deposited in many tissues, including the liver, brain, eyes and kidney. Symptoms are mainly due to liver disease and to degenerative changes in the basal ganglia. Serum [ceruloplasmin] is nearly always low, but it is not clear how this relates to the aetiology of Wilson's disease.

The diagnosis may be suspected from the family history or on clinical grounds, such as liver disease in patients less than 20 years old, or characteristic neurological disease. Kayser–Fleischer rings, due to the deposition of copper in the cornea, can be detected in most patients. The following chemical tests may be valuable:

- *Serum [ceruloplasmin]* This is usually less than 0.2 g/L (reference range 0.2–0.6 g/L).
- *Serum [copper]* This is usually less than 12 µmol/L (reference range 13–24 µmol/L).
- *Urinary copper output* This is always more than 1.0 µmol/24 h (normally <0.5 µmol/24 h).
- *Liver [copper]* is always greater than 250 µg/g dry weight (reference range 50–250 µg/g dry weight). This is the most sensitive test, but it involves liver biopsy.

These tests are not 100% specific for Wilson's disease. For example, serum [ceruloplasmin] may occasionally be low in severe cirrhosis, and urinary copper output and liver [copper] may be raised in biliary cirrhosis. However, urinary copper output is valuable for case-finding among relatives, since a normal result virtually excludes Wilson disease.

Abnormalities of other chemical tests are often present in Wilson's disease. There is usually evidence of renal tubular damage, with a generalised (overflow) amino aciduria, glycosuria and phosphaturia and, in advanced cases, renal tubular acidosis.

Alcoholic liver disease

Chronic overindulgence in ethanol is a common cause of liver disease including fatty liver, cirrhosis and alcoholic hepatitis.

The diagnosis of alcohol abuse is difficult, but the following tests may be of value:

1 *GGT and mean cell volume (MCV) of erythrocytes* Alcohol induces the synthesis of GGT by the liver, but as a single test for the recognition of chronic alcohol abuse serum GGT lacks sensitivity. The diagnostic value of serum GGT measurements can be increased by measuring the MCV of erythrocytes as well, and the finding of both a slight macrocytosis and an increased serum GGT activity provides probably the best routinely available combination of measurements for detecting alcohol abuse.

2 *Carbohydrate-deficient transferrin (CDT)* In patients with alcohol-induced liver disease, transferrin in serum has a reduced carbohydrate (sialic acid) content. Serum [CDT] is increased in about 90% of patients who drink more than 60 g of alcohol per day.

3 *Blood ethanol.*

Non-alcoholic fatty liver disease (NAFLD) and non-alcoholic steatohepatitis (NASH)

The increasing worldwide problem of obesity (see p. 236) has led to an increase in the problem of fatty injury to the liver, a condition termed non-alcoholic fatty liver disase (NAFLD). The condition is estimated to affect 20–30% of the adult population in developed countries with an obesity problem. It is characterised by fatty change in the hepatocytes, without significant inflammation or fibrosis in its uncomplicated form. Diagnosis is typically made on the basis of mild elevations in serum ALT and GGT, the former typically less than three times the upper reference range, in the presence of other evidence of insulin resistance (raised or high normal fasting glucose; obesity with central adiposity; typical lipoprotein changes of insulin resistance (p. 191)). The diagnosis may be assisted by imaging studies such as upper abdominal ultrasound scanning which confirms fatty change to the liver. Biopsy is the only proven method for accurate diagnosis but is not without significant risk. Although individuals with NAFLD may not be strictly diabetic, the condition is associated with future increased risk of diabetes and is likely to be a marker for cardiovascular disease. Accordingly, therapies to reduce the problem, including lifestyle issues such as weight loss and raising exercise levels, should be stressed.

A small number of individuals with NAFLD progress to a more serious problem called non-alcoholic steatohepatitis (NASH) which is accompanied by inflammation and fibrosis and can further progress to cirrhosis. It seems that steatosis itself can provoke chronic inflammation, probably by increased NF-κB (nuclear factor-κB) transcription factor activation with release of inflammatory cytokines such as tumour necrosis factor-α. Identifying individuals with NASH does require liver biopsy, and attempts have been made to identify the higher risk patient with fatty change who may have progressed to NASH and where biopsy may be indicated. The criteria used for biopsy have included age more than 45 years, type 2 diabetes with BMI greater than 30 and an AST/ALT ratio of more than 1.

Even with a diagnosis of NAFLD (or NASH), there is no specific therapy, either surgical or medical, which has been demonstrated by any rigorous clinical evaluation to affect outcomes such as cirrhosis or hepatocellular carcinoma. The focus is on managing diabetes risk by exercise, weight reduction and management of cardiovascular risk.

Other causes of liver disease

These include haemachromatosis (p. 259), paracetamol poisoning (p. 285) and pregnancy (p. 175)

Ascites

Liver disease is the most common cause of ascites. If a diagnostic paracentesis is performed, the appearance of the fluid (blood-stained, bile-stained, milky, etc.) should be noted, and fluid [total protein] should be determined.

Transudates and exudates

Ascites with a fluid [protein] less than 30 g/L is called a *transudate*. It is usually associated with non-infective causes such as uncomplicated cirrhosis, in which there is a combination of back-pressure effects and low serum [albumin]. However, fluid [protein] may be greater in some of these patients, and 30 g/L is not a reliable diagnostic cut-off point.

Ascites with a fluid [protein] much in excess of 30 g/L is called an *exudate*. It usually indicates the presence of infective conditions such as tuberculous peritonitis, malignant disease or pancreatic disease. If pancreatic disease is thought to be the cause, fluid amylase activity should be measured; a serosanguinous fluid with a high amylase activity will help to confirm the diagnosis. If hepatoma is suspected, serum and ascitic fluid [AFP] may both be considerably increased.

Keypoints

- Bilirubin, ALT, ALP, GGT, albumin and PT are often requested as a group of tests to determine whether liver disease is present and to give some indication of aetiology. Normal results do not exclude liver disease.
- In jaundiced patients, unconjugated hyperbilirubinaemia is usually due to haemolysis or Gilbert's syndrome. Bilirubin is absent from the urine and urinary [urobilinogen] is increased in haemolysis.
- In conjugated hyperbilirubinaemia and in some patients in whom liver damage is insufficient to cause hyperbilirubinaemia, large increases in ALT suggest hepatocellular damage, caused by drugs, toxic agents or infection. On the other hand, marked elevations in GGT and ALP suggest cholestasis. Chemical tests do not distinguish intrahepatic from post-hepatic cholestasis.
- Serum [albumin] provides a fairly good index of the progress of chronic liver disease, but is of less value in acute liver disease, due to its half-life of ~21 days. The PT provides a better index of rapid progression of liver damage.

Case 13.1

A 13-year-old boy was taken by his mother to see the GP because he had been feeling hot for the previous 2 days and had been complaining that his muscles ached. He had eaten little for the previous 2 days. On examination, the doctor found that the boy was pyrexial (38.4 °C) and appeared jaundiced.

There was no abdominal pain or tenderness, lymphadenopathy or enlargement of the spleen or liver. Urobilinogen was within normal limits in urine, and there was no detectable bilirubin in the specimen. The doctor requested liver function tests, which were as follows:

Serum	Result	Reference range
Albumin	45	35–50 g/L
ALP activity	180	40–125 U/L
ALT activity	30	10–50 U/L
Bilirubin, total	60	3–16 µmol/L
GGT activity	35	10–55 U/L

Five days later, the boy had recovered. He had no fever and his jaundice had gone, but serum [bilirubin] was still elevated at 30 µmol/L, as was the ALP activity at 175 U/L. The reticulocyte count and other haematological investigations had all been normal on both occasions. What is the most likely diagnosis, and how would you explain the abnormal results among the liver function tests?

Comments: This patient has Gilbert's syndrome. This was revealed when he developed a flu-like illness and went off his food. Caloric restriction in these patients can be used as a test to unmask the latent mild hyperbilirubinaemia. The absence of bilirubin in the urine showed that the hyperbilirubinaemia was due to increased plasma [unconjugated bilirubin], and the normal reticulocyte count excluded haemolytic anaemia as the cause.

The raised ALP activity was of bone origin, expected in a child of this age entering puberty when there is rapid bone turnover. The serum GGT activity was normal, which helped to confirm this explanation.

Case 13.2

A 40-year-old housewife complained to her GP of generalised severe itching during the previous 9 months. She had no other symptoms, and she said that her alcohol consumption was small (2–3 U/week). On clinical examination, she was slightly jaundiced, and bilirubin was detected in the urine. The results of liver function tests were as follows:

Serum	Result	Reference range
Albumin	38	35–50 g/L
ALP activity	450	40–125 U/L
ALT activity	60	10–50 U/L
Bilirubin, total	60	3–16 µmol/L
GGT activity	150	10–55 U/L

Comments: This patient has cholestatic jaundice. Her pruritus is caused by the retention of bile salts. The presence of serum anti-mitochondrial antibodies in high titre indicated that the diagnosis was primary biliary cirrhosis, one of the causes of intrahepatic cholestasis. Retention of bile salts within the liver is liable to cause hepatocellular damage, which could account for the increased serum ALT activity in this patient.

Case 13.3

A GP was called to see a 21-year-old female student who had been complaining of a flu-like illness for 2 days. The illness had become worse, with symptoms of fever, vomiting and abdominal tenderness in the right upper quadrant. On examining the patient, the doctor found that she was pyrexial and jaundiced. The liver was enlarged and tender. On questioning her, the doctor found that she had recently returned from a long holiday in Asia.

A sample of urine appeared dark, and bilirubin was present and urobilinogen was increased. A blood sample was taken for liver function tests, the results of which were as follows:

Serum	Result	Reference range
Albumin	40	35–50 g/L
ALP activity	190	40–125 U/L
ALT activity	560	10–50 U/L
Bilirubin, total	110	3–16 µmol/L
GGT activity	60	5–35 U/L

What is the most likely diagnosis?

Comments: The results and presenting features are characteristic of hepatitis caused by an infective agent. The presence of bilirubin in the urine showed that there was a conjugated hyperbilirubinaemia, and the markedly elevated serum ALT activity and increased urinary urobilinogen indicated that the jaundice was hepatocellular in origin.

Both serum ALP activity and GGT were slightly elevated, indicating that there was some degree of intrahepatic cholestasis.

Possible causes could include hepatitis A, B, C, Epstein–Barr virus, etc. In this case, the serum contained a high titre of antibodies to hepatitis A.

Case 13.4

A 68-year-old retired labourer presented complaining of loss of weight, tiredness and loss of appetite. He had lost 19 kg during the previous 3 months, but had been eating normally up until 3 weeks previously. He had experienced no pain, but on questioning admitted to drinking moderately for most of his life. He also stated that he had been passing dark urine for some time and that his stools were quite pale.

The examination showed a tired, thin man with jaundice. There was a palpable mass in the right upper quadrant of the abdomen, with no tenderness. The results of the liver function tests were

Serum	Result	Reference range
Albumin	32	35–50 g/L
ALP activity	632	40–125 U/L
ALT activity	55	10–50 U/L
Bilirubin, total	90	3–16 µmol/L
GGT activity	200	10–55 U/L

Urine analysis showed the presence of bilirubin, and urobilinogen was undetectable. Faecal occult blood was positive. α-Fetoprotein in plasma was not increased.

What is the most likely diagnosis?

Comments: The pale stools, presence of bilirubin and lack of urobilinogen in the urine, accompanied by high serum activities of ALP and GGT, suggest that the patient has cholestatic jaundice. The abdominal mass and positive faecal occult blood suggest that a tumour of the biliary tract or the pancreas may be responsible. Hepatoma was unlikely, as α-fetoprotein was negative.

Ultrasound showed a large abdominal mass and dilated intrahepatic and extrahepatic bile ducts. A CT scan suggested that there was a tumour at the head of the pancreas that was obstructing the common bile duct.

Case 13.5

A 23-year-old man was admitted to hospital with fulminant hepatorenal failure. He was jaundiced, with marked abnormalities in his liver function tests. There was also clear evidence of intravascular haemolysis. He had been experiencing vague abdominal discomfort over the past 3 years and, over this time, his liver function tests had been normal with the exception of ALT, which was found to be consistently elevated at 80 U/L (reference range 10–50 U/L).

Abdominal ultrasound showed a picture consistent with cirrhosis, with no evidence of biliary obstruction. Blood cultures, anti-mitochondrial and anti-nuclear antibodies were negative, as were tests for hepatitis B surface and core antibodies. There was no history of drug abuse, and paracetamol was not detected in the serum.

A liver biopsy revealed inflammatory and fatty changes, and stained heavily for copper. Serum ceruloplasmin was slightly decreased at 0.14 g/L (reference range 0.2–0.6 g/L).

What is the likely diagnosis? How would you confirm this?

Comments: The man has Wilson's disease (p. 205). The diagnosis was confirmed by finding a decreased serum [ceruloplasmin] of 0.14 g/L (reference range 0.2–0.6 g/L). The usual clinical manifestations of the disease are caused by excessive copper deposition, particularly in the liver and brain. The biochemical defect is present at birth, but symptoms typically appear in older children, adolescents and young adults. Most patients present with hepatic or neurological dysfunction. The haemolysis is thought to be due to the sudden release of copper from the liver, which damages the erythrocytes. About 30% of patients present with features of chronic hepatitis. Most, but not all, patients have Kayser–Fleischer rings. About 15% of patients with active hepatic involvement have normal serum ceruloplasmin concentrations; this is thought to be due to hepatic inflammation, which leads to an increase in ceruloplasmin production as part of the acute-phase response that may be sufficient to bring values into the reference range.

Patients presenting with fulminant hepatic failure usually die unless a liver transplant can be performed. In other patients, treatment with a low copper diet and penicillamine to chelate and increase urinary copper excretion usually leads to a good prognosis.

Chapter 14

Gastrointestinal tract disease

Biochemical tests play a relatively minor role in the investigation of GI tract disease, and a number of previously well-established investigations have now become obsolete. In general, microbiological investigations, radiological investigations, endoscopy and biopsy procedures have more to offer. This chapter briefly discusses the principles and limitations of biochemical and immunological tests that are currently available for the investigation of GI tract disease and also highlights some newer tests that are likely to become widely used in the future. The tests that have proved most valuable and reliable for the investigation of some conditions are given in Table 14.1.

Stomach

Peptic ulcer

Most disorders of gastric function are best assessed initially using radiological investigations and endoscopy. Most peptic ulcers are associated with *Helicobacter pylori* infection which weakens the protective mucous coating of the stomach and duodenum. The organism is present in the mucosa and is protected from stomach acidity by the cre-

Lecture Notes: Clinical Biochemistry, 8e. By G. Beckett, S. Walker, P. Rae & P. Ashby. Published 2010 by Blackwell Publishing.

ation of a more neutral microenvironment through the secretion of large amounts of urease and the subsequent conversion of urea to ammonia and carbon dioxide. This reaction forms the basis of the urea breath test to detect *H. pylori* infection. In the few patients who present with atypical or recurrent peptic ulceration that is resistant to treatment with H_2 antagonists, proton pump inhibitors and antibiotics to eradicate *H. pylori*, biochemical tests to quantify plasma [gastrin] may be of value.

Tests for *H. pylori* infection

Urea breath test

This non-invasive test relies on the urease activity of *H. pylori* to detect active infection. The patient ingests either ^{13}C- or ^{14}C-labelled urea, and urease, if present, hydrolyses urea into ammonia and isotopically labelled carbon dioxide. Carbon dioxide is absorbed from the gut and subsequently expired in the breath where it can be trapped and quantified. This breath test is used both for the identification of patients with active infection and for establishing the effectiveness of treatment.

Serological tests

Patients infected with *H. pylori* develop antibodies to the organism that can be detected by serological testing. While serological tests are used to identify patients who have been infected with the

Table 14.1 The principal examples of biochemical tests described in this chapter for the investigation of GI tract disease

Condition to be investigated	Biochemical investigations
Peptic ulcer	
Helicobacter pylori	^{13}C urea breath test
	Antibodies to *H. pylori*
Zollinger–Ellison syndrome	Plasma [gastrin]
Acute pancreatitis	Serum amylase activity
Chronic pancreatic insufficiency	Faecal elastase
Intestinal malabsorption	
Coeliac disease	Anti-tissue transglutaminase IgA
Bacterial colonisation	Glucose hydrogen breath test
Bile acid malabsorption	Serum 7α-hydroxy-4-cholesten-3-one
Inflammation (any cause)	Faecal calprotectin
Verner–Morrison syndrome	Plasma [VIP]
Carcinoid syndrome	Urinary 5-hydroxyindoleacetic acid
Laxative abuse	Urine laxative screen

organism, they are less helpful in confirming its eradication because of the slow reduction in antibody titres.

Faecal antigen testing

Enzyme immunoassays can be used to detect the presence of *H. pylori* in stool specimens.

Gastrin

Gastrin is a polypeptide released by the G cells in the gastric antrum and duodenum and is a potent stimulator of gastric acid production. Its release is normally inhibited if the gastric pH is low, but circulating levels are increased in patients with chronic hypochlorhydria. Thus, plasma [gastrin] may be elevated as a physiological response to achlorhydria or hypochlorhydria due to gastritis, treatment with H_2 antagonists, proton pump

inhibitors, pernicious anaemia or previous vagotomy. Increased plasma [gastrin] may also be found in patients with hypercalcaemia or following gastric surgery, as a result of which the antral mucosa may have become isolated from gastric contents. The most important clinical application for the measurement of gastrin is in the investigation of patients with gastric acid hypersecretion thought to be caused by a gastrinoma (Zollinger–Ellison syndrome).

Zollinger–Ellison syndrome

This syndrome is due to a gastrinoma, that is, neoplasia of either pancreatic gastrin-producing cells or gastric gastrin-producing cells, the former being the more common site. Approximately 60% of gastrinomas are malignant and 30% occur as part of the MEN syndrome (type I) (Table 16.8; p. 251). Increased gastrin production leads to chronic hypersecretion of gastric acid, which in turn causes peptic ulceration and sometimes diarrhoea and fat malabsorption leading to steatorrhoea. The steatorrhoea is thought to be due to high [H⁺] in the intestinal lumen; this inhibits the action of pancreatic lipase. In some patients, an isolated simple duodenal ulcer or diarrhoea may be the presenting feature.

The diagnosis of gastrinoma is based on the detection of an unequivocally elevated fasting plasma [gastrin] in the presence of gastric acid hypersecretion. Patients should not be receiving proton pump inhibitors or H_2 receptor blockers at the time of measurement. Provocative testing may be necessary in about 15% of patients where the basal plasma [gastrin] concentration is normal or only slightly increased and gastrinoma is suspected. The preferred test involves the IV injection of secretin which usually produces a 2-fold increase in plasma [gastrin] in patients with gastrinoma, while no change occurs in patients with G-cell hyperplasia.

The pancreas

The pancreas is a complex gland with important endocrine and exocrine functions. Its principal endocrine role relates to the regulation of glucose metabolism through the secretion of insulin and glucagon from the islets of Langerhans, and is discussed elsewhere in this volume (Chapter 6). Pancreatic juice is produced by the exocrine tissue and released into the duodenum where it is mixed with partially digested food. It is an alkaline fluid that contains a mixture of enzymes essential for protein, carbohydrate and lipid digestion. Secretion is induced in response to nervous stimuli, but mainly by the hormones secretin and cholecystokinin-pancreozymin (CCK-PZ). These are secreted by the small intestine in response to the entry of food.

Acute pancreatitis

Acute pancreatitis is commonly associated with gallstones or alcoholism; vascular and infective causes have also been recognised. Confirmation of the clinical diagnosis mainly depends on serum amylase activity measurements. Serum [calcium] may fall considerably in severe cases of acute pancreatitis, but sometimes not for a few days; it probably falls as a result of the formation of insoluble calcium salts of fatty acids in areas of fat necrosis.

Serum amylase

Amylase in serum arises mainly from the pancreas (P-isoamylase) and the salivary glands (S-isoamylase). Serum P-isoamylase activity is a more sensitive and more specific test than total amylase for the detection of acute pancreatitis, but total serum amylase activity is most often measured and is usually, but not always, greatly increased in acute pancreatitis.

Serum amylase activities greater than 10 times the normal value are virtually diagnostic of acute pancreatitis. Maximum values of more than five times the upper reference limit are found in about 50% of cases, but are not pathognomonic of acute pancreatitis, since similarly high values sometimes occur in the afferent loop syndrome, mesenteric infarction and acute biliary tract disease, as well as in acute parotitis.

Smaller and more transient increases may occur in almost any acute abdominal condition (e.g. per-

forated peptic ulcer), or after injection of morphine and other drugs that cause spasm of the sphincter of Oddi. Moderate increases have also been reported in patients with DKA. In patients with acute pancreatitis, serum amylase activity usually returns to normal within 3–5 days.

Macro-amylasaemia

In this rare disorder, part of the serum amylase activity circulates as a high molecular weight form which, unlike normal amylase, is not cleared by the kidney. The diagnosis may be made when the increased serum amylase activity is found to be persistent and accompanied by a normal urinary amylase activity.

Chronic pancreatitis

Impaired secretion of pancreatic enzymes may not be evident until the disease is advanced, but may then give rise to malabsorption, especially steatorrhoea. Tests involving the analysis of bicarbonate and enzyme activity in duodenal aspirate were previously regarded as the gold standard for assessing exocrine pancreatic function. However, they require a high degree of technical expertise and are time consuming, expensive and uncomfortable for the patient, and have now been replaced by pancreatic imaging techniques. The direct measurement of pancreatic elastase in faeces is now regarded as the most useful biochemical test of exocrine pancreatic secretion.

Faecal elastase

Elastase is a pancreas-specific enzyme that is not degraded during intestinal transport. Concentrations in faeces are 5–6 times higher than those of duodenal fluid, and low levels are associated with pancreatic insufficiency. Although patients with modest degrees of pancreatic insufficiency cannot be reliably identified, its diagnostic sensitivity in patients with severe disease is high. False-positive results may be observed in some patients with watery diarrhoea.

Faecal elastase is not affected by pancreatic enzyme replacement therapy and is a convenient test to perform since only a single stool sample is required. It is recommended as the test of first choice in the investigation of patients presenting with diarrhoea thought to be of pancreatic origin.

Small intestine and colon

Tests of absorptive function

Carbohydrate absorption

With the widespread availability of small bowel histology, previously established non-invasive tests for investigating the absorptive capacity for carbohydrates have been discontinued in many centres. For example, the xylose absorption test, which was used to investigate the ability of the intestine to absorb monosaccharides, is now available only in a minority of laboratories. Similarly, the measurement of intestinal permeability by quantifying the absorption and urinary excretion of an oral mixture of disaccharide (lactulose) and monosaccharide (rhamnose) is now rarely performed in routine clinical practice. Other than demonstrating that an abnormality may exist, these tests are non-specific and non-diagnostic and will not be considered further

Disaccharidase deficiency
Disaccharidase deficiency may be exhibited as intolerance to one or more of the disaccharides – lactose, maltose or fructose. The defect may be congenital or acquired. The most reliable way of specifically diagnosing disaccharidase deficiency is to measure enzyme activity in small intestinal biopsy specimens. Many gastroenterologists advocate monitoring the symptomatic response to a low dairy diet as the most reliable test for lactase deficiency, which is the most common of the disaccharidase deficiencies.

Fat absorption

The faecal fat test, which involves 3- or 5-day collections of stools for the measurement of unabsorbed fat, has traditionally been used to assess fat absorption. However, due to difficulties relating to the inherently unpleasant nature of the test, inadequate sample collection, lack of analytical quality control and standardisation, and the limited diagnostic information provided by a positive result, many laboratories are abandoning the use of this test and it can no longer be recommended.

Triglyceride (triolein) breath test
This test avoids the difficulties and unpleasantness of collecting faeces over several days. Following digestion and absorption of an oral dose of [^{14}C] triolein (the marker is in the fatty acid component), part of the fatty acid is metabolised to $^{14}CO_2$, which is then excreted in expired air. A high $^{14}CO_2$ excretion is associated with normal fat absorption, whereas $^{14}CO_2$ excretion is low in patients with fat malabsorption. Despite the simplicity of this test, it is rarely requested and is not widely available. Breath tests have a low sensitivity for mild or moderate malabsorption.

Amino acid absorption

Certain specific disorders of amino acid transport affect both intestinal and renal epithelial transport. In Hartnup disease, there is impaired transport of neutral amino acids, and deficiency of some essential amino acids (especially tryptophan) may occur. In cystinuria (p. 60), the dibasic amino acids (cystine, ornithine, arginine and lysine) are affected; however, there is no associated nutritional defect, despite the fact that lysine is an essential amino acid. These disorders are investigated by examining the pattern of amino acids excreted in the urine by chromatography.

Bile acid absorption

Bile acids are essential for the absorption of dietary fats. The primary bile acids are formed in the liver, conjugated with glycine and taurine, and then excreted in bile. Together with phospholipids, bile salts form micelles, which render dietary fats soluble; bile salts also promote the action of pancreatic lipase and co-lipase, and solubilise the products of lipolysis and allow them to be absorbed.

Table 14.2 Malabsorption due to insufficient bile salts

Reason for bile salt insufficiency	Examples of causes of the insufficiency
Impaired synthesis of bile acids	Cirrhosis of the liver
Impaired delivery of bile acids to the intestine (due to obstruction to the outflow of bile)	Gallstones, carcinoma of the head of the pancreas
Impaired delivery of bile acids to the enterohepatic circulation	
Impaired absorption of bile acid conjugates from the terminal ileum	Ileal disease (e.g. Crohn's disease), resection of the terminal ileum
Impaired ability of the liver to clear bile acid conjugates from the portal blood and to secrete them again into the bile	Cholestasis associated with hepatic cirrhosis
Deconjugation of bile acid conjugates in the upper small intestine (reducing their effective concentration intestine at the site of fat absorption)	Bacterial colonisation of the upper small intestine (the 'stagnant gut syndrome')

Bile salts are mostly reabsorbed in the terminal ileum through an active process and then transported back to the liver where they are re-excreted in bile, completing the enterohepatic circulation. Insufficient bile acids may give rise to malabsorption of fat (Table 14.2).

Fat-soluble vitamins (A, D, E and K) share absorptive mechanisms with other dietary lipids. Malabsorption of fat-soluble vitamins, which is most commonly manifest as vitamin D deficiency (p. 81), occurs in conditions causing fat malabsorption.

Tests of terminal ileal function

Disease or resection of the terminal ileum results in a reduction of absorptive capacity and a loss of bile acids into the colon where they may inhibit sodium reabsorption and cause water secretion and diarrhoea.

Evidence of bile acid malabsorption can be obtained by the measurement of the serum metabolite 7α-hydroxy-4-cholesten-3-one, an intermediate in the bile acid biosynthetic pathway (Figure 14.1), which is increased in the presence of increased bile acid turnover. While this test is not widely available at present, it has the potential to replace the more expensive [75Se]homotaurocholate (75Se-HCAT) test in which the percentage retention of an oral dose of this synthetic γ-emitting bile salt is estimated by whole body scanning, 7 days after its administration.

Bacterial colonisation of the small intestine

The small intestine is usually sterile. However, when there is stasis (e.g. blind loop, stricture) or a colonic fistula or, occasionally, when immune mechanisms are impaired, anaerobic bacteria colonise the intestine. This often causes fat malabsorption, due at least partly to excessive deconjugation of bile acid conjugates by the bacteria and the premature passive reabsorption of the resulting unconjugated bile acids. This leads to a relative deficiency of bile salts in the intestinal lumen and decreased micelle formation. Vitamin B_{12} deficiency may also develop due to its consumption by the bacteria.

Investigations

- *Culture of small bowel aspirate* The definitive diagnosis of bacterial colonisation of the small intestine requires intubation for the collection of specimens, on which microbiological procedures are then performed.
- *Glucose hydrogen breath test.* This is based on the ability of some bacteria to ferment carbohydrates with an end-product of hydrogen, which is not produced by mammalian cells. The hydrogen produced in the gut by bacterial action following an oral glucose load is absorbed from the intestine and transported to the lungs where it is excreted in expired air and can be measured. While the sensi-

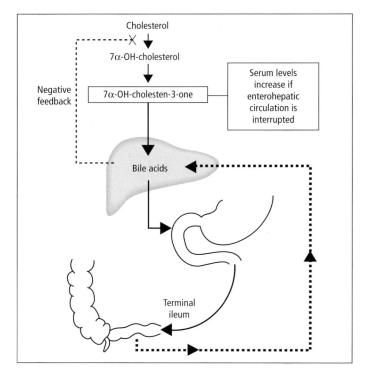

Figure 14.1 Bile acid biosynthesis increases if its enterothepatic circulation is interrupted, leading to an increase in the serum concentration of the biosynthetic intermediate 7α-OH-cholesten-3-one.

tivity of the test is poor compared with the culture of a small bowel aspirate, it is of value if a positive result is obtained.

Reabsorption of water and inorganic constituents

About $8\,L$ of intestinal secretions are produced each day, and if these are not largely reabsorbed, fluid and electrolyte disturbances will develop rapidly. Reabsorption takes place not only in the jejunum and ileum, but also in the colon. Acute and severe disturbances may occur in patients following surgery, especially operations on the GI tract, and losses of K^+ often become very large.

Non-surgical intestinal causes of electrolyte imbalance include severe diarrhoea (e.g. due to cholera, in which there is a defect in Na^+ reabsorption in the jejunum).

Serological tests for coeliac disease

Coeliac disease is an autoimmune disorder triggered by a sensitivity to gliadin and is the most common small bowel enteropathy in the Western world. Screening studies indicate that the overall prevalence in European populations is approximately 1% athough many cases may remain undiagnosed because of the diversity of symptoms associated with the disease. First-degree relatives of an affected patient have an increased risk of the disease and there is also an association with other autoimmune disorders such as type 1 diabetes and autoimmune thyroiditis.

Serological testing for coeliac disease is now the most frequently requested laboratory invesigation in patients with GI disturbances. It is also included in practice guidelines for the investigation of iron deficiency anaemia and in some clinical protocols for monitoring patients with other autoimmune disorders.

Circulating antibodies to tissue transglutaminase (tTG) are found in patients with coeliac disease and testing for anti-tTG IgA is the first line investigation of choice. The assay is readily automated and has superseded the more technically demanding test for anti-endomysium IgA which is also present. Anti-tTG IgA has a high sensitivity and specificity for coeliac disease and is useful both in screening and in monitoring the response to treatment. A small intestinal biopsy remains the gold standard in making the final diagnosis.

IgA deficiency

It should be noted that selective IgA deficiency occurs in 1:500 of the general population and in approximately 2–3% of patients with coeliac disease. To avoid false-negative serum IgA antibody tests total IgA levels should be measured in all patients undergoing initial screening. In IgA-deficient patients, anti-tTG IgG should be measured.

Gastrointestinal inflammation

Calprotectin is a calcium-binding protein derived from activated neutrophils as a result of inflammation and is elevated in faeces when pathology resulting in an inflammatory process occurs in the intestine. It is resistant to degradation in the gut and its measurement in faeces has a high sensitivity and specificity for organic disease. Highest levels are found in inflammatory bowel disease and bacterial infection, but faecal calprotectin may also be increased in cancer of the colon and stomach, colonic polyps and diverticular disease. In contrast, faecal calprotectin is normal in patients with irritable bowel syndrome in which there is no identifiable pathology in the intestine.

The measurement of faecal calprotectin provides a useful non-invasive method of identifying patients with organic disease who require further GI investigations. A negative result suggests that organic disease is unlikely and may reduce the need for endoscopy in some patients. Currently, the calprotectin assay is available in specialised centres only, but its use will undoubtedly become more widespread.

Faecal occult blood

Testing for faecal occult blood (FOB) is now firmly established as a tool for screening asymptomatic populations for bowel cancer, and it results in a 16% reduction in the relative risk of colorectal cancer mortality. The success of screening programmnes depends on the standardisation of specimen collection and the optimisation of laboratory analysis which is performed in specialist screening centres only.

In contrast, in a more acute setting, FOB testing is now regarded as too insensitive for use in the investigation of patients with iron deficiency anaemia or with symptoms of bowel cancer. Current practice guidelines state unambiguously that FOB testing is not recommended for the investigation of symptomatic patients and should not influence clinical decision making. A negative FOB test does not exclude either chronic gastrointestinal blood loss or cancer, and can provide false reassurance resulting in delayed diagnosis.

The investigation of malabsorption and diarrhoea

Efficient digestion and absorption require the stomach, pancreas, hepatobiliary system and small intestine all to be functioning normally. Severe defects in the function of any one of these organs may cause intestinal malabsorptive disease; the patient may complain of diarrhoea or weight loss. The causes of carbohydrate, protein and amino acid, and lipid malabsorption are summarised in Table 14.3. Most of these have been referred to in this chapter, but a few are considered elsewhere in this volume.

Clinical diagnosis

First, it is important to consider the history of the patient's illness and the findings on physical examination, and to formulate a provisional diagnosis and list the differential diagnoses.
• *Pancreatic disease* may cause malabsorption of protein, fat or carbohydrate, due to deficiency of digestive enzymes.

Table 14.3 Examples of the ways in which GI diseases cause malabsorption

Dietary constituent	Disease of the GI tract	Why malabsorption may occur
Generalised malabsorption	Coeliac disease	Villous atrophy
Polysaccharides	Chronic pancreatitis	Amylase deficiency
Disaccharides	Intestinal mucosal defect	Disaccharidase deficiency
Proteins	Chronic pancreatitis	Pancreatic peptidase deficiency
Amino acids	Intestinal mucosal defect	Specific amino acid transport abnormalities
Lipids	Chronic pancreatitis	Lipase and/or co-lipase deficiency
	Insufficient bile salts	Micelle formation impaired
	Gastrinoma	High intestinal [H+] inhibits pancreatic lipase
	A β-lipoproteinaemia	Transfer of lipids to plasma impaired

In addition to the above, any generalised intestinal disease is liable to cause malabsorption of all dietary constituents.

• *Biliary disease* may cause malabsorption of fat and fat-soluble vitamins, due to lack of bile acids.
• *Intestinal mucosal disease* may affect digestion or transport, or both, of many dietary constituents, and reabsorption of bile acids. The effects may be general, or relatively specific.
• *Bacterial colonisation of the small intestine* may cause a functional deficiency of bile acids, and so interfere with absorption of fats. It may also interfere with the digestion of protein or absorption of amino acids, and decrease the availability of water-soluble vitamins.

Initial investigations

• *Microbiological examination*, including stool microscopy and culture, should always be performed before biochemical tests are requested whenever an infectious cause of a GI disorder needs to be excluded.
• *A faecal specimen* should be inspected; this may suggest that the patient has steatorrhoea.
• *Preliminary biochemical investigations on blood specimens* should include urea and electrolytes, albumin and other 'liver function tests', calcium and CRP. Preliminary haematological investigations (Hb, full blood count, vitamin B$_{12}$, folate and ferritin) should also be performed.

Further investigations

• *Radiology* (e.g. barium meal, barium enema), *endoscopy* (e.g. gastroscopy, duodenoscopy, ERCP,

colonoscopy) and *mucosal biopsy* (e.g. duodenal biopsy) may be indicated.
• *Coeliac serology* Anti-tTG IgA.
• *Tests of pancreatic function*, for example faecal elastase.

Several other biochemical abnormalities may occur in association with intestinal malabsorption, and require appropriate investigation and treatment. These include:
• *Vitamin* deficiency.
• *Defects in calcium absorption* that may cause rickets or osteomalacia.
• *Malabsorption of iron* This may cause iron deficiency anaemia. Mixed deficiencies of vitamin B$_{12}$, folate and iron may also occur.
• *Malabsorption of protein* Reduction in serum [albumin] most often results, but hypogamma-globulinaemia may be marked.

Factitious diarrhoea

Factitious diarrhoea is becoming increasingly common in tertiary referral centres, and a high index of clinical suspicion may be necessary to prevent extensive needless investigation. Possible laxative abuse should be investigated in a specialist laboratory by screening a random urine sample for over-the-counter laxatives including the colonic stimulants bisacodyl and senna. If possible, the urine sample should be collected at a time when the patient is known to have diarrhoea. It should be remembered that patients may use laxatives intermittently and that a single negative result does not exclude this diagnosis.

Osmotic laxatives such as magnesium sulphate also may cause diarrhoea when used inappropriately, and an elevated faecal osmotic gap may provide a clue to their use. The faecal osmotic gap is calculated by measuring the sodium and potassium concentrations in faecal water and then doubling their sum to account for anions. This figure is then subtracted from an assumed osmolality of 290 mosm/kg which has been shown to give a close approximation to intracolonic osmolality.

Carcinoid tumours and the carcinoid syndrome

Carcinoid tumours arise in the gut or in tissues derived from the embryological foregut (e.g. thyroid, bronchus). The most common sites are the terminal ileum and the ileocaecal region. The tumours produce vasoactive amines which, because of the venous drainage of the tumours, are usually carried directly to the liver and there inactivated. Symptoms are only likely to occur either when the tumour has metastasised to the liver, or when the tumour drains into the systemic circulation (e.g. bronchial adenoma of the carcinoid type).

Most carcinoid tumours secrete excessive amounts of 5-hydroxytryptamine (5-HT; serotonin), which is metabolised and excreted in urine as 5-hydroxyindoleacetic acid (5-HIAA). Atypical carcinoid tumours secrete excessive amounts of 5-hydroxytryptophan (5-HTP) and relatively little 5-HT; they may also secrete histamine. Whereas only about 1% of dietary tryptophan is normally metabolised to 5-HTP, 5-HT and 5-HIAA, in the carcinoid syndrome, as much as 60% of dietary tryptophan is metabolised along this hydroxyindole pathway.

The *carcinoid syndrome* is usually associated with tumours of the terminal ileum and extensive secondary deposits in the liver. The main presenting features include flushing attacks, abdominal colic and diarrhoea, and dyspnoea, sometimes associated with asthmatic attacks. Valvular disease of the heart is often present. Carcinoid tumours can give rise to severe hypoproteinaemia and oedema, even in the absence of cardiac complications. There may also be signs of niacin deficiency, due to major diversion of tryptophan metabolism away from the pathway leading to niacin production (p. 230). Some carcinoid tumours produce ACTH or ACTH-like peptides, and may cause Cushing's syndrome (p. 136) in the absence of the symptoms commonly associated with the carcinoid syndrome.

Biochemical investigation of 5-HT metabolism

Measurement of 5-HIAA excretion in a 24-h urine specimen is the most widely performed investigation; the output is usually greatly increased. Bananas and tomatoes contain large amounts of 5-HT; they should not be eaten the day before or during the urine collection.

Timing of urine collection If attacks are frequent, the time of starting the collection is unimportant. If attacks are less often than daily, the patient should be instructed to wait and begin the collection when the next attack occurs.

GI hormones and Verner–Morrison syndrome

A number of GI hormones with various hormonal and local effects have been identified (Table 14.4). Excess amounts of these GI peptides are secreted by rare tumours. These tumours can often be identified by finding raised levels of the corresponding peptide in plasma. For example, in the Verner–Morrison syndrome, hypersecretion of vasoactive intestinal peptide (VIP) causes severe watery diarrhoea and hypokalaemia.

Table 14.4 Examples of GI peptides

Peptide and GI location	Probable functions
Gastric antrum and duodenum	
Gastrin (in cells called the G cells)	Stimulates gastric H^+ production. Also trophic to gastric mucosa
Duodenum and jejunum	
Secretin	Stimulates water and HCO_3^- secretion from the pancreas
CCK*	Stimulates secretion of enzymes by the pancreas, and contraction of the gallbladder
Glucose-dependent insulinotrophic peptide (GIP)[†]	Stimulates postprandial release of insulin, inhibits gastric acid secretion
Motilin	Stimulates intestinal motor activity
Pancreas	
Pancreatic polypeptide	Inhibits enzyme release from the pancreas, and relaxes the gallbladder
Ileum and colon	
Enteroglucagon	Increases small intestinal mucosal growth and slows the rate of intestinal transit
All areas of the GI tract	
VIP*	Secretomotor actions, also vasodilatation, and relaxation of intestinal smooth muscle

* CCK and VIP are examples of peptides found both in the GI tract and in the CNS.

† GIP is also known as gastric inhibitory polypeptide.

Keypoints

- At present, biochemical tests play a relatively minor role in the investigation of patients with suspected GI disorders.
- Plasma [gastrin] is raised in about 70% of patients with gastrinoma, while abnormal acid secretion is demonstrable in most patients. A raised [gastrin] is also found in patients with achlorhydria and hypochlorhydria.
- Serum amylase activities more than 10 times the normal value are virtually diagnostic of acute pancreatitis, and values greater than five times the normal value are suggestive of the disease. Moderate increases in serum amylase occur in many acute abdominal conditions.
- The measurement of faecal elastase is the preferred biochemical test of exocrine pancreatic function and is helpful in the investigation of patients with diarrhoea thought to be of pancreatic origin.
- Faecal fat estimation provides only limited diagnostic information and should be abandoned.
- Coeliac serology is used as an initial screen for jejunal malabsorption.
- Faecal calprotectin is a sensitive indicator of GI tract inflammation; a negative result may eliminate the need for further expensive investigation.
- Urinary 5-HIAA excretion is usually greatly increased in patients with the carcinoid syndrome.

Case 14.1

A 26-year-old woman was referred to the GI clinic with a 3-month history of abdominal discomfort and intermittent watery diarrhoea. Initial blood tests, including U&Es, liver function tests and CRP, did not show any significant abnormality although it was noted that the serum [potassium] was at the lower limit of the reference range. Haematological indices were normal. A screen for coeliac disease involving the measurement of anti-tTG IgA was also negative, as was a stool culture.

Measurement of electrolytes in the faecal water and calculation of the faecal osmotic gap (290 − 2 × (faecal [sodium] + faecal [potassium])) yielded the following results: *(continued on p. 221)*

Case 14.1 (continued)

Faecal	Result
Sodium	17 mmol/L
Potassium	12 mmol/L
Osmotic gap	232 mmol/kg

What conclusions may be drawn from these results?

Comments: A faecal sodium concentration of <60 mmol/L and a faecal osmotic gap >100 mmol/kg suggests that the diarrhoea was due to the presence of an osmotically active substance. Further investigation demonstrated that the concentration of magnesium in the faecal water was 63 mmol/L (reference cut-off 45 mmol/L), indicating that the diarrhoea was likely to be factious in origin and due to the ingestion of a magnesium-containing laxative.

In secretory diarrhoea associated with colonic stimulants or hormonal causes (e.g. a VIP-producing tumour), the osmotic gap is low (<50 mmol/kg) and the faecal sodium is generally >90 mmol/L.

Case 14.2

A 49-year-old man presented with a history of weight loss and chronic abdominal pain which was sometimes exacerbated by eating. He had experienced episodes of diarrhoea and had been passing greasy foul-smelling stools, which were difficult to flush. He consumed up to a bottle of whisky per day. Biochemical testing showed that U&Es were within reference limits. Other results were as follows:

Serum	Result	Reference range
Calcium	1.83	2.10–2.60 mmol/L
Albumin	29	35–50 g/L
ALP	183	40–125 U/L
ALT	36	10–50 U/L
Bilirubin	16	3–16 µmol/L
GGT	269	51–55 U/L
Amylase	251	<100 U/L
Random glucose	16	<11.1 mmol/L

Comment on these results. What is the most likely diagnosis?

Comments: When a patient presents with chronic abdominal pain associated with steatorrhoea but without a previous history of acute pancreatitis, the usual diagnostic problem is to distinguish between chronic pancreatitis and carcinoma of the pancreas. The modestly raised serum amylase is not diagnostic of pancreatic disease since similar levels may be found in other abdominal disorders such as perforated peptic ulcer or cholecystitis.

An ultrasound examination and CT scan revealed dilation and calcification of the main pancreatic duct and was consistent with the diagnosis of chronic pancreatitis. The subsequent demonstration of a low level of faecal elastase (76 µg/g faeces; reference range >200 µg/g faeces) confirmed that the exocrine pancreatic secretory function was inadequate. It is likely that the cause of this patient's disease was long-term alcohol abuse and that this was responsible for the elevation of serum GGT through hepatic enzyme induction. The elevation of ALP was found to be due to the bone isoenzyme, suggesting that fat malabsorption had led to vitamin D deficiency, osteomalacia and a low serum [calcium]. The elevated random plasma glucose is consistent with clinical diabetes that tends to occur relatively late in the course of chronic pancreatitis.

Case 14.3

A 12-year-old boy who had been diagnosed with type 1 diabetes 6 years earlier was generally unwell and now complained of intermittent episodes of diarrhoea. Initial biochemical investigations did not reveal any electrolyte disturbances or abnormalities of liver function, and haematological parameters were within reference limits. Coeliac serology results were as follows:

Serum	Result	Reference range
Anti-tTG IgA	<0.07	0.1–7.9 AU
Total IgA	<0.1	0.8–4.5 g/L
Anti-tTG IgG	>100	0.1–5.9 U/mL

Comment: This case illustrates the importance of checking total IgA levels when anti-tTG IgA is requested. Here the anti-tTG IgA result was unreliable because the patient was IgA deficient and it was essential that anti-tTG IgG antibodies were measured. The elevated anti-tTG IgG result suggested a diagnosis of coeliac disease which was confirmed by duodenal biopsy showing severe flattening of the villi and extensive loss of the brush border. The co-existance of coeliac disease and type 1 diabetes in this patient is consistent with the recognised increase in the prevalence of coeliac disease in patients with other autoimmune disorders.

Chapter 15

Nutrition

Introduction

In worldwide terms, nutritional disorders are responsible for much morbidity and mortality. The three main categories of nutritional disorder are:

- *undernutrition,* which is dominated by insufficient food energy, producing the features of starvation
- *malnutrition,* which is deficiency of one or more of the essential nutrients
- *obesity,* which is excessive positive energy balance.

Disease is also possible as a result of nutrient excess (e.g. iron overload, alcohol excess) or the effect of potentially toxic agents in food (e.g. favism, an acute haemolytic anaemia due to sensitivity to the fava bean).

Nutritional issues, directly or indirectly, impinge upon many of the tests undertaken in clinical biochemistry. Many analytes are altered by nutritional status. For example, diet exerts important short-term effects on serum [triglyceride] and plasma [glucose], and longer term effects on serum [cholesterol]. Certain inborn errors of metabolism may demand special diets, which are monitored biochemically (e.g. phenylalanine in PKU). Less obviously, diagnostic tests may only be valid if certain nutritional requirements are met. For example, measurement of 5-HIAA requires exclusion of rich sources of serotonin from the diet (p. 219), screening for hypercalciuria requires an adequate calcium intake, etc. Laboratory measurements are also necessary in the management of patients receiving nutritional support, especially total parenteral nutrition (TPN), and in the assessment of malabsorption (e.g. faecal elastase). Suspected nutritional deficiencies, ranging from possible iron deficiency to vitamin or trace metal deficiencies, also require specialist laboratory tests.

In this chapter, the first section considers the principal nutritional constituents, including the clinical significance and measurement of vitamins and trace elements. This is followed by a section on nutritional support and finally a section on the contrasting problems of protein-energy malnutrition (PEM) and obesity.

Principal dietary constituents

The nutrients in food can be subdivided into the following categories:
- Energy (in the form of carbohydrate and fat)
- Protein (as a source of nitrogen and essential amino acids)
- Major minerals (notably potassium, sodium, magnesium, calcium)
- Micronutrients (13 essential vitamins and a number of trace elements).

Lecture Notes: Clinical Biochemistry, 8e. By G. Beckett, S. Walker, P. Rae & P. Ashby. Published 2010 by Blackwell Publishing.

Food also contains non-nutrients. These include, for example:

- Fibre
- Substances present as additives or arising from food production (e.g. preservatives, colouring, fungicides used to preserve fruit, growth hormones used in animal husbandry)
- Other non-nutritive substances which may add flavour, smell, colour, etc. to food.

Carbohydrates

The major source of dietary energy is normally provided by carbohydrate, in the form of sugars (e.g. sucrose, lactose) or digestible polysaccharides; the major food polysaccharide is starch, found in cereals, root vegetables and legumes. Non-digestible polysaccharides contribute to dietary fibre. Carbohydrates are not essential nutrients, but insufficient carbohydrate intake leads to ketosis. The energy supplied is 4 kcal/g. Dietary carbohydrate in excess of the body's energy needs can be converted by the liver to fat. Stored carbohydrate is limited to muscle and liver glycogen, with the latter's store depleted 18–24 h after starvation. Complex carbohydrates contribute to the indigestible fibre content of the diet.

Fats

Dietary fat consists largely of triglycerides, with small amounts of other constituents (e.g. cholesterol). The National Food Survey (2000) showed that in Britain, on average, 35% of total energy was taken as fat and 48% was carbohydrate. Since the energy content of fat is greater than that of carbohydrate (~9 kcal/g, compared with 4 kcal/g for protein and for carbohydrate), the *weight* of dietary fat is substantially less than for carbohydrate on this diet.

Triglycerides contain saturated or unsaturated fatty acids, or both. Saturated fats are typically animal in origin, with epidemiological evidence that they predispose to cardiovascular disease possibly by raising LDL-cholesterol. Unsaturated fats are principally of plant or fish origin and tend to lower LDL-cholesterol and be cardioprotective,

particularly in the case of the ω-3 unsaturated fatty acids found in fish oils (e.g. eicosapentenoic acid).

In terms of daily intake, the current recommendation for fat intake in the UK is that energy intake from fat should ideally be no more than 30% of total calorie intake with no more than a third provided as saturated fat.

Linoleic and linolenic acids comprise the 'essential' free fatty acids required for membrane synthesis and serving as precursosrs for prostanoid biosynthesis Arachidonic acid is also essential but can be made *in vivo* from linoleic acid.

Proteins

Dietary protein from both animal and plant sources is required as a source of nitrogen and the essential amino acids (eight of the 20 amino acids used in protein synthesis are essential). The carbon skeleton of the amino acids can also be a source of energy, and protein normally provides about 11–14% of total calories on a 70–100 g protein diet; the minimum requirement is 40 g of protein of good biological value. Vegetable protein may be deficient in one or more of the eight essential amino acids, but this deficiency can be overcome by complementation, whereby a combination of cereals and legumes together provide protein of good biological value. As with carbohydrate, the energy supplied is 4 kcal/g.

Trace elements

More than 20 elements are known to be essential in animal nutrition. Of these, seven are 'bulk' elements (Na, K, Ca, Mg, Cl, S and P) and the rest are referred to as trace elements, present in tissues at less than 100 ppm. Table 15.1 lists some data about those that are known as *essential* trace elements.

The clinical importance of iron (e.g. in haem), iodine (in thyroid hormones) and cobalt (in cobalamin) is well established. Clinical syndromes associated with deficiency of copper, selenium, zinc, chromium, manganese and molybdenum have all been described, and these six elements will be considered here. The effects of iodine and iron defi-

Table 15.1 Trace elements essential to the human body

Essential trace element	Approximate total adult body content concentration	Daily oral intake (recommended for adults)*	Serum
Chromium	<6 mg	0.1 mg	<20 nmol/L
Cobalt	1 mg	As vitamin B$_{12}$	<10 nmol/L
Copper	100 mg	1.2 mg	12–26 μmol/L
Iodine	10–20 mg	0.15 mg	<5 nmol/L[†]
Iron	4–5 g	Males: 10 mg	14–32 μmol/L
		Females: 10–50 mg[‡]	10–28 μmol/L
Manganese	10–20 mg	3 mg	<20 nmol/L
Molybdenum	10 mg	0.2 mg	<15 nmol/L
Selenium	15 mg	0.1 mg	<4 nmol/L
Zinc	1–2 g	7–10 mg	10–20 μmol/L

* Much smaller amounts of inorganic trace elements are required if these are being provided as part of TPN.

† The total concentration in iodine-containing compounds in serum, mainly contained in the thyroid hormones, is 250–600 nmol/L; only 5 nmol/L is present as inorganic iodide.

‡ 10–20 mg/day in the reproductive period; 20–50 mg/day during pregnancy.

ciency are described elsewhere (pp. 118 and 258). Deficiency of *inorganic* cobalt has not been reported in man.

Deficiencies of essential trace elements usually arise in association with PEM, or with other abnormal nutritional states (e.g. TPN, neonatal feeds, synthetic diets). Specific inherited disorders in trace element handling are rare. Excessive losses, especially in association with severe and chronic GI diseases, may also cause deficiency.

Methods of assessing essential trace element deficiency are not straightforward and depend upon specialised techniques available in a limited number of laboratories. Moreover, plasma concentrations may not necessarily reflect actual nutritional status for a particular trace element, where intracellular levels may be more relevant. Despite these limitations, plasma values are often taken to indicate a specific deficiency. Changes in concentration may also reflect changes in concentration of plasma proteins that bind the metals. Diagnosis is often only made retrospectively on the basis of a clinical condition likely to have given rise to deficiency, occurring in association with clinical symptoms that can be attributed to the lack of trace elements, and which responds to treatment with the appropriate supplementation.

Zinc, copper and selenium

These micronutrients are more commonly monitored than other trace elements in the assessment of nutritional status, largely because of established deficiency syndromes associated with them.

Table 15.2 summarises some of the known function of these micronutrients and the causes and consequences of deficiency.

Absorption of zinc from the intestine appears to be controlled in a manner similar to that of iron (p. 255), with sequestration of zinc in enterocytes, as metallothionein, and transfer of some of this to the plasma; the rest is lost when the enterocytes are sloughed. Zinc is mostly transported bound to albumin, α$_2$-macroglobulin and transferrin. Specimens of blood for zinc measurement are affected by feeding and venous stasis; serum [zinc] may fall by as much as 20% after meals and levels should be assessed under fasting conditions. The body does not store zinc to any appreciable extent in any organ; urinary excretion is fairly constant at 10 μmol/24 h, with re-excretion into the gut being the main route for adjusting the amount excreted. Zinc excretion can, however, increase in trauma and catabolic states as an accompaniment to muscle protein catabolism and increase the risk of zinc deficiency. Injury, surgery, infection and a

Table 15.2 Known functions of zinc, copper and selenium, and causes and consequences of deficiency

Micronutrient	Function	Reason for deficiency	Clinical consequences (where known)
Zinc	Structural/cofactor role for several enzymes (e.g. alkaline phosphatase, carbonic anhydrase, enzymes of nucleic acid synthesis)	Dietary deficiency uncommon but observed with malnourishment and artificial nutrition. May be precipitated by alcoholism, with higher incidence reported in the elderly, in pregnancy and lactation	Dermatitis, immune deficiency, poor wound healing
Selenium	Structural component of several enzymes where it is incorporated into protein as selenocysteine. Includes anti-oxidant enzymes such as glutathione peroxidase and thioredoxine reductase, and other enzymes such as type I iodothyronine 5-deiodinase. Se deficiency is often assessed by measurement of glutathione peroxidase activity of red cells.	Rare but found in association with low Se content in soil, possibly artificial nutrition	Cardiac and skeletal myopathy. Possible increased risk of atheroma and some cancers
Copper	Required for the action of several enzymes: superoxide dismutase (anti-oxidant); tyrosinase (melanin synthesis); dopamine hydroxylase (synthesis of noradrenaline); cytochrome c oxidase (energy generation); lysyl oxidase (cross-linking collagen). Circulates as ceruloplasmin (see p. 205)	Rare but in association with artificial feeding and malnutrition in infants fed exclusivley cow's milk. High Zn intake can precipitate Cu deficicency (via metallothionein synthesis, which chelates Cu)	Microcytic anaemia, neutropenia. Osteoporosis

variety of acute illnesses are often accompanied by a fall in serum [zinc] due to the stimulation of hepatic metallothionein synthesis; this is one of the many components of the acute-phase response (p. 240). Measurement of CRP may point to an acute-phase response as the cause of a low serum zinc. Zinc levels may also fall in malignant disease or chronic liver disease without clinical zinc deficiency.

Other trace elements

Chromium may be involved in glucose homeostasis; a chromium complex present in brewer's yeast ('glucose tolerance factor') is able to improve glucose tolerance in some diabetics. Malnourished infants may develop severe glucose intolerance that improves with chromium supplementation. In adults, a syndrome presenting with weight loss, peripheral neuropathy and marked insulin-insensitive glucose intolerance has been described that improves with chromium supplementation.

Manganese is a component of certain metalloenzymes, and manganese ions activate a large number of other enzymes, for example those involved in the synthesis of glycosaminoglycans, cholesterol and prothrombin. Despite this extensive range of enzyme requirements for manganese, true deficiency in humans appears to be very rare.

Molybdenum is a component of xanthine oxidase and some other metallo-enzymes. Its deficiency has been reported to cause xanthinuria, with low serum [urate] and low urinary uric acid output.

Vitamins

Vitamins are all organic compounds that, as originally defined, cannot be synthesised in the human body and must be provided in the diet. They are essential for the normal processes of metabolism, including growth and maintenance of health. It is now known that the body is able to produce part or even all of its requirements for some of the vitamins, for example vitamin D from cholesterol and niacin from tryptophan. Table 15.3 summarises some data concerning both water-soluble and fat-soluble vitamins.

Table 15.3 The vitamins

Vitamin	Outline of the principal functions	Recommended daily amounts	Some effects of deficiency
Fat-soluble vitamins			
Vitamin A (retinol)	Vision, epithelial cell function	0.7 mg (males) 0.6 mg (females)	Night blindness, keratomalacia
Vitamin D (cholecalciferol)	Intestinal absorption of calcium, bone formation	7–8.5 μg for children 5 μg for adults (10 μg in pregnancy/lactation)	Rickets and osteomalacia
Vitamin E (tocopherols)	Antioxidant, membrane stability	4–8 mg, as γ-tocopherol	Haemolytic anaemia
Vitamin K (phytomenadione)	Hepatic synthesis of prothrombin	150 μg	Coagulation defects
Water-soluble vitamins			
Thiamin (vitamin B_1)	All the vitamins that comprise the group of B vitamins act as coenzymes or prosthetic groups for various enzymes that are important in intermediary metabolism	0.5 mg/1000 kcal or 1 mg (whichever is the greater)	Beri-beri, cardiac myopathy
Riboflavin (vitamin B_2)	See above	0.6 mg/1000 kcal or 1.2 mg	Cheilosis, stomatitis (as for vitamin B_1)
Niacin	See above	6.6 mg/1000 kcal or 13 mg (as for vitamin B_1)	Pellagra
Pyridoxine (vitamin B_6)	See above	2.2 mg (males) 2.0 mg (females)	Dermatitis, stomatitis, CNS symptoms
Biotin	See above	15 μg/1000 kcal (50 μg/1000 kcal children)	Anorexia, in dermatitis
Folic acid	See above	200 μg (300 μg in pregnancy)	Megaloblastic anaemia
Cyanocobalamin (vitamin B_{12})	See above	3 μg	Megaloblastic anaemia
Vitamin C (ascorbic acid)	Collagen formation	40 mg	Scurvy, anaemia

Deficiency may arise from inadequate diet, impaired absorption, insufficient utilisation, increased requirement or increased rate of excretion. Vitamin deficiency develops in stages:

1 *Subclinical deficiency,* in which there is depletion of body stores. These are normally relatively large in the case of fat-soluble vitamins (e.g. A and D) and vitamin B_{12}, but small in the case of other water-soluble vitamins.

2 *Overt deficiency,* which is usually accompanied by other evidence of malnutrition (e.g. PEM).

Biochemical investigations help to confirm the diagnosis of some overt vitamin deficiency diseases, and may allow the diagnosis to be made at an earlier stage. Several types of biochemical tests are available, of which only some will be applicable to the investigation of suspected deficiency of a particular vitamin. The vitamin may be directly measured in whole blood, plasma or serum, erythrocytes, leucocytes or tissue biopsy specimens. Alternatively, direct measurement of the vitamin or one of its major metabolites in urine is possible. In general, plasma concentrations of vitamins do not necessarily reflect the vitamin status of the body. Measurements of vitamins in cells generally give a much better indication of the body's vitamin status. Plasma levels usually fall before cellular and tissue levels fall, but low or undetectable plasma levels can occur in the absence of deficiency. Conversely, recent dietary intake can cause the plasma concentrations of vitamins to fluctuate markedly, even in severe deficiency. However, a sustained high plasma [vitamin] usually excludes a deficiency state.

Alternative approaches to assessment of vitamin status focus on the cofactor function of the vitamin. These include cofactor saturation tests in which the activity of the enzyme is measured *in vitro* before and after the addition of the enzyme's vitamin cofactor or prosthetic group. Clinical suspicion of a vitamin deficiency can also be corroborated by observing a response to the relevant vitamin supplementation; however, in the absence of measurements, the level of certainty is lower.

Deficiency of fat-soluble vitamins

Vitamin A

This vitamin is present in the diet as retinol. It can also be derived from dietary β-carotene, some of which is hydrolysed in the intestine to form retinol. A rich source is liver, although leafy vegetables and some fruits also provide the vitamin in large amounts. After absorption, followed by esterification in the mucosal cells, the ester is transported in the blood by retinol-binding protein. Specific binding proteins on cell membranes are involved in the uptake of vitamin A ester from plasma into the tissues. The vitamin is stored in the liver, mainly as its ester.

The active form of vitamin A, 11-*cis*-retinal, is necessary for rod vision, and its deficiency can cause night blindness. Another form, retinoic acid, induces differentiation of epithelial cells. Vitamin A deficiency predisposes to GI and respiratory tract infections and leads to night blindness and, if severe, to keratinisation of the cornea, corneal ulceration and, ultimately, blindness. Serum [vitamin A] may be decreased in states of severe protein deficiency, due to lack of its carrier protein, and may then increase if the protein deficiency is corrected.

Laboratory measurement is carried out by determination of serum [vitamin A], but this provides only limited information about the state of the tissue stores.

Vitamin D

The formation and metabolism of vitamin D are described on p. 73. Rickets in infancy and childhood, and osteomalacia in adults are the main forms of vitamin D deficiency (p. 83).

Vitamin E

Eight related tocopherols and tocotrienols possess vitamin E activity; they have antioxidant properties, and protect against oxidant (free radical) damage to polyunsaturated fatty acids in cell membranes.

Vitamin E deficiency is a rare complication of prolonged and severe steatorrhoea, and of prolonged parenteral nutrition. Altered red cell membrane stability can lead to haemolytic anaemia in children, while skeletal muscle breakdown may be responsible for the raised serum CK activity observed in both adults and children. Neurological consequences have also been described. Deficiency is investigated by measuring plasma [vitamin E].

Vitamin K

Vitamin K is not only found in liver and leafy vegetables (as K_1 or phylloquinone) but is also synthesised by colonic bacteria (as K_2 or menaquinone). It is necessary for the post-translational modification in proteins of glutamate side chains by γ-carboxylation. The presence of a second carboxyl group on the glutamate side chain confers phospholipid-binding properties on the modified protein in the presence of Ca^{2+}. Proteins containing γ-carboxyglutamate include certain clotting factors (II, VII, IX and X) and the bone matrix protein, osteocalcin.

Vitamin K deficiency is most often due to treatment with anticoagulants (e.g. warfarin); it leads to reduced levels of the vitamin K-dependent coagulation factors and, hence, to haemorrhage. Deficiency may also arise in obstructive jaundice, and levels may be low in the newborn (leading to haemorrhagic disease of the newborn). Tests to assess vitamin K status include the PT – an important test in the investigation and management of jaundiced patients (p. 199) and of those on anticoagulant treatment.

Deficiency of water-soluble vitamins

Ascorbic acid (vitamin C)

Vitamin C deficiency leads to scurvy which is characterised by perifollicular haemorrhages, swollen gums with loosened teeth, bruising, spontaneous haemorrhages and anaemia. Frank scurvy rarely occurs nowadays, but its subclinical form is by no means uncommon, especially among elderly people living alone. Ascorbic acid is a water-soluble anti-oxidant which maintains iron in the reduced (ferrous) form and which is essential to the activity of lysine and prolyl oxidase which cross-link collagen. Rich sources include citrus fruits, blackcurrants and potatoes.

Plasma [ascorbate] measurements provide a poor index of tissue stores. Leucocyte ascorbate measurements provide a reasonable assessment of tissue stores of ascorbate, but difficulties in obtaining leucocytes uncontaminated by other cellular elements mean that the buffy layer, consisting of leucocytes and platelets (and a few erythrocytes), is normally examined instead. Leucocytes and platelets take up ascorbate against a concentration gradient, and may retain most of their ascorbate even when plasma [ascorbate] has fallen to undetectable levels. Buffy layer [ascorbate] falls at about the same time as clinical evidence of scurvy appears, and seems to give a good indication of the body's stores of the vitamin. In clinical practice, suspicion of vitamin C deficiency may prompt a trial of vitamin C supplementation without formal measurement of vitamin C status.

Thiamin (vitamin B_1)

Dietary thiamin is readily absorbed and phosphorylated to its active form in the liver. Rich sources include wheat germ, yeast, legumes, nuts and some meats. As its derivative, thiamin pyrophosphate (TPP), thiamin is important as a coenzyme in carbohydrate metabolism, being necessary for oxidative decarboxylation reactions (e.g. conversion of pyruvate to acetyl-CoA) and transketolation reactions. Deficiency is associated with generalised malnutrition and is found in chronic alcoholism; it can lead to mood changes (depression, irritability), defective memory, peripheral neuropathy and, in more extreme cases, to beri-beri with cardiac failure. Severe and acute deficiency leads to Wernicke's encephalopathy, with memory loss and nystagmus; it is essential to supply adequate amounts of thiamin during re-feeding when requirements are increased.

Erythrocyte transketolase provides a specific and sensitive index of tissue [thiamin] and is the chemical measurement of choice for investigating possible thiamin deficiency. Enzyme activity is measured in red cell haemolysates before and after the addition of TPP.

Riboflavin (vitamin B$_2$)

The nucleotides of riboflavin are the prosthetic groups of many enzymes involved in electron transport, and riboflavin is essential for normal oxidative metabolism (e.g. as a cofactor for cytochrome c reductase and succinyl-CoA dehydrogenase).

Deficiency is typically in association with other nutrient deficiency. The findings include angular stomatitis, cheilosis and skin and eye lesions. Deficiency usually occurs as part of a mixed state involving several vitamins of the B complex, often including thiamin as well. Dietary sources include liver, kidney and milk products.

The activity of glutathione reductase in haemolysed erythrocytes, measured before and after the addition of flavin–adenine dinucleotide (the FAD effect), is a test for riboflavin deficiency.

Niacin

This term includes nicotinic acid and its amide (collectively referred to as niacin). Nicotinamide is a component of nicotinamide–adenine dinucleotide (NAD) and its phosphate (NADP); these are coenzymes of many dehydrogenases. The body's requirements for nicotinamide are met partly by dietary niacin, but a substantial part normally comes from metabolism of tryptophan.

Deficiency can be caused by an inadequate dietary intake. Maize protein is a poor source of tryptophan, and contains a bound form of niacin that is unavailable to the body. It may also be caused by conditions in which large amounts of tryptophan are metabolised along abnormal pathways (e.g. carcinoid syndrome, p. 219), and an acute deficiency can be precipitated by isoniazid treatment. Severe deficiency leads to pellagra, characterised by dermatitis (typically exposed skin parts), diarrhoea and mental changes, including dementia in chronic deficiency. Chemical methods for detecting niacin deficiency measure its excretion in urine or the excretion of its metabolites.

Folic acid

The active form is tetrahydrofolic acid which functions as a coenzyme in the transport of one-carbon units from one compound to another, and is essential for nucleic acid synthesis. Deficiency leads to impaired cell division, especially manifest as a pancytopenia, with defective red cell maturation (megaloblastic anaemia); folate deficiency is one of the common vitamin deficiency states in humans arising from malabsorption, increased requirement (e.g. pregnancy) or excessive losses (e.g. dialysis) or a combination. A large, multicentre Medical Research Council trial demonstrated that folic acid supplementation reduces the occurrence (or recurrence) of NTDs (spina bifida, anencephaly and encephalocoele) by about 70%; the vitamin should be started by the mother before conception. Methods of investigation include serum [folate] and erythrocyte [folate]. Good sources are liver, kidney and fresh vegetables.

Other water-soluble vitamins

The term vitamin B$_6$ includes pyridoxine, pyridoxal, pyridoxamine and their 5-phosphate derivatives. Good sources are liver and cereals (whole grain). The active form of the vitamin, pyridoxal phosphate (PP), is the prosthetic group of many enzymes, including the aminotransferases – ALT and AST – and amino acid decarboxylases. Deficiency of vitamin B$_6$ is rare and nearly always occurs as part of a mixed deficiency of the B vitamins.

As a test for suspected pyridoxine deficiency, the activity of ALT or AST in haemolysed erythrocytes can be determined before and after the addition of PP (the PP effect).

Biotin serves as a coenzyme for carboxylase reactions, including those catalysed by pyruvate carboxylase and acetyl-CoA carboxylase. Deficiency in man has been reported during TPN, and very rarely in association with excessive consumption of raw egg white, which contains the biotin-binding protein, avidin. Deficiency symptoms include dermatitis, alopecia, mental depression, nausea and vomiting.

Dietary deficiency of cyanocobalamin or vitamin B$_{12}$ is rare but found in vegans (the vitamin is largely obtained from animal sources). The usual cause is pernicious anaemia where autoimmune disease is associated with loss of intrinsic factor, required for absorption of the vitamin. Deficiency leads to a megaloblastic anaemia and, additionally, may be associated with demyelination, particularly of the spinal cord, with neurological defects. Deficiency is usually diagnosed by haematological examination of blood and bone marrow specimens, and is confirmed by measuring serum [vitamin B$_{12}$] and by investigating vitamin B$_{12}$ absorption from the intestine before and after the administration of intrinsic factor (the Schilling test).

Assessment of nutritional status

This depends upon a combination of history, clinical examination and biochemical assessment. History or clinical examination alone are often sufficient in a severely malnourished patient. A good dietary history, which may require detailed recording of food and drink intake over a 7-day period, is very valuable and may identify generalised malabsorption or a specific nutritional problem.

Nutritional measures include body weight and height (for determination of BMI), skin-fold thickness as a measure of subcutaneous fat, and mid-arm muscle area (derived from mid-arm muscle circumference and triceps skinfold thickness) as a measure of skeletal muscle mass. Physical examination can also expose signs of malnutrition (e.g. bleeding gums in scurvy; dermatitis in niacin deficiency). Bioelectrical impedance can be measured to determine total body water content, fat and fat-free mass. Estimates of muscle mass can be based on 24-h urinary creatinine or 3-methylhistidine excretion; both methods depend on the accuracy of urine collections. Nitrogen losses can be determined indirectly by measurement of 24-h urinary urea excretion.

Biochemical tests to assess overall nutritional status are of very limited value. Serum albumin concentration is sometimes used but is a poor measure of nutritional state as it is affected by renal and liver disease as well as nutrition. Moreover, levels can fall rapidly as part of the acute-phase response, while malnourished patients may display acceptable albumin levels for weeks (since reduced formation is accompanied by reduced catabolism). Other 'nutritional' proteins such as retinol-binding protein or transferrin offer little advantage over albumin.

In contrast, specific biochemical measurements of vitamins or trace elements may be helpful in nutritional assessment and confirm an underlying deficiency suspected on clinical grounds.

Nutritional support

Nutritional support is essential in the presence of severe undernutrition and malnutrition. Patients in hospital may be undernourished and also benefit.

Patients who are severely ill with sepsis, multiple trauma or extensive burns may develop a marked negative nitrogen balance, demanding nutritional support. Other indications include unconsciousness, clinical cachexia, radiotherapy or chemotherapy, major resection for malignancy, renal failure, post-operative management of major surgery and complications of surgery, or any circumstances in which the GI tract is not available or is unable to support nutrition (e.g. severe inflammatory bowel disease, gut resection, fistula). At one extreme this support may take the form of TPN, where all nutritional needs are met via an IV route. As far as possible the enteral route should be used, which is both safer and less costly than the parenteral route. Where a patient is unable to eat, the feed can be provided via a nasogastric tube or via a gastrostomy or jejunostomy if feeding is likely to be longer.

Energy requirements vary depending upon build, level of activity and, in sick patients, on whether they are pyrexial or catabolic (e.g. after trauma or major surgery). Basal energy requirements can be calculated on the basis of sex, weight, height and age, and adjusted for activity, hypercatabolism, etc.

Energy is provided by either carbohydrate or fat. A more physiological approach is to use a mixture of carbohydrate and fat. The calorific value of carbohydrate of 4 kcal/g contrasts with the 9 kcal/g of fat. If the diet is administered as a liquid feed (either enterally or parenterally), inclusion of fat means that a smaller volume can be used to deliver the energy requirements.

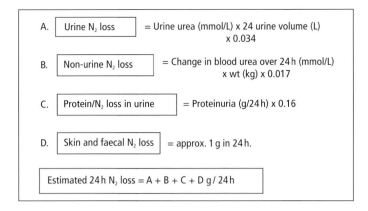

A. | Urine N₂ loss | = Urine urea (mmol/L) x 24 urine volume (L)
x 0.034

B. | Non-urine N₂ loss | = Change in blood urea over 24 h (mmol/L)
x wt (kg) x 0.017

C. | Protein/N₂ loss in urine | = Proteinuria (g/24 h) x 0.16

D. | Skin and faecal N₂ loss | = approx. 1 g in 24 h.

Estimated 24 h N₂ loss = A + B + C + D g / 24 h

Figure 15.1 Calculation of nitrogen losses (and, therefore, nitrogen requirements) from 24-h urinary urea measurement.

Nitrogen is provided by protein and/or amino acids in the diet, and a balanced feed should provide the essential amino acids required for health. Protein also has a calorific value similar to that of carbohydrate. In general, protein intake should normally provide 10–15% of the energy requirements and can be calculated on that basis. Utilisation of amino acids also depends upon the overall adequate provision of calories to meet energy requirements. Where necessary (e.g. in parenteral nutrition (p. 232), nitrogen requirements can be matched to the overall nitrogen losses. Figure 15.1 shows how 24-h urinary urea measurement can be used to determine the overall nitrogen losses.

Micronutrients will also be needed and are provided on the basis of available evidence at the recommended dietary allowance (RDA), either as a balanced diet, or as actual constituents of defined feeds used for enteral or parenteral nutrition.

Water requirements must also be met, taking into account insensible losses plus the minimal volume to allow adequate renal excretion. In general, around 2 L will be required, but the actual figure will vary depending upon other potential fluid losses, the presence of pyrexia, renal function, etc. Similarly, basic electrolyte requirements will vary depending upon actual daily losses, renal function, baseline deficiencies, etc. This is discussed further under parenteral nutrition.

Methods of nutritional delivery

With respect to hospitalised patients, nutritional support can be provided by oral feeding, using tube feeding into the gut (nasogastric, nasoduodenal, gastrostomy or jejunostomy, small bore tubes) or by parenteral nutrition.

While oral feeding is the most desirable (and safest) route it may not be possible in the presence of oral pathology, with swallowing difficulties or in the anorexic or unconscious patient. In this situation, tube feeding provides a good alternative – it is cheaper and safer than parenteral nutrition, while allowing delivery of all nutritional requirements. It is also physiological, in the sense that nutrients are absorbed into the portal circulation. It also helps maintain the integrity of the gut. Problems of tube blockage or oesophageal erosion may occur.

Parenteral nutrition

Some of the indications for parenteral nutrition are listed in Table 15.4. It is particularly indicated in the short bowel syndrome or in the presence of fistula formation involving the GI tract. Most IV feeding is complete, providing all essential nutrients exogenously, and it is then known as TPN. Nutrients are delivered (typically via a central vein) at a pre-defined rate using an appropriate pump and delivery set, usually from a large bag containing all the prescribed ingredients and over a 24-h

Table 15.4 Principal indications for total parenteral nutrition

Short bowel syndrome
Radiation enteritis
Acute pancreatitis
Prolonged ileus
Severe inflammatory bowel disease (especially fistula
  formation)
Hypermetabolic states (e.g. severe burns, sepsis)

Table 15.5 Total parenteral nutrition: typical composition of a standard feed

Nitrogen	12–14 g (as amino acids)
Fat	900 kcal (as 500 ml of 20% fat emulsion)
Glucose	1000 kcal (as 1.25 L of 20% dextrose)
Sodium	70–100 mmol
Potassium	60–100 mmol
Calcium	5–10 mmol
Magnesium	5–10 mmol
Phosphate	30 mmol
Trace elements	Present
Vitamins	Present (water soluble and fat soluble)
Volume	2.5–3 L

It is emphasised that the above table represents a suitable standard regime only. Individual patients may have requirements that differ considerably from those listed above.

period. Administration of parenteral nutrition via a peripheral vein is unusual, though possible for short periods. The energy which can be delivered by the peripheral route is limited because hyperosmolar glucose and amino acid solutions are irritant and can lead to thrombophlebitis; it is for this reason that the central vein route is preferred. TPN is also used in the home in some patients who require constant support through this route (e.g. short bowel syndrome) and may then be delivered during the overnight period.

Composition of the feed

Table 15.5 lists the typical composition of an adult feed over a 24-h period. More accurate assessment of energy requirements depends upon estimated expenditure, which relates to height, weight and age, as well as factors such as pyrexia, mobility and whether or not the patient is hypercatabolic. Nitrogen requirements can be estimated from 24-h urine urea losses. The electrolyte requirements illustrated are 'typical' but would be adjusted according to individual need, and may, for example, be increased in the presence of excessive electrolyte losses (e.g. diarrhoea) or reduced with renal disease, cardiac failure or advanced liver disease. Micronutrient requirements would vary less on an individual basis but could be adjusted to meet specific deficiencies.

1 *Energy content* The complete IV feed must provide adequate calories, typically 1800–2000 kcal/24 h; more may be required in some circumstances (e.g. after severe burns). Calories are normally provided as a mixture of carbohydrate (glucose) and fat. In order to provide 1000 kcal as glucose, it is necessary to use *hypertonic* solutions,

since about 5 L of 5% dextrose would be needed in order to provide 1000 kcal, whereas the same amount of energy could be provided with 1.25 L of 20% dextrose. Fat, administered as an emulsion, has a higher energy content than glucose, such that 500 mL of a 20% fat emulsion provides about 900 kcal. The fat emulsion should also provide essential fatty acids.

2 *Nitrogen content* The commercially available solutions contain all the essential amino acids. The prescription is normally in the range 12–14 g nitrogen/24 h. Some patients require less nitrogen (e.g. small, elderly patients), while others require more (e.g. hypercatabolic patients with severe burns, multiple trauma).

3 *Electrolyte content* The requirements for Na^+ and K^+ over the 24-h period must be stated on each day's prescription. Typically, the Na^+ requirement will be 70–100 mmol/24 h, but more will be needed in the event of excessive losses of Na (e.g. severe diarrhoea, fistula), and less where there is Na^+ retention (e.g. renal disease, congestive cardiac failure). Potassium requirements are more variable. Intracellular repletion, or the administration of glucose and insulin, may increase demands for K^+, whereas requirements will be very small in renal failure or where there is extensive tissue break-

233

down. A stable patient probably requires 60–100 mmol K$^+$/24 h.

4 *Vitamins and minerals* The requirements for calcium and phosphate depend on individual needs of patients, but average requirements are about 5–10 mmol/24 h for calcium and 30 mmol/24 h for phosphate. The magnesium requirement is normally about 5–10 mmol/24 h. Trace metals and both water-soluble and fat-soluble vitamins are also added to the feed.

5 *Fluid volume* This is dictated by clinical circumstances, but 2.5–3 L/24 h meets the requirements for most patients (less in the elderly). Depending upon the particular energy prescription, a certain minimum volume will be required to deliver the prescribed number of calories.

Biochemical monitoring of patients on total parenteral nutrition

The proper monitoring of patients on TPN requires attention to fluid balance, temperature, regular weighing (where feasible) as well as regular biochemical and haematological measurements (the latter includes full blood count and clotting measurements). This section considers the biochemical measurements that should be made which are as follows:

- Measurement of serum urea, creatinine, Na$^+$, K$^+$ and total CO$_2$ concentrations daily until the patient is stable with accurate records of fluid balance. Where there are potentially large electrolyte losses (e.g. via a fistula after surgery on the GI tract, the diuretic phase of acute renal failure), knowledge of (a) the fluid [K$^+$] and [Na$^+$] and (b) the volume of the fluid lost assist in the interpretation of abnormal serum electrolyte values and can help decide on the amount of K$^+$ and Na$^+$ to be added to the feed.
- Glucose should be measured at least daily and sometimes more often until the patient is stable.
- CRP measurement twice weekly can be useful on account of the infection risks associated with the feeding line.
- Serum calcium (and albumin, to assist interpretation of the calcium, p. 75), phosphate and magnesium should be measured about 2 or 3 times

weekly until stable and in the absence of severe derangements of these analytes.

- Mild derangements in 'liver function tests' are sometimes observed during TPN, and these tests (p. 196) should also be carried out twice weekly
- Trace element monitoring (principally copper, zinc and selenium) require baseline measurement and every 2–3 weeks initially. Iron, ferritin, vitamins B$_{12}$ and folate are also measured at about the same frequency as the trace elements. Individuals on longer term nutrition – including home TPN – would also have assessment of vitamin status (especially vitamin D) and other trace elements such as manganese.
- Regular measurement of other proteins (i.e. in addition to albumin) can be used to assess nutritional status but is of limited value.
- Twice-weekly 24-h urine collections should be made so that nitrogen losses can be estimated from the urea excretion; these figures are inevitably underestimates, due to incomplete urine collections and the failure to take into account other routes of nitrogen loss. Moreover, the proportion of urinary N as urea varies with the acid–base status. If proteinuria is significant, these losses must also be determined and taken into account. Despite these drawbacks, the estimated nitrogen losses help to decide whether the nitrogen content of the feed is sufficient to maintain a positive nitrogen balance.

Complications of total parenteral nutrition

This section will concentrate on the biochemical complications, though it is important to remember that infective problems, in particular, can arise from the TPN delivery system itself. An important and potentially serious complication of TPN is sepsis introduced via the catheter, and blood and other cultures may be required. Catheter care and the stipulation that, except in extreme emergencies, the catheter must be used *exclusively* for the administration of the feed are important concepts in feeding patients by the parenteral route. Thrombosis and embolism at the site of delivery are occasional complications

The principal biochemical complications are:

• Electrolyte disturbances. For example, hypokalaemia can arise when losses or requirements exceed supply. Conversely, hyperkalaemia may arise, especially in patients with renal disease or those with metabolic acidosis. Hyponatraemia is relatively common and may reflect the underlying metabolic response to trauma/surgery with raised vasopressin levels, though it may also arise if sodium and water losses are excessive and not matched by intake, or in the presence of sodium and water retention with oedema and ascites (e.g. heart failure, liver failure). Assessment of fluid balance and clinical condition usually allows these different causes to be distinguished. Hypernatraemia may reflect water deficiency or, sometimes, excess sodium intake in the feed.

• Glucose intolerance is a relatively common problem, especially in the older individual, and often reflects the high glucose feeds and a balance of insulin lack/stress hormone increase (e.g. associated with sepsis and the catabolic state) which favour hyperglycaemia. Insulin infusion may be necessary. Conversely, sudden cessation of the high glucose feed can lead to a rebound hypoglycaemia.

• Liver function test abnormalities are also described. Fatty liver disease and steatohepatitis are recognised with associated liver function test abnormalities and may reflect increased fat production within the liver from carbohydrate. A cholestatic picture is also possible, especially in the absence of any enteral feeding. In general, the liver function test and liver changes appear to be reversible, though children are more susceptible to more longer term problems, as are adults on longer term TPN.

• Hypocalcaemia and hypomagnesaemia can reflect inadequate intake, and magnesium, in particular, can be lost with sodium and potassium if fluid losses are excessive. Low phosphate frequently reflects the increased phosphate requirements associated with tissue growth and repair (see 'The re-feeding syndrome' below).

The re-feeding syndrome

This is a potentially serious condition which especially arises when a more severely malnourished patient is re-fed too quickly. It is not restricted to parenteral nutrition. In a malnourished individual there is an adaptation to poor carbohydrate supply which includes increased ketone body formation and utilisation, low insulin and low basal metabolic rate (BMR). The sudden availability of plentiful glucose will stimulate insulin and a switch to glucose utilisation, with increased requirements for phosphate, potassium and magnesium which move into the cell under the influence of insulin. Thiamin requirements are also raised (e.g. for pyruvate dehydrogenase activity on the glucose oxidation pathway). The consequences can be life-threatening, with hypokalaemia, hypophosphataenia and hypomagnesaemia, and neurological and cardiovascular problems associated with thiamin deficiency.

Patients at risk include:
• Low BMI ($<16\,kg/m^2$)
• Chronic malnutrition (including kwashiorkor and marasmus)
• Anorexia nervosa
• Malnutrtion with pre-existing hypomagnesaemia, hypokalaemia (e.g. severe, chronic alcoholism).

Calories should be introduced gradually with adequate supplies of potassium, phosphate, magnesium and thiamin, and careful biochemical monitoring.

The nutrition team

It cannot be emphasised too strongly that nutritional support is a multidisciplinary affair. Clinical biochemistry has a crucial role to play in advising on the selection of tests, recording the results and advising on the metabolic complications that might arise. Ideally, a nutrition team includes representatives from clinical biochemistry, microbiology, pharmacy, dietetics and nursing, in addition to one or more clinicians (often surgeons), all of whom should have a special interest in nutrition. As well as advising on policy in this costly area, such a team should be able to offer expert advice and be competent to audit nutritional care.

Major nutritional problems

This section will consider two contrasting nutritional problems which, on a worldwide scale, are both common and important. These are PEM and obesity.

Protein-energy malnutrition (PEM)

This arises from insufficient food, anorexia, persistent vomiting or regurgitation, or malabsorption. It may also be seen where the BMR is increased (severe infections, thyrotoxicosis), in cancer cachexia and other illnesses. The severity of undernutrition is assessed by clinical and dietary history, supplemented by appropriate anthropometric measurements and biochemical tests (see section on Nutritional assessment) and the BMI, defined as weight/(height)^2 (expressed in kilograms and metres, respectively). The acceptable range of BMI is 20–25.

A range of biochemical abnormalities may be found. Blood glucose may be low, with a corresponding increase in plasma free fatty acids and ketone bodies (with associated mild metabolic acidosis). Plasma [glucagon] and [cortisol] levels increase at the expense of a reduced [insulin]. Reverse T3 increases at the expense of normal T3. Creatinine excretion diminishes.

PEM in children leads to a spectrum of diseases. Nutritional marasmus is the childhood version of severe starvation, and is typically found in cases where the child is weaned early onto dilute cow's milk formula. Weight is less than 60% of the standard weight, and there is often evidence of vitamin and other nutrient deficiencies, with associated chronic infections. In kwashiorkor, the diet is low in protein, but may be relatively satisfactory in carbohydrate intake (e.g. a child weaned onto diets such as yam, cassava or diluted cereal). The insulin levels may be less affected (since carbohydrate is present), with diversion of amino acids from the viscera to muscles, leading to impaired albumin synthesis by a fatty liver (with reduced lipoprotein export). The low albumin leads to the characteristic hypoalbuminaemic oedema found in this condition.

Obesity

The most common nutritional disorder in affluent societies is defined as an excess of body fat. Obesity is stated to occur at a BMI of 30 and gross obesity at a BMI of 40 or above. In general, it arises from an excess of calorie intake over expenditure. The problem may be multifactorial, with socioeconomic factors, age, sex and heredity all contributing. Occasionally, obesity is found in association with specific disorders such as hypothyroidism, Cushing's syndrome, hypogonadism or hypopituitarism, and rarely with monogenetic disorders such as leptin deficiency (see below). Biochemical measurements may all be normal, but simple obesity shows an association with type 2 diabetes (p. 92), hyperlipidaemia (typically, mixed), hyperuricaemia and sometimes fatty liver with mild derangements in liver function tests.

The metabolic and other problems associated with obesity have led to the concept of a condition termed the metabolic syndrome which carries increased risk of cardiovascular disease. There are various definitions of this condition which differ in detail but are broadly similar. For example, the International Diabetes Federation defines the condition on the basis of central adiposity plus any two of four factors (fasting triglyceride ≥1.7 mmol/L; HDL-cholesterol <1.03 in males or <1.29 in females; a blood pressure of ≥130/85; a fasting glucose of ≥5.6 mmol/l). Central obesity is determined by the waist circumference (generally >90 cm in men and >80 cm in women). The precise aetiology of the metabolic syndrome is unknown but central obesity and insulin resistance are certainly important factors. Moreover, the clinical utility and pathogenesis of the condition have been questioned and may offer no benefit over and above established means of cardiovascular risk estimation (such as the Framingham Risk Score).

A major concern is the increasing prevalence of obesity which is rising to epidemic proportions such that around 25% of the adult population in the UK are clinically obese. The increase has been especially prominent in men age 55–64, with 36% of men in this age range defined as obese.

Indeed, the problem is replacing malnutrition and infectious diseases as the most significant health problem worldwide. The rise in obesity is almost certainly multifactoral but reflects a combination of calorie intake above requirements ('junk foods') and inactivity. The lack of education on nutritional matters has also come in for criticism.

In recent years, there has been increasing research in the area of obesity and appetite control and this was particularly stimulated by the discovery of the hormone leptin, a 16-kDa hormone which is secreted by adipose tissue. The discovery of leptin followed the investigation of the cause of the severe obesity seen in the genetically obese ob/ob mouse. When a recombinant leptin was administered to the ob/ob mouse, it reversed the abnormalities of obesity, hyperphagia, diabetes and hyperinsulinaemia. Leptin itself has a structural homology to members of the cytokine family and appears to be expressed exclusively in adipose tissue. The leptin receptor which is also a member of the cytokine receptor superfamily is highly expressed in the brain and particularly in hypothalamic nuclei which are known to have a role in appetite control. Although obesity and severe hyperphagia result from the absence of leptin signalling, the evidence is principally that leptin in normal physiology acts as a sensor of peripheral nutrient stores to signal to the brain to activate or suppress the neurohumoural and reproductive responses to starvation. In obese humans, plasma leptin is generally high. This has led to the suggestion that 'leptin resistance' might contribute to cases of human obesity. However, this is controversial and the central nervous system (CNS) regions which respond to leptin may be optimally set to respond at the very low levels of leptin which are seen in nutritionally deprived states. In other words, the high plasma leptin levels, on average, in obese individuals are a consequence of the obesity rather than a cause.

Treatment of obesity, in the absence of rare specific causes, is directed at individual lifestyle issues, though population-based strategies which promote healthy eating also have a place.

Further Reading

Ayling, R. and Marshall, W. (2007) *Nutrition and Laboratory Medicine*. ACB Venture Publications.

British Heart Foundation Statistics website (http://www.heartstats.org/homepage.asp?id=6)

Keypoints

- Nutritional disorders are common and are important on a worldwide basis. Broadly speaking, three disorders are recognised: undernutrition, malnutrition and obesity.
- Clinical biochemical tests may be required for nutritional assessment, particularly measurement of certain vitamins, inorganic ions, trace elements. Plasma proteins (e.g. albumin, transferrin) have limited usefulness.
- Patients receiving TPN require regular biochemical monitoring. In the uncomplicated patient: daily serum [urea], [creatinine], [Na], [K], [total CO_2], [glucose]; twice weekly serum [calcium], [phosphate], [magnesium] and liver function tests; twice weekly 24-h urine collections to assess nitrogen requirement.
- Nutritional status often affects the measurement or interpretation of laboratory tests in clinical biochemistry.

Case 15.1

A 56-year-old female with chronic alcoholism is admitted for observation after sustaining a head injury after a fall. Examination reveals peripheral oedema and tachycardia. Sensation is markedly reduced in all limbs distally in a glove and stocking distribution and the patient appears ataxic, confused with a slight horizontal nystagmus.

What type of nutritional deficiency might account for the findings in this woman and how might you confirm your suspicions?

Comments: This woman displays the clinical features of thiamin deficiency. This is a recognised complication in a proportion of alcoholics and reflects low thiamin intake, impaired absorption and possibly accelerated destruction of thiamin diphosphate. The principal manifestations of thiamin deficiency affect the cardiovascular and nervous systems. Patients may develop peripheral vasodilatation, retention of water and sodium, and a biventricular heart failure. The tachycardia and peripheral oedema are expected findings in relation to the cardiovascular problems of thiamin deficiency. In the nervous system, a peripheral neuropathy may be found and is shown in this patient in the reduced sensation. The CNS may also be involved, and the clinical features of ataxia and nystagmus support CNS involvement. Confirmation of the diagnosis is best made by measuring the activity of the enzyme transketolase in red cells. This is a thiamin-dependent enzyme and the native activity is measured, followed by determination of the increment in activity on addition of exogenous thiamin. An enhancement in transketolase activities by >15% by added thiamin is good evidence for thiamin deficiency.

Case 15.2

A 42-year-old male visits his GP with a history strongly suggestive of angina on exertion. The GP records a weight of 125 kg and a height of 1.6 m. Waist circumference is 120 cm. His blood pressure is elevated at 175/105. A blood sample is sent to the laboratory and shows a fasting glucose of 6.8 mmol/L, a cholesterol of 7.2 mmol/L, triglycerides of 6.2 mmol/L and a HDL of 0.6 mmol/L.

What is the likely condition in this man which underlies his ischaemic heart disease. What are the criteria used to diagnose this particular condition?

Comments: This patient has the features of the metabolic syndrome (see p. 236). Although the fasting glucose does not reach a level diagnostic for diabetes mellitus, a glucose tolerance test would be recommended. His problem of angina and probable ischaemic heart disease is likely to progess unless attention is paid to correcting these problems, by a combination of lifestyle or drug-related means. In this type of patient, a lifestyle approach which concentrates on weight loss and nutrition can have a major impact on successfully managing his ischaemic heart disease.

Case 15.3

A 53-year-old female with a BMI of 21 undergoes small bowel resection for a volvulus after an acute surgical admission and subsequently requires home parenteral nutrition to meet her nutritional needs. A feed is prescribed which takes into account her calorie and nitrogen requirements, and provides suitable daily amounts of electrolytes and water as well as micronutrients. Despite this, biochemical monitoring of serum reveals a phosphate of 0.3 mmol/L, a magnesium of 0.4 mmol/L and a potassium of 3.0 mmol/L. The sodium is 132 mmol/L with a creatinine of 38 mol/L. Plasma glucose is 8.2 mmol/L.

Can you explain these findings? What changes would you make to her feed, if any? Are there any other biochemical measurements which might be helpful at this stage, bearing in mind that she has short bowel syndrome and is likely to require home parenteral nutrition?

(continued on p. 239)

Case 15.3 *(continued)*

Comments: The patient already has a low BMI prior to her surgery and, at the time of introduction of parenteral nutrition, is likely to be underweight. Her reduced muscle bulk is likely to be reflected in the low serum creatinine of 38 mmol/L. The introduction of nutrients by means of parenteral nutrition will stimulate the laying down of new cellular material which requires electrolytes such as phosphate, magnesium and potassium to be incorporated into the new cell structure. This anabolic utilisation of these electrolytes would be stimulated by the simultaneous infusion of glucose and the insulin response elicited. The low serum levels of these electrolytes almost certainly reflects their incorporation into cellular material and indicates that the parenteral feed could be adjusted to provide more of these electrolytes. Mild hyponatraemia is quite a common finding in patients undergoing parenteral nutrition and is not, in itself, an indication to increase the sodium content of the feed. Assessment of the urine sodium excretion in a 24-h urine collection can establish whether or not sodium administration is adequate. Similarly, a raised plasma glucose is also not an uncommon finding in the face of the high glucose load administered as a component of the parenteral feed. Levels would need to be monitored, although a value of 8.2 mmol/L would not necessarily be an indication for insulin administration on the basis of a single, isolated reading.

Chapter 16

Trauma, inflammation, immunity and malignancy

Plasma contains over 300 proteins. Many of these have a specific biochemical role, and organic disease may result when their concentration in plasma is reduced. Conversely disease processes such as trauma, infection and inflammation may themselves lead to changes in the concentration of a wide range of plasma proteins. Some plasma proteins, including most enzymes and tumour markers, have no known function in blood, and arise as a result of cell death or tissue damage. The measurement of some specific proteins, however, may have a valuable clinical role in monitoring progression of a disease or response to therapy. Table 16.1 lists examples of commonly measured plasma proteins.

Many laboratories do not measure serum [total protein] as part of a general profile, as a fall in the concentration of one protein may be masked by a coincident or compensatory increase in another.

Electrophoresis separates the proteins into five broad fractions – albumin, α_1-globulins, α_2-globulins, β-globulins and γ-globulins (Figure 16.1); each of the globulin fractions consists of a mixture of many proteins. Serum protein electrophoresis has limited diagnostic value except in the detection and quantification of the paraproteins found in multiple myeloma (see Figure 16.1 and later text).

Changes in plasma proteins in trauma, infection and inflammation – 'the acute-phase response'

Following trauma, infection, inflammation, burns, etc., the body responds by initiating a series of mechanisms that lead to:

- Acute haemodynamic changes.
- A rapid fall in the concentration of some plasma proteins (e.g. albumin, transferrin).
- An increase in the concentration of several specific proteins some hours after the injury. These proteins are the acute-phase proteins, and are listed in Table 16.2.

The cytokines and a host of vasoactive substances are important mediators of the acute-phase response. The rapid decrease in concentration of certain proteins appears to result from loss of plasma protein into the extravascular space, due to increased vascular permeability caused by vasoactive substances, including cytokines, prostaglandins and histamine. The increase in the acute-phase plasma proteins results from increased synthesis and release, which appears to be mediated by interleukin-6.

Lecture Notes: Clinical Biochemistry, 8e. By G. Beckett, S. Walker, P. Rae & P. Ashby. Published 2010 by Blackwell Publishing.

Table 16.1 Examples of plasma proteins commonly measured for the diagnosis and monitoring of disease

Proteins and their electrophoretic mobility	Principal function(s)	Used in the detection or investigations of disease
Albumin	Colloidoncotic pressure, transport functions	Malnutrition, malignancy, liver, kidney and GI disease
α₁-Globulins		
α₁-Fetoprotein	Unknown	NTDs, tumour marker
α₁-Protease inhibitor (API)	Anti-protease	API deficiency
Prothrombin	Blood clotting	Coagulation screen; liver function test
α₂-Globulins		
Ceruloplasmin	Copper transport	Wilson's disease
Haptoglobin	Hb binding	Haemolytic disorders
α₂-Macroglobulin	Anti-protease, transport	Proteinuria (e.g. selectivity investigations)
β-Globulins		
C-reactive protein	Defence	Infection, inflammation
β₂-Microglobulin	Defence	Monitoring myeloma, renal failure
Transferrin	Iron transport	Iron deficiency/excess
γ-Globulins		
Igs (IgG, IgA, IgM, etc.)	Defence	Liver disease, infections, autoimmune disease, paraproteinaemias, etc.

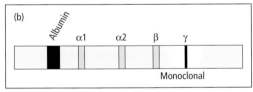

(a) Normal serum
Albumin α1 α2 β γ

(b) Monoclonal
Albumin α1 α2 β γ

Figure 16.1 Separation of serum proteins by electrophoresis. The upper figure (a) shows the pattern in a normal serum sample. The lower figure (b) shows the typical discrete band found in the γ-globulin region in patients with myeloma.

Table 16.2 Examples of acute-phase proteins that increase

Protein	Function	Increase
C-reactive protein	Binds extracts of pneumococcal cell walls	↑↑↑↑
Anti-protease inhibitors	Protease inhibitor	↑↑↑
Ceruloplasmin	Copper transport. Superoxide scavenger	↑↑↑
α₁-Acid glycoprotein	Tissue repair?	↑↑
Fibrinogen	Clotting	↑↑
Haptoglobin	Binds Hb	↑

Albumin, pre-albumin and transferrin fall.

Table 16.3 Causes of hypoalbuminaemia

Artefact	Physiological	Pathological
Dilution of sample – sample taken from drip arm	Pregnancy	Impaired synthesis, malnutrition, malabsorption, chronic liver disease, analbuminaemia
	Recumbency	Excessive loss from kidney, GI tract or skin
		Overhydration
		Increased capillary permeability – hypoxia, sepsis, etc.
		Increased metabolism – injury, sepsis, malignancy, etc.

Albumin

Albumin is quantitatively the most important contributor towards maintaining the colloid oncotic pressure of plasma, and hypoalbuminaemia may lead to the development of oedema. Increased albumin concentrations are found in dehydration and if excessive venous stasis is applied during venepuncture. Hypoalbuminaemia may arise due to a number of reasons in addition to the acute-phase response (Table 16.3).

Hypoalbuminaemia

Pathological causes include:
- *Reduced synthesis*, due to liver disease (p. 199), malnutrition and intestinal malabsorptive disease, if these are severe and prolonged.
- *Altered distribution*, due to increased capillary permeability, which enables plasma to leak into the extravascular compartment (e.g. severe burns), or to serous effusion (e.g. ascites), when there is sequestration of proteins.
- *Increased catabolism*, as a result of injury (e.g. major surgery or trauma), infection or malignant disease.
- *Abnormal losses*, The liver can normally replace up to 5 g/day. Greater albumin losses (which may involve losses of other proteins besides albumin) may occur in nephrotic syndrome, GI tract disease and in burns or certain skin diseases.
- *Overhydration*, which is usually iatrogenic.
- *Artefact* due to taking a blood sample from a site close to an IV infusion. This should always be considered (Table 16.3).

Analbuminaemia

This is a rare disorder in which plasma [albumin] is usually less than 1.0 g/L. However, there may be no symptoms or signs – not even oedema – due to compensatory increases in plasma [globulins].

Bisalbuminaemia

Albumin variants occur in the healthy population, and heterozygotes for some variant albumins may express two gene products, which appear as two bands on electrophoresis. This is known as *bisalbuminaemia*, and has no pathological significance.

C-reactive protein (CRP)

This protein is a β-globulin, originally named after a property of serum that had been obtained from acutely ill patients, which caused the precipitation of a polysaccharide (fraction C) from pneumococcal extracts. CRP binds strongly to certain lipids, particularly phospholipids. It seems that CRP is somehow involved in the body's response to foreign materials. CRP increases in infection and inflammatory disease processes (up to 20- to 30-fold) and is widely measured as an alternative or adjunct to the less sensitive erythrocyte sedimentation rate (ESR). CRP measurements using a sensitive assay have been used for risk assessment in patients with ischaemic heart disease.

α_1-Protease inhibitor (α_1-anti-trypsin) (API)

Proteases such as trypsin, chymotrypsin, elastase and thrombin are continually being released into the blood in small amounts from a number of sources, including the pancreas, leucocytes and intestinal bacteria. API is one of several plasma proteins that inhibit the activity of these proteases, particularly neutrophil elastase, and may function to limit proteolytic activity at sites of inflammation. Interest in API principally relates to the association between certain diseases of the lung and liver and API deficiency due to genetic polymorphism.

Clinical consequences of the genetic polymorphism of API

Many allelic genes code for API, the alleles being given the general designation PI (protease inhibitor), and more than 90 genetic variants have been described, some of which result in marked decreases in API activity. The most common allele has been named M, with the usual homozygote being PI^{MM} (the MM type). The two most commont mutations that give rise to API deficiency are the PI^Z and PI^S alleles. Individuals who are homozygous for the PI^Z or PI^S alleles are prone to the following diseases.

Pulmonary emphysema

About 1% of patients with emphysema have API deficiency PI^{SS} or PI^{ZZ}, but this percentage is much higher in young patients. When associated with API deficiency, emphysema tends to manifest itself in the 20–40 year age group. Smoking seems to be a strong predisposing factor for the development of the disease in these patients, possibly because particles in smoke stimulate phagocytic activity, with the local release of proteases.

Hepatic disorders

Neonatal jaundice, usually presenting as a predominantly cholestatic picture, is common in PI^{ZZ} individuals. Although the jaundice may resolve, there is usually progression to hepatic cirrhosis. In about 20% of children with cirrhosis, the hepatic disorder can probably be attributed to API deficiency. In adults, cirrhosis and hepatoma are associated with the Pi^{ZZ} phenotype.

Phenotyping of API by isoelectric focusing is desirable in all cases in which plasma API levels are low or borderline, so that appropriate genetic counselling can be given to affected individuals or to their family members. Genotyping can also be used to investigate relatives of patients with API deficiency and also for antenatal screening.

The immunoglobulins and disease

The Igs are a group of structurally related proteins that function as antibodies; they are synthesised by the plasma cells of the lymphoreticular system.

The basic Ig molecule is made up of four polypeptide chains consisting of a pair of identical heavy chains (M_r 50–75 kDa each) and a pair of identical light chains (M_r 22 kDa each) linked by disuphide bridges. There are five principal types of heavy chain (γ, α, μ, δ and ε) and two types of light chain (κ and λ). Every Ig can be assigned a formula that indicates its composition, according to its types of chain (e.g. $\alpha_2 \lambda_2$, $\gamma_2 \kappa_2$, etc). The antigen-combining sites are between the adjacent light and heavy chains (Figure 16.2).

The immunoglobulin classes

Three major classes of Ig (IgG, IgA and IgM) and two minor ones (IgD and IgE) have been recognised; the

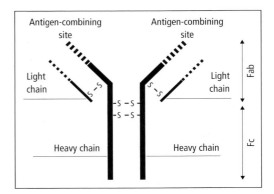

Figure 16.2 The Ig molecule, which consists of two identical pairs of heavy and light chains, held together by disulphide bonds (shown as –S–S). The molecules can be split by papain into three components; these are the two antigen-binding fragments (Fab), each of which has one binding site, and the crystallisable fragment (Fc). The variable regions of the Ig molecule are shown as interrupted lines. The heavy chains are one of five types (γ, α, μ, δ or ε), and the light chains are one of two types (κ or λ).

Table 16.4 Some features of the major classes of the Igs

Feature	IgG	IgA	IgM
Average molecular mass	146 kDa	160 kDa	875 kDa
Plasma concentration	5.0–13.0 g/L	0.5–4.0 g/L	0.3–2.5 g/L
Light chain type	κ or λ	κ or λ	κ or λ
Heavy chain type	γ	α	μ
Structure of protein	$\gamma_2\kappa_2$ or $\gamma_2\lambda_2$	$\alpha_2\kappa_2$ or $\alpha_2\lambda_2$	$(\mu_2\kappa_2)_5$ or $(\mu_2\lambda_2)_5$
Plasma half-life	21 days	6 days	5 days
Immune response	Secondary	Local, secretory	Primary
Present in secretions	Trace	Yes	Trace
Transplacental passage	Yes	No	No

type of heavy chain determines the class. Table 16.4 lists several features of the major classes. Both light and heavy chains have 'constant' and 'variable' sections. The 'constant' portion varies little within each particular chain type, whereas the variable portion (which is associated with the antigen-combining site) is different for each Ig, even within a single chain type. The variable portion is responsible for the specificity of the antibody.

• *IgG immunoglobulins* comprise the major antibody of the secondary immune response and are formed particularly in response to soluble antigens such as toxins and the products of bacterial lysis. They are widely distributed in the ECF, and cross the foetoplacental barrier.

• *IgM immunoglobulins* in plasma are pentamers of the basic Ig structure linked around a J chain polypeptide. They tend to be formed especially in response to particulate antigens, such as those on the surface of bacteria. In the presence of complement, IgMs are very effective in producing lysis of these cells. Following an antigenic stimulus, IgM formation usually precedes IgG formation, and IgMs are thought to provide an early defence mechanism against intravascular spread of infecting organisms.

• *IgA immunoglobulins* as they occur in plasma, are monomers. However, over 50% of IgA synthesis occurs in lymphoreticular cells under the mucosa of the respiratory and alimentary tracts. Here dimeric 'secretory IgA' is synthesised and secreted into the alimentary or respiratory tract and may form part of the defence mechanism against local infections.

• *IgD immunoglobulins* are present in minute amounts in plasma. They are also often present, with monomer IgM, on the surface of B lymphocytes. They are probably concerned with antigen recognition and with the development of tolerance.

• *IgE immunoglobulins* bind to cells such as the mast cells of the nasopharynx. In the presence of antigen (allergen), an antigen–antibody reaction leads to the release of histamine and other amines and polypeptides from the mast cell, giving rise to a local hypersensitivity reaction.

Immunoglobulin deficiencies

Identification of Ig deficiencies requires quantification of specific classes of Ig. Low concentrations of Igs may be due to a variety of causes.

Physiological causes

The concentrations of IgM and IgA in serum are low at birth and gradually rise until adult levels are achieved at approximately 1 year and 10 years, respectively. IgG is high at birth due to transplacental passage of maternal IgG. After birth IgG falls due to loss of maternal IgG but then gradually rises again until adult values are found after 1 year.

Inherited deficiencies of immunoglobulin synthesis

Hypogammaglobulinaemia and, rarely, *agammaglobulinaemia* are conditions in which there is defective production of IgG, IgA and IgM. Children develop severe, recurrent bacterial infections when over the age of 1. The most common is IgA deficiency which has an incidence of approximately 1:400.

Acquired deficiencies of immunoglobulin synthesis

Secondary hypogammaglobulinaemia is much more common than the inherited deficiencies. It may occur in lymphoid neoplasia (e.g. chronic lymphatic leukaemia, Hodgkin disease, multiple myelomatosis), in 'toxic' disorders or certain types of drug therapy, in protein-losing syndromes (e.g. nephrotic syndrome), and in prematurity and delayed maturity.

Hypergammaglobulinaemia (polyclonal – diffuse)

Liver disease, infection and autoimmune disease gives rise to stimulation of B lymphocytes and an increased production of γ-globulin, which on serum protein electrophoresis is revealed as a broad (diffuse) band (Figure 16.1). The increase may affect all the Ig classes, or it may affect predominantly one class. The antibodies produced are heterogeneous. Quantitation of the separate Ig classes is occasionally helpful in diagnosis. In most cases, however, the cause of the diffuse increase in plasma [total Ig] is apparent. The measurement of antibodies to specific antigens is of value (e.g. hepatitis surface antigens). Multiple discrete bands (oligoclonal bands) or, rarely, a single discrete band may occur in the λ-globulin region in response to an antigenic stimulus.

Hypergammaglobulinaemia – (monoclonal – discrete – paraproteinaemia)

A paraprotein is a monoclonal Ig or light chain produced by a clonal population of B cells. They are often identified as a discrete Ig band on electrophoresis of serum (figure 16.1). Plasma cell disorders are often associated with multiple myeloma and malignant lymphoid tumours, but benign causes are also described. The detection of a paraprotein in blood or urine requires further investiga-tion to determine whether the paraproteinaemia is malignant or benign (see below).

Myeloma, lymphoid malignancies and paraproteinaeimea

Malignant paraproteinaemias occur in multiple myeloma, plasmacytoma, malignant lymphoid tumours (chronic lymphocytic leukaemia, amyloidosis) and heavy chain disease. The prevalence of paraproteinaemia rises with age, and is about 3% in the geriatric population.

Multiple myeloma is the most common clinically important disorder associated with a paraprotein and is due to malignant proliferation of plasma cells which leads to bone destruction, impaired immune function, hyperviscosity, amyloidosis and renal impairment. The disorder often presents as bone pain (associated with lytic areas on X-ray), pathological fractures, bleeding or bruising, anaemia, recurrent infection or symptoms of hypercalcaemia. The diagnosis can be confirmed by finding an increased number of plasma cells in bone marrow and observing lytic lesions on X-ray.

Most myelomas produce complete Ig molecules, usually IgG, and the amount produced is often proportional to the tumour mass. Excessive amounts of Ig fragments (light chains or parts of heavy chains) are also produced in about 85% of cases. Dimers of light chains (M_r 44 kDa) are usually found in urine, and are called 'Bence Jones' proteins. In about 10–20% of cases of myeloma (usually the less differentiated – termed 'light-chain disease' or 'Bence Jones myeloma'), excess light chains may be the only abnormality in serum.

Measurement of serum free light chains is becoming more widely available and allows the quantification of free κ and free λ light chains secreted by plasma cells; such measurments may eventualy remove the need to measure free light chains in urine.

Waldenström macroglobulinaemia usually follows a more prolonged course than multiple myeloma. There is proliferation of cells that resemble lymphocytes rather than plasma cells. They produce complete IgM molecules and often an excess of light chains. Increased plasma [IgM] causes

Table 16.5 Diagnostic criteria for MGUS, asymptomatic and symptomatic myeloma

	MGUS	**Asymptomatic myeloma**	**Symptomatic myeloma**
Monoclonal protein	In serum <30 g/L	In serum >30 g/L	In serum >30 g/L and/or in urine
Bone marrow	Clonal plasma cells <10%	Clonal plasma cells >10%	Clonal plasma cells >10% or plasmacytoma
Evidence of organ/tissue impairment	No evidence of other B-cell proliferative disorders	No myeloma-related organ/tissue impairment	Any myeloma-related organ/tissue impairment

increased plasma viscosity, which tends to make the circulation sluggish, and thromboses are common.

Heavy-chain disease (Franklin disease) comprises a group of rare conditions in which heavy-chain fragments corresponding to the Fc portion of the Igs are synthesised and excreted in urine. Abnormal production of α and γ heavy chains is the most common derangement.

Amyloidosis is a heterogenous group of clinical conditions characterised by systemic deposition of protein fibrils. Amyloid fibrils may occur as a secondary complication of plasma cell malignancies.

Monoclonal gammopathy of unknown significance (MGUS)

Often a paraprotein is found on electrophoresis in patients who have no symptoms and it may be unclear if this is due to early malignant disease or a benign disorder. MGUS is present in approximately 2% of individuals over 50 years of age and 3% of patients over 70. It is defined by a low concentration of paraprotein (<30 g/L), less than 10% of bone marrow plasma cells and the absence of myeloma-related organ or tissue damage (Table 16.5). In MGUS the overall rate of progression to myeloma is in the order of 1% per year; long-term follow-up is thus required.

Investigation of paraproteinaemia

All patients in which paraproteinaemia has been identified should be refered for specialist review. Chemical, haematological and radiological investigations, and lymph node biopsy, are all of value

Table 16.6 Clinical features and investigations in suspected multiple myeloma

> **Clinical features**
> Bone pain, hypercalcaemia, fatigue, anaemia, infection, renal impairment, hyperviscosity
> **Investigations**
> *Diagnosis*
> Paraprotein band in serum and urine
> Serum free light chains.
> Lytic lesions on bone X-ray
> Bone marrow biopsy shows abnormal plasma cells
> *Progress and management*
> [Paraproteins]
> Hypercalcaemia – bone involvement
> Raised creatinine and urea, low eGFR – impaired renal function
> Raised β_2-microglobulin – impaired renal function, tumour burden, prognostic indicator
> Low Hb – tumour burden, marrow depression
> Low non-paraprotein Igs – predisposition to infection

when investigating cases of suspected paraproteinaemia and in their follow-up (Table 16.6).

Initial investigations

Electrophoresis of serum and concentrated urine should be performed, followed by immunofixation to confirm the type of any monoclonal band. Any paraprotein observed should be quantified by densitometry. Immunofixation is also indicated in patients where there is a strong suspicion of myeloma but in whom electrophoresis is negative. On finding a paraprotein, the most important diagnostic decision is whether the condition is MGUS, asymptomatic or symptomatic myeloma (Table 16.5)

Serum protein electrophoresis shows a single discrete band, usually in the γ-globulin region but occasionally in the β-globulin or α$_2$-globulin region, in over 90% of patients in whom there is overproduction of complete Ig molecules; the concentrations of the other Igs may be reduced. Occasionally, a band due to the presence of light chains may be observed. Plasma must *not* be used, since the fibrinogen band may obscure or mimic paraproteins. Quantification of serum free light chain concentrations and the κ:λ ratio can be used as an alternative to quantifying urinary light chains (see below)

Urine protein electrophoresis on a fresh early-morning urine sample is usually needed to demonstrate Bence Jones protein; its small size (M_r 44 kDa) means that it is cleared rapidly by the kidney. If Bence Jones protein is detected, the monoclonal nature of the light chains can be confirmed by immunofixation. In multiple myeloma, the light chains are nearly always dimers of type κ *or* type λ, but not a mixture of the two. Most cases of myeloma and many cases of macroglobulinaemia have Bence Jones proteinuria. In light-chain disease, there is Bence Jones proteinuria but usually no serum paraprotein component.

Further investigations

If a paraprotein is found, further chemical measurements should usually be performed, including the following.

1 *Non-paraprotein Ig*. The serum concentrations of these Igs should be measured, to assess the likelihood of intercurrent infection.

2 *Plasma [β$_2$-microglobulin]*. This provides a good index of prognosis, presumably because plasma [β$_2$-microglobulin] depends both on the turnover of tumour cells and on renal function. High (>6 mg/L) levels indicate a poor prognosis.

3 *Plasma [creatinine]* and eGFR to assess renal (glomerular) function. Myeloma is commonly associated with both glomerular and tubular dysfunction.

4 *Plasma [calcium]*. This may be raised due to increased release of calcium from bone.

5 *Plasma ALP* activity is usually normal or only slightly raised, as osteoblastic activity is not increased in multiple myeloma.

6 *Plasma [urate]*. This may be raised due to increased cell breakdown, especially after cytotoxic therapy. Urate deposition may cause renal damage in myeloma.

7 *Haemoglobin and full blood count*. Anaemia is quite common.

Cryoglobulins

These are Igs that precipitate when cooled to 4 °C and redissolve when warmed to 37 °C and may result in a clinical syndrome of systemic inflammation caused by cryoglobulin-containing immune complexes. They occur in a number of diseases associated with both diffuse and discrete hypergammaglobulinaemia. Cryoglobulinaemia may be classified as follows:

- *Type I cryoglobulinaemia*, is the result of a monoclonal Ig, usually IgM, or light chains and is thus found in some cases of lymphoproliferative disorders.

- *Types II and III cryoglobulinaemia* contain rheumatoid factors (RFs), which are usually IgM and are associated with inflammatory conditions such as systemic lupus erythematosus, viral infection and Sjorgren syndrome. These RFs form complexes with the Fc portion of polyclonal IgG. Types II and III cryoglobulinaemia represent 80% of all cryoglobulins

If cryoglobulin determinations are to be performed, blood needs to be collected into a warmed syringe without anti-coagulant, and maintained at 37 °C until the serum for cryoglobulin investigation has been separated from the cells.

Malignancy and tumour markers

Tumours may secrete a wide range of substances into blood, including hormones, enzymes and tumour antigens, which are collectively referred to as tumour markers. Table 16.7 lists the tumour markers that are in common use.

Tumour markers can be used in a number of ways, including the following.

1 *Monitoring treatment and detecting recurrence of disease* These are the most useful roles for tumour markers. An example of how sequential

Table 16.7 Tumour markers commonly used in clinical practice

Malignancy	Marker	Follow-up	Diagnosis	Prognosis	Screening
Choriocarcinoma	hCG	Yes	Yes	Yes	Yes
Colorectal	CEA	Yes			
Germ cell	hCG	Yes	Yes	Yes	
Germ cell	AFP	Yes	Yes	Yes	
Hepatoma	AFP	Yes	Yes		Yes
Myeloma	Paraprotein	Yes	Yes	Yes	
Ovarian	CA-125	Yes	Yes	Yes	
Prostatic	PSA	Yes	Yes		?
Thyroid, medullary	Calcitonin	Yes	Yes		Yes
Thyroid, follicular, papillary	Thyroglobulin	Yes			

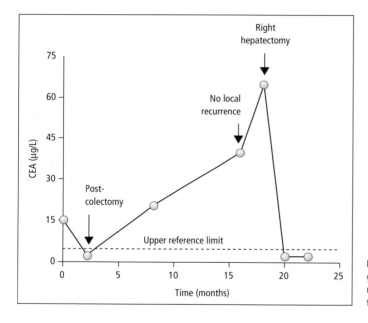

Figure 16.3 Carcinoembryonic antigen (CEA) levels in a 68-year-old man who presented with a colonic tumour.

measurements of a tumour marker can be used to monitor treatment is shown in Figure 16.3. For all tumour markers it should be recognised that concentrations within the reference range do not exclude malignancy. Furthermore a rise in the tumour marker concentration within the reference range should raise the suspicion of tumour recurrence.

2 Diagnosis Tumour markers provide an aid to diagnosis, but only when used in conjunction with clinical and radiological evidence. Often,

tumour marker concentrations may be increased in clinical conditions not associated with malignancy.

3 Screening With a few exceptions, tumour markers are of little value in screening for asymptomatic disease, but in some specific instances may be used to screen high-risk groups. Examples include measuring [calcitonin] after pentagastrin stimulation (p. 252) to screen close relatives of patients with medullary carcinoma of the thyroid, and hCG, which is used to screen for choriocarcinoma in women who have had a hydatidiform mole.

4 *Prognosis* Tumour markers can only be used for prognosis on the few occasions when the plasma concentration correlates with tumour mass. For example, hCG is used in choriocarcinoma, IgG in paraproteinaemia, and AFP and hCG in testicular tumours.

Examples of tumour markers used in clinical practice

Colorectal cancer

Carcinoembryonic antigen (CEA) is a high molecular weight glycoprotein and its measurement remains the most widely used marker as an aid to prognosis, surveillance and monitoring treatment with chemotherapy. CEA measurements appear to define a subgroup of node-negative patients of Duke B colon cancer patients that have poor prognosis and could benefit from adjuvant chemotherapy. Post-operative CEA levels should return to normal following successful surgical resection. Failure to do so suggests residual or metastatic disease. Serial monitoring with CEA can detect recurrent disease with a sensitivity of approximately 80% and specificity of approximately 70%, and provides an average lead-time of about 5 months. Patients monitored frequently with CEA have an improved 5-year survival rate, and CEA testing is often carried out every 2–3 months for at least 3 years after the initial diagnosis. Monitoring the response to chemotherapy using CEA is also desirable, with measurements being taken every 2–3 months of active treatment. A clinically significant rise in CEA can be regarded as an increase of 30% over the previous value and such a rise should prompt a repeat measurement within 1 month. Smaller but persistent incremental rises in [CEA] should also prompt further investigation. It should be remembered that [CEA] is increased in a variety of benign conditions including hepatitis, cirrhosis, inflammatory bowel disease, pancreatitis, bronchitis and smoking.

CEA is raised in only 30–50% of patients at the time of diagnosis and is thus not recommended for screening. Recently the use of faecal occult blood has been introduced as a screening test in asymptomaic subjects.

Ovarian cancer

The only tumour marker to have a well-defined role in ovarian carcinoma is the cancer antigen CA-125. The antigen is a high molecular weight glycoprotein found on the endothelium of the fallopian tubes, endocervix, endometrium and also in the normal ovary and the mesothelial cells of the pleura, pericardium and peritoneum. Serum [CA-125] is elevated when there is vascular invasion, tissue destruction and inflammation associated with malignancy. It is increased in over 90% of women with advanced ovarian cancer disease and also in 40% of patients with advanced intra-abdominal malignancy. The serum [CA-125] can be increased during menstruation and pregnancy and also in other benign conditions such as endometriosis, peritonitis and cirrhosis, especially if ascites is present. There is no clear role for CA-125 in screening, diagnosis or prognosis, but changes in serum [CA-125] can be used as a relatively reliable marker of response to treatment and disease progression. Inhibin A appears to be very sensitive for detecting granulose cell tumours of the ovary and monitoring treatment, but such measurements are not widely available. Other markers for ovarian cancer have been suggested but remain largely experimental.

Prostatic cancer

The glycoprotein *prostate-specific antigen* (PSA) is used as a tumour marker to aid diagnosis and for monitoring purposes in patients with prostatic cancer. Men without prostatic cancer have PSA in their serum and the concentration rises with age; age-related reference ranges are useful. Levels are also increased in benign prostatic hypertrophy, lower urinary tract infections and after trauma to the prostate or following digital rectal examination. The value of screening the general population is controversial and currently being investigated in a number of large clinical trials particularly as there are uncertainties about the efficacy of various treatment strategies for early prostatic cancer. Approximately 50% of men with prostatic cancer who have a PSA between 4 and 10 μg/L will have disease outside the prostate. Although a PSA of more than 4 μg/L requires further investigation, it should be appreciated that about 15% of men diagnosed with prostatic cancer will have a PSA of between 3 and 4 μg/L. Bone metastases are unlikely in patients with a PSA of less than 4 μg/L. PSA is of value in monitoring the response to therapy.

Most PSA circulates in plasma bound to α_1-anti-chymotrypsin, but a small fraction circulates unbound to any protein (free PSA). Patients with prostatic cancer appear to have a higher ratio between α_1-anti-chymotrypsin–PSA complex and free PSA than patients with benign hypertrophy, and this ratio may thus be useful in discriminating between patients with benign disease and those with malignancy.

Breast cancer

The tumour marker CA 15-3 can provide prognostic information, and serial measurement have the potential to detect recurrent disease and for monitoring treatment. This marker may become more important when more effective treatments are developed to treat metastatic disease. Her2/neu is a 185 kDa cell surface receptor protein which is a member of the epidermal growth factor receptor family. It is expressed in small amounts on the plasma membrane of normal cells. The protein appears to be involved in the growth and spread of breast cancer cells, and about 25% of patients have high levels of the protein. The presence of Her2/neu suggests an aggressive tumour and appears to provide a prognostic indicator. Patients who have HER2/neu-positive tumours may respond to treatment with herceptin – a monoclonal antibody directed to the HER2/neu protein.

Germ-cell tumours

Patients presenting with a lump in the testes or a malignancy of unknown origin should have the concentration of serum AFP and hCG measured. If raised due to secretion by the tumour, these measurements can also be used to monitor treatment. However, only about 75% of non-seminomatous germ-cell tumours and a minority of patients with seminoma or dysgerminoma secrete these markers. The markers provide indicators for prognosis as well as being a valuable tool for monitoring treatment.

Choriocarcinoma

About 50% of cases of choriocarcinoma follow a hydatidiform mole pregnancy, and hCG is used to screen these women. This is also used to assess prognosis and response to treatment.

Hepatoma

Patients with cirrhosis, haemachromatosis and persistent infection with hepatitis B and C are at high risk of developing hepatocellular carcinoma. Measurement of serum [AFP] on a regular basis (every 6–12 months) appears to be of value to allow early detection of tumour. Serum [AFP] is increased in many patients with cirrhosis, but a concentration in excess of 500 μg/L is almost diagnostic of malignancy. Patients with concentrations greater than 50 μg/L require further investigation. Serum [AFP] is of value for monitoring treatment and follow-up.

Pancreatic tumours

CA 19-9 has been used to monitor treatment in patients with adenocarcinoma of the pancreas. However, its value is limited by the fact that there are no effective treatments available for the disease.

Cholangiocarcinoma

Increases in CA 19-9 are found in patients with sclerosing cholangitis. If patients with this condition subsequently develop cholangiocarcinoma then the serum [CA19-9] shows a rapid rise to very high values.

Thyroid cancer – papilliary and follicular

Patients with these diseases are usually treated by total thyroidectomy followed by ablative doses of radioiodine. Thyroxine is then prescribed at doses that suppress TSH to concentrations of less than 0.01 mU/L with a view to impairing the growth of any residual tumour. Many of these tumours synthesise and secrete thyroglobulin, and the measurement of serum [thyroglobulin] is of value in monitoring progression of the disease, and in assessing response to treatment. Measurement of [thyroglobulin] has no role in the diagnosis of thyroid cancer since elevated concentrations are found in many thyroid disorders other than malignancy. In patients who have been treated with total thyroidectomy and ^{131}I ablation, a serum [thyroglobulin] greater than 2µg/L is highly suggestive of residual or recurrent tumour, but could also indicate persistence of a remnant of normal thyroid tissue. The sensitivity of serum thyroglobulin measurements for detecting recurrence is enhanced by an elevated TSH concentration. Therefore, serum [thyroglobulin] should preferably be measured when the serum TSH is more than 30 mU/L; this can be achieved by either withdrawal of T4 or administering recombinant TSH (Thyrogen). Endogenous thyroglobulin antibodies are common in patients with thyroid cancer and these may interfere with the assays and render thyroglobulin results unable to be interpreted. Therefore, thyroglobulin results should be interpreted with the knowledge of the thyroglobulin antibody status of the patient.

Thyroid cancer – medullary carcinoma of the thyroid (MCT)

This tumour of the parafollicular, calcitonin-producing cells (C cells) of the thyroid gland accounts for about 10% of thyroid cancers. Non-familial cases account for 80% of all cases of MCT. The familial form of the disease may occur in conjunction with neoplasia of other endocrine tissues, a syndrome known as MEN. A description of MEN is given in Table 16.8. Developments in the molecular genetics of MCT that include RET proto-oncogene mutation testing have facilitated a rational framework for management and screening of family members. The use and interpretation of such molecular diagnostics is difficult and requires careful application in individual patients and their families.

Plasma [calcitonin] is often greatly increased in patients with MCT, but plasma [calcium] is usually normal. A raised plasma [calcitonin] may occur in other conditions, including Hashimoto thyroiditis, chronic renal failure and diseases associated with transformed neuroendocrine cells (e.g. carcinoid tumours and phaeochromocytoma). It is important to get a baseline [calcitonin] in patients in order that response to therapy (usually thyroidectomy and central node dissection) and follow-up can be assessed. Lifelong follow-up is recom-

Table 16.8 Characteristic tumours in the MEN syndromes

MEN I	MEN IIa	MEN IIb
Hyperparathyroidism (95%)	Medullary carcinoma of the thyroid (100%)	Medullary carcinoma of the thyroid (100%)
Tumours secreting: (50%)	Phaeochromocytoma (30%)	Phaeochromocytoma (45%)
Gastrin	Hyperparathyroidism (50%)	Associated abnormalities:
Insulin		Mucosal neuroma (100%)
Glucagon		Marfan habitus (65%)
Vasoactive intestinal polypeptide (VIP)		Megacolon
Pancreatic polypeptide		
Carcinoid tumours (30%)		
Pituitary tumours (40%)		

Values in parentheses show the percentage of patients having the condition.

mended. The response to primary surgery can be assessed clinically, and by the measurement of serum [calcitonin]. The presence of an elevated but stable [calcitonin] level post-operatively may be managed conservatively. Progressively rising levels should trigger imaging for further staging. In the absence of recurrent symptoms, appropriate intervals are 6–12 months. The use of a pentagastrin-stimulated calcitonin test should be considered as a screening test where there is strong presumptive evidence of inherited disease but no mutation in the RET gene has been found. In patients with MCT, plasma [calcitonin] increases by 2–5 times above the basal level following combined calcium and pentagastrin administration, whereas normal subjects show little or no response.

Keypoints

- Albumin is the protein with the highest concentration in plasma. Hypoalbuminaemia may be caused by reduced synthesis in the liver, altered distribution, increased catabolism, abnormal losses or overhydration.
- Following trauma, infection, etc., there is an acute-phase response, with increased plasma [C-reactive protein], [fibrinogen], [haptoglobin], [ceruloplasmin] and [α_1-protease inhibitor] and decreased concentrations of some other plasma proteins, including albumin.
- Individuals who are homozygous for the Pi^Z or Pi^S allele of α_1-protease inhibitor are more likely to develop pulmonary emphysema and hepatic disease.
- On serum electrophoresis, a discrete Ig band (paraprotein) is highly suggestive of multiple myeloma, particularly if Bence Jones protein is detected in urine. On finding a paraprotein, the most important diagnostic decision is whether the condition is MGUS, asymptomatic or symptomatic myeloma.
- Tumour markers are of value in monitoring treatment and detecting recurrent disease. They are often of little value in screening for asymptomatic disease (except in high-risk groups) or in determining the prognosis.

Case 16.1

A 70-year-old man complained to his doctor of back pain that he had had for several months, and of feeling generally unwell. He appeared pale and he was tender over the lumbar spine. His urine contained protein (1 g/L) and his ESR was very high (90 mm in the first hour). The following abnormalities were reported:

How would you interpret these results, and what further chemical investigations would you request in this patient?

Serum	Result	Reference range
Albumin	32	35–50 g/L
Calcium	2.72	2.1–2.6 mmol/L
ALP	90	40–125 U/L
Creatinine	180	60–120 µmol/L
Total protein	84	60–80 g/L
IgA	<0.4	0.8–4.5 g/L
IgG	37	6–15 g/L
IgM	<0.2	0.35–2.90 g/L

Comments: Serum and urine protein electrophoresis would both be indicated. The serum pattern showed a discrete band in the γ-globulin region, with marked reduction of the other Igs, and urine electrophoresis revealed the presence of Bence Jones protein, subsequently identified as of the λ type. The diagnosis of multiple myeloma was confirmed on X-ray examination (which demonstrated osteolytic lesions in the skull, vertebral column, ribs and pelvis) and by the finding of atypical plasma cells in the bone marrow.

(continued on p. 253)

Case 16.1 *(continued)*

Hypercalcaemia is present in about 30% of patients with multiple myeloma, and about 50% show some evidence of impaired renal function at the time of presentation; this is associated with a poor prognosis. Some serum paraproteins are not detected using the usual immunological methods even though they may be present in high concentration. Serum electrophoresis is thus a more reliable test than immunological methods for screening for paraproteinaemia in symptomatic patients.

Case 16.2

A 73-year-old man presented to his doctor, complaining of back pain and increasing problems with passing urine. The following results from chemical tests were found:

What is the likely diagnosis?

Serum	Result	Reference range
Prostate-specific antigen	70	<4 mg/L
Albumin	38	35–50 g/L
ALP activity	200	40–125 U/L
ALT activity	35	10–50 U/L
Bilirubin total	10	2–17 µmol/L
GGT activity	35	10–55 U/L

Comments: The man is likely to have metastatic prostatic cancer. Although there is overlap in the levels of PSA seen in men with benign prostatic hypertrophy and prostatic cancer, the high levels of PSA found in this patient are usually seen only in patients with metastatic disease.

The elevated ALP in the presence of normal GGT and other liver function tests also suggest metastatic spread to bone.

Examination of the prostate per rectum disclosed an enlarged and hard prostate, and tissue obtained during a transurethral resection demonstrated the presence of tumour.

Case 16.3

A 50-year-old male lecturer presented to his doctor, complaining of tiredness, abdominal discomfort and poor appetite. He had worked in Africa in the past, where he had contracted Hepatitis B and had become a carrier. On examination, he was jaundiced and his liver was enlarged. Urine was positive for both bilirubin and urobilinogen.

The following results were found:

Serum	Result	Reference range
Albumin	34	35–50 g/L
ALP activity	400	40–125 U/L
ALT	150	10–50 U/L
Bilirubin total	60	2–17 µmol/L
GGT activity	150	10–55 U/L
α_1-fetoprotein	3000	Not detectable kU/L

What is the likely diagnosis?

(continued on p. 254)

Case 16.3 *(continued)*

Comments: The patient has a primary hepatocellular carcinoma. This is a relatively uncommon malignancy in the developed world, but common in China, South-East Asia and parts of Africa as a result of the high incidence of Hepatitis B in these regions. Chronic carriers of the virus have an increased risk of developing the malignancy. The liver function tests show a mixed pattern of cholestasis, probably arising from the tumour, and hepatitis, arising from the chronic hepatitis. The very high concentration of α_1-fetoprotein is highly suggestive of hepatocellular carcinoma, but levels of up to about 500 kU/L can be found in some patients with non-malignant hepatobiliary disease.

Case 16.4

A 54-year-old female shop assistant presented to the endocrine clinic for annual follow-up. She had been diagnosed 9 years earlier with a small focal papillary carcinoma of the thyroid that had been treated by partial thyroidectomy with no radioiodine ablation. She was taking thyroxine and had remained well with no evidence of recurrent disease.

At annual follow-up the following results were found:

Serum	Result	Reference range
TSH	4.0	0.2–4.5 mU/L
FT4	13	9–21 pmol/L
Thyroglobulin	5	µ/g/L

(Anti-thyroglobulin antibodies were negative)

How would you interpret these results?

Comments: The patient has been taking inadequate doses of thyroxine. The aim of T4 therapy in patients with papillary carcinoma of the thyroid is to suppress TSH to undetectable concentrations; this has not been achieved in this patient. Compliance should be verified and if an increase in T4 dose is required. In patients who have undergone total thyroidectomy and in whom TSH is 0.01 mU/L, thyroglobulin should be <2 µg/L. This patient has residual thyroid tissue (she only has had a partial thyroidectomy) and she has detectable circulating TSH that will stimulate thyroglobulin production from the thyroid remnant. It is thus impossible to determine from these results if the thyroglobulin is originating from the thyroid remnant or a recurrent tumour. Thyroglobulin was later found to be undetectable when the patient's TSH was <0.01 mU/L and no further action was required other than continued annual follow-up.

Chapter 17

Disorders of iron and porphyrin metabolism

Iron is an essential element present mainly in the porphyrin complex, haem, and in iron storage proteins, ferritin and haemosiderin. Haem, which is present in haemoglobin, myoglobin and cytochromes, is formed by the insertion of ferrous iron, Fe^{2+}, into protoporphyrin (Figure 17.1) which itself is synthesised by a complex chain of reactions (see Figure 17.3). In this chapter, we discuss the disorders of iron and porphyrin metabolism and consider some abnormal derivatives of haemoglobin.

Iron metabolism

The adult human possesses about 70 mmol (4 g) of iron. Iron balance is regulated by alterations in the intestinal absorption of iron. There is only a limited capacity to increase or decrease the rate of loss of iron.

Dietary iron and iron absorption

The normal intake of iron is about 0.2–0.4 mmol/day (10–20 mg/day). Good sources are liver, fish and meat. Normally, about 5–10% of dietary iron is absorbed by an active transport process. Most absorption occurs in the duodenum. The rate of

Lecture Notes: Clinical Biochemistry, 8e. By G. Beckett, S. Walker, P. Rae & P. Ashby. Published 2010 by Blackwell Publishing.

absorption is controlled by physiological and dietary factors:

- *State of iron stores in the body* Absorption is increased in iron deficiency and decreased when there is iron overload. The mechanism is unclear.
- *Rate of erythropoiesis* When this rate is increased, absorption may be increased even though the iron stores are adequate or overloaded.
- *Contents of diet* Substances that form soluble complexes with iron (e.g. ascorbic acid) facilitate absorption. Substances that form insoluble complexes (e.g. phytate) inhibit absorption.
- *The chemical state of the iron* Iron in the diet does not usually become available for absorption unless released during digestion. This depends, at least partly, on gastric acid production; Fe^{2+} is more readily absorbed than Fe^{3+}, and the presence of H^+ helps to keep iron in the Fe^{2+} form. Iron in haem (in meat products) can be absorbed while still contained in the haem molecule.

Iron transport, storage and utilisation

After being taken up by the intestinal mucosa, iron is either (1) incorporated into ferritin and retained by the mucosal cells, or (2) transported across the mucosal cells directly to the plasma, where it is carried mainly combined with *transferrin* (Figure 17.2). Iron retained by mucosal cells is lost from the body when the cells are sloughed. Mucosal cell retention is influenced by the body's iron status,

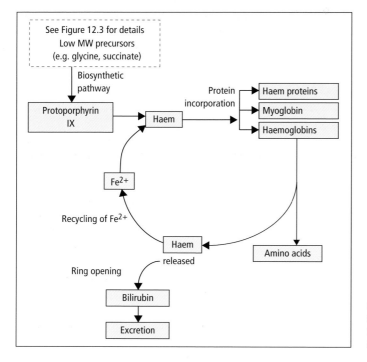

Figure 17.1 Schematic diagram illustrating the formation of haem, its incorporation into haem proteins and subsequent metabolism to bilirubin.

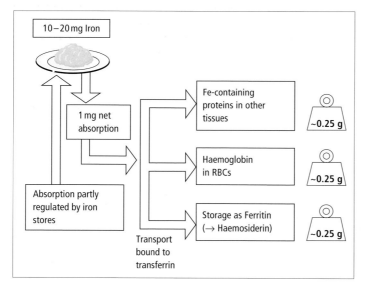

Figure 17.2 Summary of the absorption, transport and utilisation of iron. Total body iron stores (g) for the main iron-containing proteins as shown on the right side of the figure.

being reduced in iron depletion and increased in states of iron overload.

The total iron circulating bound to transferrin is normally about 50–70 µmol (3–4 mg). Iron in plasma is taken up by cells and either incorporated into haem or stored as ferritin (or haemosiderin, probably formed by the condensation of several molecules of ferritin). Iron released by the breakdown of Hb, at the end of the erythrocyte's life, is normally efficiently conserved and later reused.

Iron excretion and sources of loss

Iron excreted in the faeces is principally exogenous, that is, dietary iron that has not been absorbed by the mucosal cells and transported into the circulation. In males, there is an average loss of endogenous iron of about 20 μmol/day (1 mg/day) in cells desquamated from the skin and the intestinal mucosa. Females may have additional losses due to menstruation or pregnancy. Urine contains negligible amounts of iron.

Laboratory assessment of iron status

This is necessary in the investigation of iron deficiency states and iron overload. The following tests are used (for reference ranges, see Table 17.1).

Serum iron

This is of limited diagnostic value, since levels fluctuate widely in health. Much of this variation

appears to be random, but some specific causes can be recognised:

1 *Diurnal variation,* with higher values in the morning.

2 *Menstrual cycle,* with low values just before and during the menstrual period.

3 *Oral contraceptives,* which cause increased serum [iron].

4 *Pregnancy,* which tends to cause increased serum [iron]. However, it is often accompanied by iron deficiency so that serum [iron] falls.

Measurements of serum [iron] do *not* provide an adequate index of iron status. Although plasma [iron] is low in iron deficiency and is raised in iron overload, these changes occur relatively late when iron stores have already become either completely depleted or seriously overloaded. In addition, serum [iron] also alters in conditions not associated with changes in iron stores. Acute infections or trauma precipitate a rapid fall in serum [iron]. Chronic inflammatory disorders (e.g. rheumatoid arthritis) and malignant diseases are also associated with low levels.

Serum [iron] determination is only required for diagnostic purposes for a few conditions, for example in suspected cases of acute iron poisoning

Table 17.1 Reference ranges for iron status

	Iron (μmol/L)	Ferritin (μg/L)	TIBC (μmol/L)	TIBC saturation (%)
Reference ranges				
Males	14–32	15–300*	45–72	20–50
Females	10–28	10–150*	45–72	15–50
Physiological changes				
Premenstrual	↓	N	N	↓
Steroid contraceptives	↑	N	↑	N
Pregnancy	Variable†	↓	↑	↓
Disease states				
Iron deficiency	↓	↓	↑	<30
Iron overload	↑	↑	N or ↓	up to 100
Infections, neoplasms	↓	↑ or N	↓	N
Hypoplastic anaemia	↑	↑ or N	N or ↓	>40

N = normal; ↑ = increased; ↓ = decreased.

* A serum [ferritin] below 20 μg/L suggests that the body's iron stores are depleted.

† See above.

and in the assessment of individuals with an increased risk of haemochromatosis.

Serum ferritin

Serum [ferritin] is closely related to body iron stores, whether these are decreased, normal or increased, whereas serum [iron] becomes abnormal only in the presence of gross abnormalities of iron storage. A low, or low normal serum [ferritin] indicates the presence of depleted iron stores. However, since ferritin is an acute-phase reactant, levels may be increased in patients with iron deficiency and concurrent inflammation, malignancy or hepatic disease, although at concentrations greater than $100\,\mu g/L$ iron deficiency is almost certainly not present.

Increased serum [ferritin] is found in iron overload, irrespective of the cause, and in many patients with liver disease or cancer. A normal serum [ferritin] virtually excludes untreated iron overload. Determination of serum [ferritin] currently provides the most useful measure of iron status widely available on a routine basis.

Serum transferrin, total iron-binding capacity and iron saturation

Normally, nearly all the iron-binding capacity in serum is due to transferrin, and about 40% of the binding sites on transferrin are occupied by iron. Transferrin has a much longer half-life than iron, and serum [transferrin] shows fewer short-term fluctuations. Transferrin levels fall in PEM, during the acute-phase response, and with infections, neoplastic disease and chronic liver disease. Synthesis increases in iron deficiency.

[Transferrin] can be measured not only directly, but also indirectly as the ability of serum protein (largely transferrin) to bind iron, the so-called TIBC of serum. The ratio of serum [iron] to [transferrin] (or TIBC) then determines the transferrin (or TIBC) saturation.

In iron-deficiency anaemia, the low serum [iron] is typically associated with an increase in transferrin concentration (and TIBC). This leads to a low saturation of transferrin (and TIBC) with iron.

Conversely, in iron overload, serum [iron] is high and transferrin is normal or low, that is, a high percentage saturation of TIBC (Table 17.1). This effect is particularly marked in haemochromatosis, in which saturation of the TIBC usually rises above 60% fairly early in the disorder.

As with serum [iron], there is little place for determining serum [transferrin] or TIBC as a routine measure of iron status. However, in the detection of early or latent haemochromatosis, serum TIBC saturation should be measured. Also, in patients being treated with erythropoietin for the anaemia of chronic renal failure, the percentage saturation of TIBC provides a better index of available iron than serum [ferritin], and it is also a better guide to the need to give iron treatment.

The serum transferrin (or TIBC) is also helpful in determining the significance of very high serum [ferritin] in patients with disordered liver function of unknown cause, in whom the differential diagnosis may be between haemochromatosis and malignancy. A high serum [ferritin] in the absence of an increased percentage saturation of TIBC indicates that cancer is more likely to be the diagnosis.

Serum transferrin receptor

A circulating form of the transferrin receptor, lacking the cytoplasmic and transmembrane domains of the intact receptor, has been identified in serum. Its concentration rises in iron deficiency following the depletion of iron stores and, because levels are unaffected by inflammation, its measurement has the potential to provide an indication of iron status in patients with anaemia associated with chronic disease. Assays for serum transferrin receptor are not yet widely available.

Iron deficiency

Worldwide, this is the most common single nutrient deficiency. The main causes (Table 17.2) are deficient intake (including reduced bioavailability due to dietary fibre, phytates, etc.), impaired absorption (e.g. intestinal malabsorptive disease,

Table 17.2 Causes of iron deficiency and excess

Iron deficiency	Iron overload
Decreased intake	*Excessive intake*
Poor diet	Oversupplementation with iron tablets
Prolonged weaning (milk: poor iron source)	Repeated blood transfusions
Malabsorption	Iron utensils (especially with acid foodstuffs)
Increased requirements	*Excessive absorption*
(in the presence of inadequate intake)	Haemochromatosis
Adolescence	
Pregnancy	
Menstruating females	
Excessive iron losses	
Menorrhagia	
GI losses	
Genito-urinary losses	
Excessive blood donations	

abdominal surgery) and excessive loss (e.g. menstrual, GI bleeding).

In patients who develop iron deficiency,
- serum [ferritin] falls, then
- serum [transferrin] and TIBC increase, after which
- serum [iron] falls, and finally
- anaemia becomes evident.

A microcytic, hypochromic anaemia is characteristic, and storage iron is absent from macrophages in the bone marrow aspirate. In general, serum [ferritin] is the best diagnostic test for iron deficiency (renal failure is one of the few exceptions, see above).

Biochemical tests may help to identify the underlying cause of iron deficiency anaemia. For example, practice guidelines recommend that where GI investigations are indicated, patients should be screened for coeliac disease (p. 216) as a possible cause of malabsorption. However, it should be noted that FOB testing should NOT be used to exclude the possibility of GI blood loss in this setting. FOB tests are not sufficiently sensitive for this purpose and a negative result can give false reassurance and may delay diagnosis (p. 217).

Iron overload

This is much less common than iron deficiency (Table 17.2). Diagnosis is not usually difficult once the possibility has been considered. Increased serum [iron] with normal [transferrin] (or TIBC) often lead to 100% saturation of transferrin (or TIBC). Serum [ferritin] is increased, often to more than 1000 µg/L. More common causes are as follows:
- Increased intake and absorption. Acute overdose, mainly occurring in children, may cause severe or even fatal symptoms, due to the toxic effects of free iron in plasma (see below). Chronic overload occurs when the diet contains excess absorbable iron (e.g. acid-containing food cooked in iron pots). Iron deposits form, for example, in the liver causing hepatic fibrosis and in the myocardium causing myocardial damage.
- Parenteral administration of iron, including repeated blood transfusions.
- Hereditory haemochromatosis.

Hereditary haemochromatosis

This autosomal recessive disorder is associated with a mutation of the *HFE* gene, which is located on chromosome 6. In 85–90% of cases, the mutation is due to a single base change that results in the substitution of tyrosine for cysteine at position 282 of the HFE protein (C282Y). Individuals homozygous for this mutation are predisposed to an unregulated increase in the intestinal absorption of dietary iron although the phenotypic expression is variable. At least 90% of symptomatic individuals are male, suggesting that iron losses in menstruation and pregnancy may protect females. Excessive iron deposits build up as haemosiderin in the liver, leading to a macronodular cirrhosis in untreated individuals. Fibrotic damage to the pancreas (with diabetes mellitus) and heart involvement are also described. Other clinical features include skin pigmentation ('bronzed diabetes'), endocrine organ involvement (testicular atrophy) and arthritis with chondrocalcinosis.

Hereditary haemochromatosis can be detected at the pre-clinical stage in affected members of a family in which an index case has occurred. In families at risk, apparently unaffected members with the susceptible genotype should have regular (e.g. twice yearly) measurements of serum [iron], [ferritin] and TIBC. The first abnormalities to appear in serum are increased [ferritin] and percentage saturation of TIBC; if either of these becomes abnormal, liver biopsy is indicated. Case finding for affected relatives is important, since treatment by phlebotomy can prevent the disease from progressing.

Iron poisoning

This is potentially life threatening, particularly in children. Early clinical symptoms, which include epigastric pain, nausea and vomiting, often with haematemesis, may settle but be followed later by acute encephalopathy and circulatory failure. Acute liver and renal failure may also develop. Treatment involves giving desferrioxamine, an iron-chelating agent, which binds the iron in plasma, and the resulting complex is excreted in urine.

Serum iron values greater than 90 μmol/L require treatment. An immediate IM injection of desferrioxamine is followed by gastric lavage, leaving desferrioxamine in the stomach.

Porphyrin metabolism

Porphyrins are tetrapyrroles, some of which are intermediates in the formation of haem. Haem itself is formed when Fe^{2+} combines with protoporphyrin IX (Figure 17.1). Most cells can synthesise haem, but liver cells and bone marrow are the most active. Inherited or acquired defects in the enzymes that are involved in haem formation can lead to overproduction of pathway intermediates, with different clinical consequences. These conditions, which are relatively rare, are collectively known as the porphyrias. Figure 17.3 summarises the haem biosynthetic pathway and the disorders that result from deficiency of specific enzymes, and indicates that the porphyrias may be classified according to their clinical presentation into acute, cutaneous and mixed forms. Only about 10–20% of patients

with the enzyme defects of hereditary porphyria ever develop symptoms, but because of the protean manifestations of the porphyrias, the diagnosis is likely to be suspected more often than it presents.

Acute porphyrias

Enzyme deficiencies that lead to an accumulation of aminolaevulinic acid (ALA) and porphobilinogen (PBG) may be associated with potentially life-threatening acute attacks of severe abdominal pain often accompanied by neurological and psychiatric symptoms. Constipation, nausea, vomiting and hypertension are other common features. Acute attacks may be precipitated by a variety of factors including a wide range of commonly prescribed drugs, endogenous steroid hormones, fasting, substance abuse and stress. Skin lesions are absent in acute intermittent porphyria (AIP), the most common of the acute porphyrias, but they may accompany acute attacks in approximately half of patients with variegate porphyria (VP) and one-third of patients with hereditary coproporphyria (HC). Cutaneous manifestations may be the sole presenting feature in VP and HC, but these patients are also at risk of acute attacks if exposed to acute precipitants. In between acute attacks, patients may be symptom free.

Laboratory diagnosis

With the exception of plumboporphyria, which is an exceedingly rare disorder that has not been reported in Britain, attacks of acute porphyria are invariably associated with an elevated urinary excretion of PBG. This relates to the reduced activity of hydroxymethylbilane synthase due to either an inherited deficiency in patients with AIP or the inhibitory effects of coproporphyrinogen III and protoporphyrinogen IX which accumulate in patients with HC and VP, respectively. Therefore, in the investigation of patients with a suspected attack of one of the acute porphyrias, a fresh random urine specimen, protected from light, should be sent to the laboratory for the quantitation of PBG (screening tests may be unreliable). A negative result excludes an acute porphyria pro-

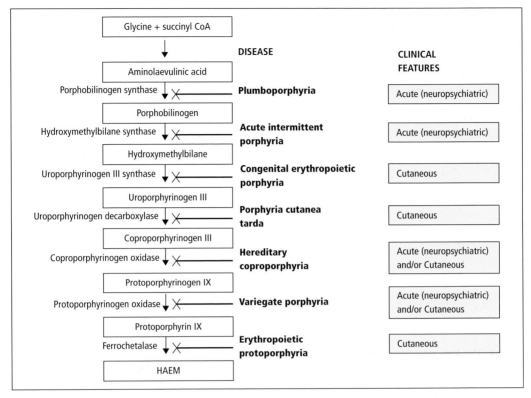

Figure 17.3 Haem synthesis. Blocks at various levels in the pathway result in the porphyrias indicated.

vided the patient is symptomatic at the time of sample collection. In between acute attacks, the excretion of PBG may return to normal. This may occur within days in patients with HC and VP but take several months following an acute episode of AIP. The identification of asymptomatic patients who are in the latent phase of their disease can be particularly difficult (see 'Family studies' below).

If PBG excretion is elevated, the acute porphyrias can be differentiated by the analysis of faecal porphyrins which are not usually elevated in AIP but show characteristic patterns in HC and VP. Initial screening tests involve the spectroscopic examination of an acid extract of faeces for porphyrins. Positive results should always be followed-up by referral to a specialist laboratory for the identification of specific intermediates. Plasma porphyrin fluorescence scanning is particularly useful in the identification of VP when porphyrin is covalently bound to plasma protein.

While the acute porphyrias are also associated with increased urinary ALA excretion, it is only necessary to quantify ALA if plumboporphyria is suspected or, possibly, in the investigation of lead poisoning (see below).

Family studies

It is most important to investigate relatives of patients with AIP, HC and VP so that gene carriers can be warned to avoid factors that may precipitate potentially fatal acute attacks. Unfortunately all of the standard biochemical investigations have limitations for identifying carrier status. PBG excretion is normal in virtually all children and in many adults with latent AIP.

Although the measurement of red cell hydroxy-methylbilane synthase activity may be helpful, because of overlap between normal subjects and patients with AIP unequivocal assignment of carrier status cannot be made. Similarly, urinary PBG and porphyrin excretion are usually unhelpful in identifying carriers of HC and VP. While an unambiguously positive pattern of faecal porphyrins or a characteristic VP porphyrin peak in plasma may identify carriers of HC and VP, negative results are inconclusive.

Genetic analysis is increasingly used in difficult cases. The gene locations of many of the porphyrias have now been identified and although a large number of mutations have been described, many are family specific and provide the opportunity for family studies.

Cutaneous porphyrias

The accumulation of porphyrins in the skin leads to photosensitivity which may present in two ways. The cutaneous manifestations of erythropoietic protoporphyria are present in childhood and include burning, itching and erythema occurring shortly after exposure to sunlight. In contrast, the skin lesions in porphyria cutanea tarda (PCT), HC, VP and congenital erythropoietic porphyria include fragile skin, subepidermal bullae, pigmentation and hypertrichosis. PCT is the most common of all the porphyrias and is usually sporadic (aetiological factors include alcohol, oestrogens, iron and chemicals), with only 10–20% of cases familial.

Laboratory diagnosis

The diagnosis of erythropoietic protoporphyria is made by demonstrating excess free protoporphyrin in red cells. The examination of both urine and faeces for excess porphyrins is essential in the investigation of patients thought to have one of the remaining cutaneous porphyrias. Initial screening tests involve the spectroscopic examination of acidified urine or an acid extract of faeces. Positive results should always be followed-up by referral to a specialist laboratory for the identification of specific intermediates. This is particularly important for the differentiation of patients with PCT from those with either HC or VP who may present with skin lesions alone but still be at risk of life-threatening acute neurological attacks.

Lead poisoning

The accumulation of lead impairs the biosynthesis of haem through its inhibitory effects on the activity of PBG synthase, coproporphyrinogen oxidase and ferrochelatase. This results in an increase in:
- *Urinary ALA and coproporphyrin* which rise as the blood lead concentration increases.
- *Red cell zinc protoporphyrin* which, in the absence of iron deficiency, represents the average exposure of the erythrocyte to lead during its lifespan.

These tests are not sufficiently sensitive to detect reliably low levels of lead exposure, and the measurement of blood lead is the method of choice for investigating environmental or industrial exposure to lead.

Abnormal derivatives of haemoglobin

These all reduce the oxygen-carrying capacity of the blood (Table 17.3). The abnormal derivatives of Hb can all be identified by means of their characteristic absorption spectra, and it is possible to measure the various derivatives quantitatively if they are present in sufficient amounts.

Methaemoglobin

This is oxidised Hb, the Fe^{2+} normally present in haem being replaced by Fe^{3+}; the ability to act as an O_2 carrier is lost. The normal erythrocyte contains small amounts of methaemoglobin, formed by spontaneous oxidation of Hb. Methaemoglobin is normally reconverted to Hb by reducing systems in the red cells, the most important of which is NADH-methaemoglobin reductase. Excess methaemoglobin may be present in the blood because of increased production or diminished ability to convert it back to Hb. If there is more than 20 g/L of methaemoglobin, cyanosis develops. Haemolysis

Table 17.3 Abnormal forms of Hb

Hb derivative	Description
Methaemoglobin	Fe^{3+} replaces Fe^{2+}. Genetic or acquired causes
Haematin	Protoporphyrin containing Fe^{3+}, released from methaemoglobin. May combine with albumin to form methaemalbumin
Sulphaemoglobin	Produced by oxidation of Hb in the presence of SH-containing compounds. Often present with methaemoglobin
Carboxyhaemoglobin	Very stable compound where CO replaces O_2 in oxyhaemoglobin. Unable to transport O_2

sometimes occurs in cases of methaemoglobinaemia, and methaemoglobin then appears in the urine, giving it a brownish colour.

Both genetically determined and acquired conditions can cause methaemoglobinaemia; the acquired group is much more common.

- *Genetic causes of methaemoglobinaemia* include, first, a group of haemoglobinopathies, collectively termed Hb M, where an amino acid substitution stabilises Hb in the Fe^{3+} form. A second group has a deficiency in the enzyme system that reduces methaemoglobin. Reducing agents (such as ascorbic acid or methylene blue) work effectively in the second group, but are ineffective in the first group.
- *Acquired methaemoglobinaemia* usually arises following the ingestion of large amounts of drugs, for example phenacetin, the sulphonamides, excess of nitrites, or certain oxidising agents present in the diet. Treatment with reducing agents is also effective in reversing acquired methaemoglobinaemia.

Sulphaemoglobin

This is formed when Hb is acted on by the same substances as those that cause acquired methaemoglobinaemia, if they act in the presence of sulphur-containing compounds, such as hydrogen sulphide that may arise from bacterial action in the intestine. Sulphaemoglobin and methaemoglobin are often present at the same time in these patients. Sulphaemoglobin cannot act as an O_2 carrier, nor can it be converted back to Hb. Because of its spectroscopic characteristics, patients with even a mild degree of sulphaemoglobinaemia are cyanosed.

Carboxyhaemoglobin (COHb)

Carbon monoxide is a colourless, odourless gas that avidly combines with the haem moiety in Hb and cytochrome enzymes. It combines at the same position in the Hb molecule as O_2, but with an affinity about 200 times greater than that of oxygen. As a result, even small quantities of CO in the inspired air cause the formation of relatively large amounts of COHb, with a corresponding reduction in the O_2-carrying capacity of the blood. This is due not only to the blocking effect of CO on O_2-binding sites, but also to a shift to the left of the oxygen dissociation curve (Figure 3.4) that occurs even when only one of the four O_2-binding sites on Hb is occupied by CO. As little as 1% CO in the inspired air can be fatal in minutes.

In general, non-smokers have COHb values of less than 1%, except in some city dwellers. However, values of as much as 10% occur in heavy smokers. Acute poisoning (smoke inhalation, faulty heaters or flues, car exhaust fumes, attempted suicides) gives rise to non-specific symptoms of lethargy, headache and nausea that may proceed to confusion, agitation and deep coma. When poisoning is suspected, COHb levels can be measured in the laboratory. Urgent treatment with 100% oxygen and, where necessary, cardiorespiratory resuscitation and treatment of cerebral oedema should be instituted. Hyperbaric oxygen is particularly helpful in the more serious cases, especially when COHb levels are 30% or more (concentrations >40% usually result in unconsciousness, and may be fatal).

Keypoints

- About 1 mg of dietary iron is absorbed daily. This is transported in blood in transferrin, and stored mainly as ferritin and haemosiderin.
- Most of the body iron is present in haem.
- The best routine measure of iron stores is serum [ferritin].
- Serum [iron] is of limited diagnostic value on its own, except in acute poisoning.
- Iron-deficiency anaemia is common and may be due to inadequate dietary iron, malabsorption or excessive blood losses.
- Iron overload is rarer. It may be due to excessive iron intake or administration, or a genetically determined increase in iron absorption (haemochromatosis).
- The acute porphyrias are potentially life threatening. Acute attacks are associated with the appearance of PBG in urine.
- The differential diagnosis of the porphyrias depends on the pattern of overproduction of haem precursors.
- Lead inhibits several stages in porphyrin synthesis. However, blood lead is the measurement of choice in suspected lead poisoning.
- Abnormal forms of the major haem protein, Hb, may interfere with blood O_2 transport.

Case 17.1

Two sisters, whose mother had recently received a diagnosis of haemochromatosis, were referred to a haematologist for assessment of their iron status and genetic testing. Both were well and asymptomatic. Initial biochemical findings were as follows:

Serum	Patient 1	Patient 2	Reference range
Ferritin	162	668	<150 g/L
Iron	33	43	10–28 µmol/L
Transferrin	1.7	2.1	2.0–4.0 g/L
Transferrin saturation	74	78	15–50%

What would you consider to be the iron status of each sister?

Comments: Chromosomal analysis indicated that both sisters were homozygous for the C282Y mutation. The younger sister, aged 32 (patient 2), showed clear evidence of increased iron stores with an elevated serum [ferritin], [iron] and transferrin saturation. She was subsequently treated by regular therapeutic phlebotomy. In contrast, the ferritin concentration suggested that the iron stores were only marginally increased in the elder sister, aged 40 (patient 1). Interestingly, this sister had been a regular blood donor for a number of years and had thereby protected herself from iron overload. No active treatment was necessary and she was subsequently reviewed on a regular basis.

Case 17.2

A 35-year-old woman was admitted to a hospital with a history of abdominal pain and vomiting. She had been constipated for 5 days and also complained of numbness in the buttocks and aching at the tops of her legs. Her condition deteriorated rapidly and she was found on the floor hallucinating. A visiting aunt mentioned that there was a family history of porphyria.

Results of initial biochemical investigations were as follows:

(continued on p. 265)

Case 17.2 *(continued)*

Analyte	Result	Reference range
Serum		
Urea	7.8	2.5–6.6 mmol/L
Na	122	135–145 mmol/L
K$^+$	3.4	3.6–5.0 mmol/L
Osmolality	256	280–295 mmol/kg
Urine		
Osmolality	556	

What do these results show? What further tests would be useful for investigating this patient for acute porphyria?

Comments: The initial biochemical results revealed marked hyponatraemia and a correspondingly low serum osmolality. The urine was relatively concentrated, suggesting inappropriate ADH secretion. A 30-fold elevation in the urinary concentration of PBG provided confirmation that the patient was experiencing an attack of one of the acute porphyrias. Faecal concentrations of porphyrin were not elevated, excluding the possibility of HC or VP. The activity of hydroxymethylbilane synthase in red cells was reduced, confirming the diagnosis of AIP. It was not possible to identify any specific precipitating factor in this case. Hyponatraemia and inappropriate ADH secretion are frequently observed in patients presenting with an acute attack of porphyria.

Case 17.3

A 27-year-old woman had become increasingly unwell over the previous 3 days and was admitted to hospital complaining of severe abdominal pains, nausea and vomiting. The diagnosis was uncertain but after 7 days her symptoms had largely resolved. Before discharge it was suggested that the patient may have experienced an attack of acute porphyia and therefore fresh samples urine and faeces were tested for PBG and porphyrins. The following results were obtained:

Analyte	Result	Reference range
Urine		
PBG	1.4	<1.5 µmol/mmol creatinine
Porphyrin	34	<35 nmol/mmol creatinine
Faeces		
Coproporphyrin	201	<46 nmol/g
Protoporphyrin	725	<134 nmol/g

Comments: Because the urine PBG was within reference limits, the patient was not having an acute porphyria attack at the time the sample was collected. However, analysis of the faecal sample showed an accumulation of proto- and coproporphryin that was consistent with a diagnosis of variegate porphyria. It was subsequently possible to retrieve an earlier urine sample that had been stored in the Microbiology Department since admission. Analysis showed an elevation of PBG, confirming that the patient had indeed experienced an acute porphyria attack around the time of admission.

  This case demonstrates (1) the importance of obtaining urine samples for PBG analysis at the time of a suspected porphyria attack and (2) that in patients with variegate porphyria, PBG excretion may return to normal rapidly following an acute attack.

Chapter 18

Uric acid, gout and purine metabolism

The clinical importance of purines rests largely on the disorders characterised by increased serum [urate]. Urate accumulation may arise from:

- Increased intake (diet)
- Increased production (either increased nucleic acid breakdown or increased *de novo* synthesis of purines)
- Decreased renal excretion
- A combination of the above.

Purine metabolism and uric acid

Purines are simple, cyclic organic molecules which are essential constituents of the nucleic acids, both DNA and RNA. The purine bases adenine and guanine comprise the 'A' and 'G' of the DNA code with the 'C' and 'T' contributed by the related pyrimidine bases, cytidine and thymine. When a ribose sugar moiety is linked to the purine base a nucleoside is formed (e.g. adenosine, made up of the purine adenine linked to ribose). The addition of a phosphate group to the ribose ring generates the corresponding nucleotide (e.g. adenosine 5-monophosphate, AMP). As such the purines are essential constituents of metabolically important compounds such as ATP.

Lecture Notes: Clinical Biochemistry, 8e. By G. Beckett, S. Walker, P. Rae & P. Ashby. Published 2010 by Blackwell Publishing.

Figure 18.1 shows that uric acid is the end-product of breakdown of the purine bases. It emphasises that the source of the purines can be from the three routes of diet, nucleic acid breakdown or *de novo* purine synthesis. Once formed, uric acid is predominantly excreted via the kidneys (~70%) with some excretion via the intestine. At physiological pH, uric acid is almost completely ionised, circulating as the urate anion.

Fig. 18.2 summarises the *de novo* synthetic route for purines from the simpe activated ribose molecule, 5-phosphoribosyl-1-pyrophosphate (PRPP). The purine ring is built onto this sugar, and the nucleotide which is first formed (IMP; see Figure 18.2) can be converted to both AMP and GMP nucleotides. It also illustrates that the pathway to uric acid can be reversed at some points (converting the free purine bases to corresponding nucleotides), the so-called salvage pathway. The nucleotides produced by the salvage pathway can be re-incorporated into nucleic acids.

Serum urate

Serum [urate] may be increased (hyperuricaemia) as a result of either excessive formation, reduced excretion or a combination of both. (Figure 18.1). Other factors can also influence these underlying routes of serum [urate] accummulation. These are:

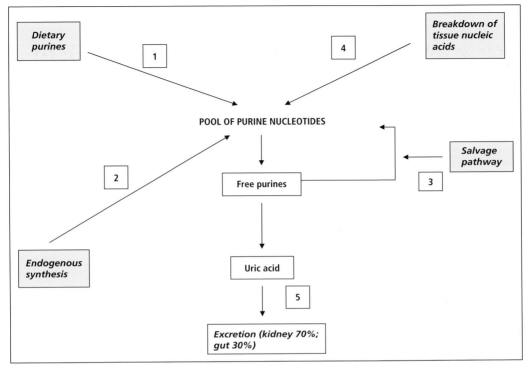

Figure 18.1 Routes to the formation of uric acid production and examples: (1) purine-rich diet (meats, seafood); (2) 5-phosphoribosyl-1-pyrophosphate synthase overactivity; (3) hypoxanthine-guanine phosphoribosyltransferase deficiency; (4) tumour lysis syndrome; (5) renal failure.

- *Sex* Serum levels are higher in males (0.12–0.42 mmol/L) than in females (0.12–0.36 mmol/L).
- *Obesity* Levels tend to be higher in the obese.
- *Social class* The more affluent social classes tend to have a higher serum [urate].
- *Diet* Serum [urate] rises in individuals taking a high-protein diet (especially meat or seafood). High alcohol consumption and fructose-containing beverages are also associated with raised serum [urate]. Dairy foods and coffee drinking appear to lower urate when examined in epidemiological studies.
- *Genetic factors*.

Hyperuricaemia (Table 18.1)

The importance of hyperuricaemia arises because of its potential to cause the condition known as gout, where joint pain and damage arise from the deposition of uric acid crystals in the joints and from the fact that uric acid crystals may be deposited in the renal tract causing renal calculi.

Solutions of monosodium urate become supersaturated when the concentration exceeds 0.42 mmol/L. However, the relationship between the presence and severity of hyperuricaemia and the development of arthritis or renal calculi is more complex than simple considerations of solubility might suggest.

Dietary factors

High purine diets. A high meat diet or one rich in seafood increases the purine load. The protein content *per se* does not appear to be responsible. For example, dairy foods have a relatively high

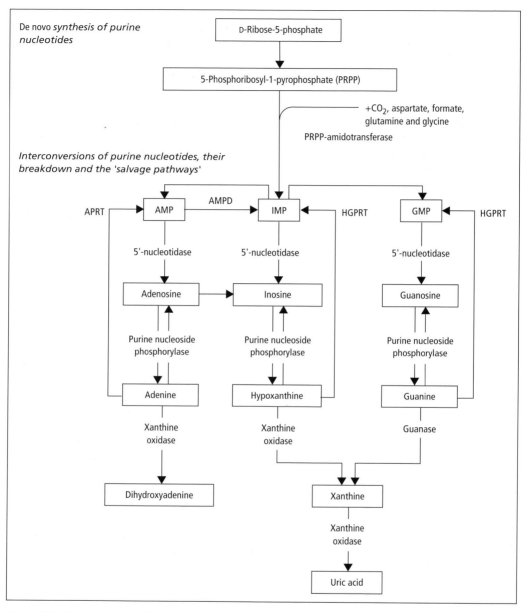

Figure 18.2 The upper part of this figure is a simplified representation of the synthetic pathway leading to the *de novo* synthesis of inosinic acid (IMP), a purine nucleotide that can then be converted to adenylic acid (AMP) and guanylic acid (GMP) by complex reactions, indicated by the upper pair of curved arrows. The lower part of the figure shows the breakdown of AMP, IMP and GMP to the corresponding purines, and their further metabolism to uric acid (the main end-product of purine metabolism) and dihydroxyadenine. It also shows, with another set of curved arrows, the salvage pathways for re-forming AMP, IMP and GMP from their corresponding purine bases, by reactions catalysed by hypoxanthine-guanine phosphoribosyltransferase (HGPRT) and by adenosine phosphoribosyl transferse (APRT).

protein content with low purine content and may actually lower serum [urate], possibly as a consequence of a uricosuric effect of protein.

● *Alcohol excess.* The image of the gout-ridden individual consuming high levels of alcohol is well known, and nutritional surveys have established a strong link between hyperuricaemia and alcohol intake. The mechanism is probably multifactorial, including an increased nucleotide breakdown, diuresis, dehydration and the influence of lactic acids and ketone bodies (arising from the effects of alcohol metabolism) in reducing [urate] excretion.

● *Fructose-containing beverages.* A possible mechanism is the consumption of ATP through the fructokinase reaction, with the ADP formed reconverted to ATP in the adenylate kinase reaction, generating AMP which serves as a precursor for uric acid (Fig. 18.2).

Endogenous overproduction of urate

A number of mechanisms are possible. For example:

● Unspecified overactivity of the pathways of nucleotide metabolism, as opposed to nucleic acid synthesis, leading to urate formation ('endogenous overproduction').

● Decreased activity of the 'salvage' pathway so that purine bases are metabolised to urate rather than re-incorporated into nucleotides and nucleic acids.

● Increased nucleic acid breakdown when cell turnover or destruction is increased.

Defective elimination of urate

Renal excretion of urate is a complex process. Except for a small fraction bound to plasma proteins, urate is completely filtered at the glomerulus; this is then mostly reabsorbed in the proximal tubule. In the distal tubule, there is *both* active secretion *and* post-secretory reabsorption at a more distal site. These processes can all be affected by disease or drugs:

● *GFR* When the GFR becomes reduced for any reason (p. 56), urate retention occurs.

● *Distal tubular secretion* Lactic acid, 3-hydroxybutyric acid and some drugs (e.g. thiazide diuretics) compete with urate for this excretory pathway. Any condition giving rise to lactic acidosis or ketosis tends to be associated with hyperuricaemia.

● *Distal tubular reabsorption* Overall, urate clearance approximates to 10% of the filtered load. Most uricosuric drugs (e.g. probenecid) act by decreasing tubular reabsorption of urate. Salicylates and many other uricosuric agents have paradoxical and dose-dependent effects on the renal tubular handling of urate. With *low* doses, salicylates mainly reduce distal tubular secretion, tending to cause hyperuricaemia. With *high* doses of salicylates, however, reduction of tubular reabsorption is the dominant effect, and there is increased urate excretion.

Gout

Hyperuricaemia is associated with *gout*, a condition characterised by recurrent attacks of monoarticular arthritis. Patients with primary gout (see below) often show deposition of urate as tophi in soft tissues. Some also develop renal stones, mainly composed of uric acid, but the incidence varies widely, largely depending on the presence of other contributory factors such as dehydration or a low urinary pH.

The risk that a previously asymptomatic individual will develop gout varies with the serum [urate]. The annual incidence is very low when serum [urate] is below 0.42 mmol/L, but rises progressively with higher concentrations. It occurs in both sexes but is unusual pre-menopausally. In individuals with hyperuricaemia, it is likely that supersaturation of urate (>0.42 mmol/L) causes crystals to accumulate in connective tissues (e.g. joints) over a long period prior to the development of symptoms.

A high serum [urate] does not always lead to gout, and the majority of patients with hyperuricaemia do not develop gout. A precipitating factor may be a sudden change in serum [urate] in either direction, perhaps precipitated by a sudden dietary

Table 18.1 Causes of hyperuricaemia and gout

Primary	Secondary
Idiopathic	*Increased production*
• Familial component • Majority show decreased urate excretion, with otherwise normal renal function • Associations with metabolic syndrome (obesity, hypertension, hypertriglyceridaemia, etc.)	• Myeloproliferative disorders • Malignancy • Tumour lysis syndrome • Psoriasis • Alcohol (nucleotide breakdown) • Fructose-containing beverages (increases AMP formation and purine breakdown)
Enzyme defects on urate pathway (rare)	*Decreased elimination*
• PRPP synthase overactivity • PRPP amidotransferase overactivity • HGPRT deficiency (salvage pathway)	• Renal failure (acute or chronic) • Lactate or ketoacid excess (metabolic acidosis) with reduced secretion of urate • Drugs, e.g. thiazide diuretics, low-dose salicylate with reduced secretion of urate • Alcohol (increases lactate and ketoacid formation)
	Excessive intake of purines
	• Purine-rich diet (high meat and seafood diet)

change or change in alcohol intake. For this reason, an acute attack of gout may not necessarily be accompanied by hyperuricaemia.

It is usual to subdivide gout into primary and seondary causes (Table 18.1).

• Primary gout typically has a familial component. The detailed causation is unclear but a reduced renal excretion relative to the serum [urate] may be the most common reason, with a minority showing increased overproduction without a clearly defined metabolic lesion. The precise genetic basis is unclear. There is also an association with hyperlipidaemia, ischaemic heart disease and metabolic syndrome, though it is difficult to disentangle the genetic and environmental factors which may be in common. There are rare forms of primary gout which arise from clearly defined and inherited metabolic enzyme defects which increase uric acid formation. Some of these are listed in Table 18.1.

• Secondary gout describes the problem in association with other disorders which secondarily increase urate formation (e.g. increased cell death

in myeloproliferative disorder) or decrease excretion (e.g. renal failure).

In practice, both primary and secondary factors may contribute. For example, the patient may have a primary predisposition to hyperuricaemia which is then compounded by alcohol excess.

Primary gout

The diagnosis is often made clinically on the basis of the distribution of the joint involvement, a past history of similar episodes (especially if responsive to colchicine) and the presence of a raised serum [urate]. By definition, secondary causes of gout should have been excluded. Not all cases are typical clinically, and it should be remembered that

• a high serum [urate] makes the diagnosis of gout probable, but not certain

• a small minority of patients with gout have a normal serum [urate] at the time of an attack.

For the definitive diagnosis of gout, it may be necessary to aspirate joint fluid during an acute attack. This is then examined microscopically, and the finding of needle-shaped urate crystals that show negative birefringence establishes the diagnosis.

Pathogenesis

The acute symptoms of gout are probably due to trauma or local metabolic changes causing crystals of monosodium urate to be shed into the joint cavity. The crystals are phagocytosed by leucocytes and macrophages and cause damage to membranes within the leucocytes. Lysosomal contents and other mediators of the acute inflammatory response (cytokines, prostaglandins, free radicals, etc.) are then released, causing both the systemic and the local acute manifestations of gout. Because the solubility of uric acid decreases with falling temperature, it is speculated that this may explain the predilection of gout to affect peripheral 'colder' joints such at the first metatarsophalangeal joint.

The progress of gout may be over many years. Patients may have asymptomatic hyperuricaemia for many years before the first acute attack. This can be followed by periods which are symptom-free but punctuated by acute attacks which may become increasingly frequent and, if unchecked, progress to chronic tophaceous gout.

Treatment

- In an acute attack, anti-inflammatory drugs (e.g. indomethacin) are usually prescribed. Colchicine is also effective during an acute attack and also has a useful prophylactic effect.
- Uricosuric drugs and allopurinol should be avoided at this stage.

Long-term treatment aims to reduce serum [urate]:

- Weight reduction is encouraged (if appropriate). High purine diets and certain drugs (e.g. thiazide diuretics) should be avoided. Alcohol restriction is encouraged.
- Uricosuric drugs (e.g. probenecid) and inhibitors of urate synthesis (e.g. allopurinol) are often required. Because acute changes in serum [urate] (increases or decreases) can precipitate attacks of gout, the uricosuric drugs and allopurinol should be avoided within several weeks of an acute attack.

- Allopurinol (an isomer of hypoxanthine) inhibits xanthine oxidase, thereby causing a fall in serum [urate] and in urinary [urate]. Levels of the more water-soluble xanthine increase.
- In patients in whom urate stones seem likely to form, a high fluid intake and alkalinisation of the urine reduce the likelihood of stone formation.

Secondary gout

Hyperuricaemia may occur as a complication of several disorders, all of which affect either urate production or excretion, or both. These conditions, although commonly causing hyperuricaemia, are only uncommonly associated with the joint manifestations of gout.

Overproduction of urate

Myeloproliferative disorders Polycythaemia rubra vera is probably the most common of these disorders, which may be associated with signs of gout; this is due to increased turnover of red cell precursors causing hyperuricaemia.

Cytotoxic drug therapy Increased rates of cell turnover cause hyperuricaemia. Renal failure may occur due to deposition of urate crystals in the collecting ducts and ureters. Maintenance of a high fluid intake and prophylaxis with allopurinol usually prevent this.

Psoriasis The hyperuricaemia is thought to be due to an increased rate of cell turnover in the skin.

Hypercatabolic states and starvation There may be both an increased rate of cell destruction and impaired urate excretion due to an associated lactic acidosis.

Defective elimination of urate

Chronic renal disease Serum [urate] rises in uraemia due to the reduced GFR, but clinical gout is very unusual.

Diuretic therapy Most effective diuretics (e.g. chlorothiazide, frusemide) cause hyperuricaemia by reducing distal tubular secretion of urate.

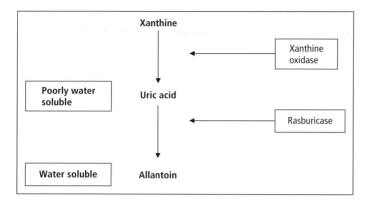

Figure 18.3 Formation of allantoin using rasburicase.

Table 18.2 Causes of a low serum [urate].

Plasma dilution
SIADH (pp. 22)
Pregnancy

Decreased formation
Xanthine oxidase deficiency
Severe liver disease
Rasburicase treatment

Increased excretion
Uricosuric drugs (e.g. allopurinol)
Fanconi syndrome

Lactate accumulation in conditions such as type I glycogen storage disease (von Gierke's disease) often cause hyperuricaemia.

Hypouricaemia

Low serum [urate] may arise as follows (Table 18.2):
• Dilutional states such as SIADH or pregnancy.
• Decreased production. This can be found in severe liver disease. Another example is the condition called xanthinuria arising from an inherited deficiency of the enzyme xanthine oxidase (which normally converts xanthine to urate). Xanthine crystals can form in the urinary tract.

• Increased excretion. This is usually in association with defective proximal tubular reabsorption (Fanconi syndrome).
• Rasburicase (Figure 18.3). This is a genetically engineered enzyme which is a urate oxidase. It converts uric acid to the water-soluble allantoin. It is especially helpful in preventing the renal and other complications of excessive urate formation in the tumour lysis syndrome (massive cell lysis such as is found during treatment of haematological malignancies). It has a short half-life but can effectively reduce serum [urate] to very low levels. Modifications of rasburicase to increase its half-life are starting to find a place in the treatment of gout.

A low serum [urate] has not usually been regarded as pathological in its own right. However, uric acid has anti-oxidant properties which may be more important than have hitherto been realised. For example, there is a literature which reports associations between low serum [urate] and a variety of neurological disorders such as multiple sclerosis and Parkinson disease. It is speculated that urate may help prevent damage to nervous tissue from oxidants such as peroxynitrite, though it is unclear if the low [urate] is a causal factor or consequence of the neurological problem.

Keypoints

- In humans, urate is the main end-product of nucleic acid and purine metabolism.
- Urate in plasma and tissue fluids is close to the limit of its solubility.
- Urate is mainly excreted in the urine.
- Serum urate may rise due to either increased production (e.g. increased cell turnover) or decreased renal excretion (or a combination of both).
- Gout is characterised by arthritis due to an inflammatory reaction to the deposition of urate crystals in joints. Urate may be deposited in connective tissue elsewhere, and urate renal stones may also form.
- Primary gout tends to be familial and most individuals demonstrate a reduced renal excretion without overt kidney disease. Rare inborn errors of urate formation may cause primary gout. The term secondary gout is applied to other disorders in which an increase in serum [urate] is a complication of the disorder itself.
- Treatment depends upon the use of drugs to reduce inflammation in the acute attack and drugs which lower serum [urate] in the chronic phase.
- Hypouricaemia is relatively unusual but has raised interest in a possible anti-oxidant function of urate.

Case 18.1

Whilst authorizing clinical results prior to release to the wards, the clinical biochemist on duty was surprised to find a serum [urate] level which was extremely low (undetectable in the laboratory analyzer). Initially, she felt that this must have been an analytical error and asked for the result to be repeated. Again, the serum [urate] was undetectable. She rang up the haematology ward to discuss this result with the Specialist Registrar. Can you suggest a likely explanation for this finding?

Comment: it turned out that the patient had an acute lymphoblastic anaemia which was being actively treated. In anticipation of possible problems arising from the excessive formation of urate (as a consequence of massive cell lysis), the patient was on treatment with rasburicase. This is a genetically engineered urate oxidase which converts uric acid to the water-soluble allantoin. It is so effective as to reduce the serum [urate] to virtually undetectable levels, hence the laboratory finding which was a correct analytical result!

Case 18.2

A 48-year-old hospital manager was admitted with severe colicky pain in his lower left lumbar region and an associated history of haematuria. He was overweight with a blood pressure of 165/105. Serum lipids on the admission sample showed triglyceride levels of 5.2 mmol/L, a total cholesterol of 7.2 mmol/L and a HDL cholesterol of 0.8 mmol/L. Serum calcium was normal but the urate was 0.75 mmol/L. Further questioning revealed an episode of severe pain in his first metatarso-phalangeal joint of his left foot while holidaying in Spain. This was treated while abroad and resolved after a few days but he could not recollect what treatment had been given. What is the likely cause of this man's condition?

Comment: The clinical history here, together with the high serum urate level, all point towards the diagnosis of primary gout. The first metatarso-phalangeal joint is the most common to be involved in first attacks of gout. The acute joint pain itself coincides with the time the patient was on holiday and possibly overindulging in alcohol and rich foods which may well have precipitated the initial episode. The high serum urate is likely to be longstanding and has led to the formation of renal stones. A history of severe lumbar pain, colicky in nature, and associated with haematuria is classical for renal colic. Where possible, examination of any stones passed or removed should be undertaken to confirm that these are composed of uric acid. There is a known association of gout with hyperlipidaemia, particularly a raised triglyceride. Additionally, associations with hypertension, obesity and IGT are also described.

Chapter 19

Central nervous system and cerebrospinal fluid

Many neurological disorders have a biochemical basis, or are associated with disturbances of metabolism. However, neurochemistry is a specialised subject that is beyond the scope of this book. Many generalised disorders of metabolism affect the CNS, for example Hartnup's disease, Wilson's disease and PKU, and these are considered elsewhere. In this chapter, we discuss the information to be gained from examining the CSF.

CSF composition

The CSF approximates to an ultrafiltrate of plasma. There are, however, differences between the relative concentrations in plasma and CSF of both low molecular mass and high molecular mass substances.

1 Low molecular mass substances
  • *Differential rates of diffusion* Dissolved CO_2 diffuses into CSF more rapidly than HCO_3^-, so CSF [H^+] (which depends on the $HCO_3^- : H_2CO_3$ ratio) may be significantly different from plasma [H^+].
  • *Effects of ultrafiltration* Bilirubin is nearly all protein bound in plasma, and normally very little crosses the blood–brain barrier. Calcium is

only partly protein bound, and Ca^{2+} readily crosses into the CSF.

2 High molecular mass substances
  • *Differential rates of diffusion* Eighty percent of CSF protein is derived from plasma proteins by passive diffusion across the blood–brain barrier, and the total concentration of CSF protein is approximately 200 times less than that of plasma. The concentration of individual proteins depends both on the permeability of the barrier and on their plasma concentrations. All plasma proteins commonly measured are present in CSF and, in general, their relative concentrations are proportional to those in plasma.
  • *Secretion of proteins* Pre-albumin is synthesised by the choroidal epithelium and is present at concentrations greater than can be achieved by passive diffusion.
  • *Receptor-mediated transfer* Desialated transferrin (Tau protein) may arise during receptor-mediated transfer of transferrin from plasma.

Examination of CSF

Appearance

CSF is normally clear and colourless. Turbidity is usually due to leucocytes, but it may be due to microorganisms. Blood-stained CSF may indicate recent haemorrhage, or damage to a blood vessel

Lecture Notes: Clinical Biochemistry, 8e. By G. Beckett, S. Walker, P. Rae & P. Ashby. Published 2010 by Blackwell Publishing.

during specimen collection. Xanthochromia (yellow colour) is most often due to previous haemorrhage into the CSF, but it may indicate that CSF [protein] is very high. The CSF may be yellow in jaundiced patients.

CSF bilirubin

Patients investigated for suspected subarachnoid haemorrhage (SAH) initially undergo a CT scan. In experienced hands, this will be positive for subarachnoid blood in 98% of patients presenting within 12 h of SAH. In patients presenting later, the blood load may have cleared and the diagnostic sensitivity of the CT scan is reduced to 50% after 1 week. However, as erythrocytes in CSF undergo lysis and phagocytosis, oxyhaemoglobin is released and is converted into bilirubin in a time-dependent manner. In CT-negative patients, the identification of bilirubin in CSF may be helpful in establishing the diagnosis.

Specimen requirements

• CSF specimens should be obtained at least 12 h after the suspected SAH.
• The specimen should be protected from light.
• The specimen should be delivered to the laboratory immediately after collection for centrifugation and spectrophotometric examination.
• If possible, a blood sample for bilirubin analysis should be taken at the same time as an aid to the interpretation of the CSF results.

Because oxyhaemoglobin can interfere with the detection of bilirubin, *in vitro* lysis of any red cells present in the CSF specimen should be avoided. Therefore:
• The least bloodstained fraction of CSF (usually the last) should be taken for spectrophotometric examination.
• CSF should not be transported by pneumatic tube in order to minimise *in vitro* haemolysis of any contaminating red cells.

Spectrophotometric examination

Visual inspection for xanthochromia is unreliable, and it is essential that a spectrophotometric scan of the CSF supernatant be performed. The presence of an increased level of bilirubin is consistent with a recent bleed into the CSF. Available evidence suggests that bilirubin may be present for up to 2 weeks following SAH. However, this can vary greatly especially in the case of small bleeds and, therefore, a negative bilirubin result cannot completely exclude SAH.

A spectral band characteristic of oxyhaemoglobin may also be present in CSF obtained from patients with SAH. However, since oxyhaemoglobin may also be released following *in vitro* haemolysis of red cells introduced during collection, its predictive value for SAH is poor and the presence of oxyhaemoglobin alone is inconclusive.

CSF glucose

Lumbar CSF [glucose] is normally 0.5–1.0 mmol/L lower than plasma [glucose], whereas CSF [glucose] in specimens obtained from the cerebral ventricles and from the cisterna magna normally differs little from plasma [glucose].

Interpretation of CSF [glucose] requires a matching plasma glucose obtained at the same time as the lumbar puncture. In hypoglycaemia, CSF [glucose] may be very low; it is raised when there is hyperglycaemia.

CSF glucose may be low or undetectable in patients with acute bacterial, cryptococcal, tubercular or carcinomatous meningitis, or in cerebral abscess, probably due to consumption of glucose by leucocytes or other rapidly metabolising cells. In meningitis or encephalitis due to viral infections, it is usually normal.

CSF total protein

Lumbar CSF protein (reference range 100–400 mg/L) is normally almost all albumin. Ventricular and cisternal CSF [protein] is lower than lumbar CSF [protein]. Much higher CSF [protein] may have no pathological significance in the neonatal period, for example lumbar CSF [protein] may then be as much as 900 mg/L.

CSF [protein] is increased in a large number of pathological conditions. Whenever it is increased, organic disease of the CNS is probably present. In acute inflammatory conditions of the CNS, the increase may be very marked due to increased capillary permeability.

In the demyelinating disorders, there is often a moderate increase in CSF [protein], usually in the range 500–1000 mg/L. Primary and secondary neoplasms involving the brain or the meninges can cause very large increases in lumbar CSF [protein] if spinal block occurs. Values over 5000 mg/L may be observed. These specimens may be xanthochromic because of the high protein content, and a protein clot may form on storage after a few hours.

CSF oligoclonal bands

CSF normally contains small amounts of IgG (reference range 8–64 mg/L), a trace of IgA and minute amounts of IgM. An increase in CSF immunoglobulin (Ig), particularly IgG, can either result from intrathecal synthesis or it can be secondary to an increase in plasma Igs and/or impairment of the blood–CSF barrier. Increased intrathecal synthesis of Ig results from the expansion of a limited number of clones of plasma cells and is associated with discrete oligoclonal bands that are present in CSF but not a paired serum.

Examination of CSF for oligoclonal bands is an essential laboratory test in the investigation of demyelinating disease. It is an integral part of making a diagnosis of multiple sclerosis where bands are seen in more than 95% of clinically definite cases. Other conditions associated with increased intrathecal IgG synthesis and oligoclonal banding include neurosyphilis, subacute sclerosing panencephalitis, polyneuritis, systemic lupus erythematosus and sarcoidosis.

The identification of oligoclonal bands by isoelectric focusing and immunoblotting of paired CSF and serum samples is now regarded as the 'gold standard' laboratory test for the detection of intrathecal synthesis of IgG. It is more sensitive than earlier quantitative approaches involving the calculation of the IgG index (CSF [IgG] : serum [IgG] ÷ CSF [albumin] : serum [albumin]). This attempts to detect intrathecal synthesis against a background of varying serum IgG and impaired CSF–blood barrier function, but at best is positive only in approximately 75% of patients who turn out to be oligoclonal band positive.

Identification of CSF

CSF rhinorrhoea is potentially serious due to the risk of infection. It may arise as a result of traumatic fracture, surgery or the erosion of bone by extracranial tumours. True CSF rhinorrhoea may be differentiated from other causes of rhinorrhoea (e.g. allergic rhinitis) by demonstrating the presence of asialotransferrin (Tau protein) which is found in significant quantities in CSF but not serum.

Case 19.1

A 43-year-old woman was referred to the neurologists by her GP. She had complained of a severe headache that had started suddenly 2 days earlier. The possibility of an SAH was considered but a CT scan did not reveal any evidence of subarachnoid blood. A lumbar puncture was performed and a sample of CSF was sent to the laboratory for spectroscopic examination.

The following trace was obtained:

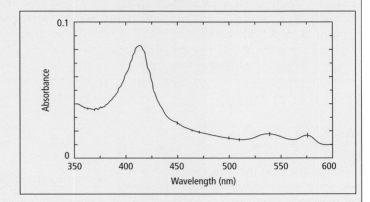

Figure 19.1 Spectrophotometric scan of CSF

What do these results show?

Comments: This trace shows that oxyhaemoglobin with a maximum absorbance at 414 nm was present in the CSF specimen received by the laboratory. However, the net bilirubin absorbance was within normal limits. If present in significant quantities, bilirubin would have been apparent as a shoulder on the oxyhaemoglobin peak between approximately 425 and 500 nm.

Since this sample was taken 48 h after the onset of the headache, bilirubin should have been present if an SAH had occurred. The presence of oxyhaemoglobin alone is of doubtful significance and is likely to reflect *in vitro* haemolysis of red cells introduced into the sample at the time of collection. The patient was discharged and remained well, although the cause of the headache was not established.

Chapter 20

Therapeutic drug monitoring and chemical toxicology

Poisoning is one of the most common causes of emergency admission to hospitals. Of the numerous potentially fatal chemicals and drugs, only a limited number is encountered in practice. It may be important to know the nature and blood levels of the poison, as this may help management and determine prognosis.

Drug therapy should usually be monitored on clinical grounds rather than on blood levels. However, for a few drugs, measurement of drug levels in blood (and occasionally genotyping or phenotyping of a particular enzyme) is essential to ensure a therapeutic effect without toxicity.

Drug abuse is an increasing social and medical problem. Urinary drug measurements have an important part to play in the management of a number of these individuals.

This chapter outlines the important role that clinical biochemistry departments play in monitoring the therapeutic use of certain drugs, investigating patients when drugs and poisons may have been taken in overdose and in screening for drugs of abuse.

Lecture Notes: Clinical Biochemistry, 8e. By G. Beckett, S. Walker, P. Rae & P. Ashby. Published 2010 by Blackwell Publishing.

Therapeutic drug monitoring

When is therapeutic drug monitoring required?

For many drugs, the dose given correlates well with a pharmacological effect, and the correct dosage can be satisfactorily determined by clinical assessment or the measurement of a biochemical response. For example, the pharmacological actions of anti-coagulants and of anti-hypertensive drugs can be assessed, and dosage adjusted, on the basis of prothrombin time and blood pressure measurements, respectively.

Measurement of plasma or blood drug levels is required:

1 For drugs that have a narrow therapeutic range, for example lithium.

2 For drugs which in overdose may produce symptoms that are similar to those of the disease being treated, for example phenytoin or ciclosporin.

3 Where the drug may produce abnormalities in hepatic or renal clearance.

4 Where drug absorption may vary with dose or other circumstances.

Table 20.1 lists the drugs for which the case for therapeutic drug monitoring (TDM) has been clearly established. Regular monitoring of patients taking these drugs is not usually required once the

Table 20.1 Therapeutic drug monitoring; examples of drugs for which it is indicated

Drug	Therapeutic range in plasma*		Time to collect blood	Half-life (h)	Reason[†]
	Level	Units			
Aminoglycoside antibiotics	Peak 5–10	mg/L	30 min to 1 h after last dose		b, c, d, e
Gentamycin/ tobramycin	Trough <2	mg/L	Just before next dose	2–3	b, c, d, e
Carbamazepine	4–10	mg/L	Just before next dose	8–24	c
	17–42	µmol/L			
Ciclosporin	700–1500	µg/L/L	2 hours after dose (C2)	6–24	c
Digoxin	0.8–2.0	ng/mL	6–18 h after last dose	36–48	a, b, c, d
	1.0–2.6	nmol/L			
Lithium	416–694	mg/100 mL	12–18 h after last dose	10–35	a, b, e
	0.6–1.0	mmol/L			
Phenytoin	10–20	mg/L	Long half-life – not critical	20–40	a, c
	40–80	µmol/L			
Tacrolimus	Varies with transplant		Just before next dose		
Theophylline	10–20	mg/L	Not critical[‡]	3–13	a, b, c, d
	55–110	µmol/L			

* For conversion factors for numerical values from mass units into molar units, see p. 323.

† Key to the reasons for performing therapeutic drug monitoring: (a) wide inter-individual variation; (b) low therapeutic index; (c) therapeutic effect or signs of toxicity difficult to recognise; (d) administration of a potentially toxic drug to a seriously ill patient; (e) very toxic in overdose.

‡ Timing of peak levels will depend on formulation, for example slow-acting preparations.

patient has been stabilised on a dose of drug that has produced the desired clinical effect.

TDM is important if there is a particular clinical problem to be addressed, such as:

1 Establishing a dose regimen when therapy has just begun, or when it needs to be changed.

2 Failure to achieve therapeutic control, although dosage is apparently adequate.

3 Loss of control in a patient previously stabilised on treatment. This may, for example, be due to partial compliance or altered metabolism.

4 To check for toxicity, especially if several drugs are being given.

When should the blood sample be taken?

When a single dose of drug is taken for the first time, plasma levels will initially rise rapidly and then decline in a curvilinear manner similar to that

shown in Figure 20.1. The characteristics of this curve provide essential details about the kinetics of the drug and the information needed to calculate the approximate dose and frequency of the drug for the desired therapeutic concentration in plasma. For any drug given at regular intervals, a steady-state relatively constant concentration in plasma is reached after about five half-lives (Figure 20.1). However, peak levels (achieved just after administration) and trough levels (achieved immediately prior to the next dose) may still be recognised. For most drugs, it is important that trough levels are adequate to achieve the desired therapeutic effect. Thus, blood samples are often withdrawn just before a dose of the drug is taken, but at any rate samples should usually be taken after the initial peak has subsided, unless toxicity is suspected.

In all cases, the time of blood sampling and of the last dose of the drug must be given.

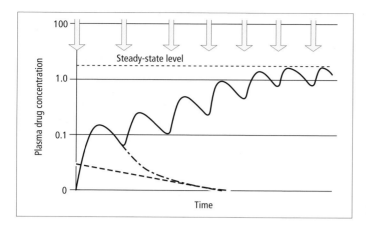

Figure 20.1 The effect on plasma drug concentration of giving repeated regular doses of a drug. As can be seen, after approximately five doses of the drug, a steady state-level is reached, with peak and trough values being found. The hatched line represents the elimination half-life and the hatched/dotted line shows the plasma drug concentration profile if a single dose of the drug had been given. Arrows show the time of each dose of the drug.

Interpretation of drug levels

Therapeutic ranges If the blood has been taken at the appropriate time, the plasma level can be compared with published therapeutic ranges (Table 20.1). These published ranges indicate the range of plasma drug levels which in the majority of the population have been shown to provide the desired therapeutic effect without a high risk of toxicity. Published ranges offer little more than guidelines, because of inter-individual variation in the clinical response to drugs.

Interpretation of a result requires:

1 *Correct timing of blood sampling in relation to the dose* If specimens are collected too soon after the start of treatment, or after dosage has been changed (i.e. before a steady-state concentration of drug has been achieved), TDM results will be misleading.

2 *Clinical information* Published therapeutic ranges cannot make allowance for the possible effects of hepatic or renal disease in individual patients, or for the consequences of drug interactions that might stem from particular prescribing combinations. For example, in patients with renal impairment, drugs will be eliminated from the circulation at a rate that may be much slower than normal. Alternatively, in patients taking drugs that result in the induction of hepatic drug-metabolising enzyme systems, the clearance of other drugs being taken simultaneously by the patient may be enhanced.

Other important issues in therapeutic drug monitoring

Free and bound drugs

Most drugs circulate partly bound to plasma proteins, the bound and unbound forms being in equilibrium. The pharmacological response is usually determined by the tissue concentration which, in turn, is related to the plasma [unbound drug]. However, plasma [free drug] is difficult to measure, and TDM depends on the measurements of plasma [total drug]. For some drugs, the concentration of drug in saliva may reflect the concentration of free drug in plasma, and salivary drug measurements are now widely used in screening for drugs of abuse.

The importance of drug metabolites

Most drugs are metabolised to inactive products, although some are inactive when taken and are converted to active drug in the liver or GI tract. For example, primidone is converted to active metabolites, principally phenobarbitone. If primidone therapy is to be monitored, plasma [phenobarbitone] is the measurement required.

A number of different analytical methods are sometimes used for measurement of a single drug (and possibly of its metabolites). This explains the differences that may be found between results from different laboratories. It also explains why some less specific methods may give rise to misleading results if there are high concentrations of *inactive metabolites* in plasma. Even specific methods may give rise to misleading results if they fail to measure *active metabolites*.

Units of measurement

Plasma drug concentrations may be expressed in mass (gravimetric) or molar units of concentration (Table 20.1). The practice of referring to numerical values of drug measurements without mentioning the units is dangerous, since it can lead to serious – and sometimes fatal – mistakes.

Specific drugs

Aminoglycoside antibiotics

These antibiotics have a very short half-life of 2–3 h if renal function is normal, but in patients with infection or renal impairment the half-life becomes prolonged (up to 100 h). In addition, tissue pools of gentamycin may become saturated if treatment is for more than a week, and then plasma levels may start to rise sharply. Gentamycin is *nephrotoxic* and *ototoxic*. Therefore, TDM is particularly important in patients with impaired renal function who receive the drug for more than 7 days, or those on high loading doses for serious infection. Peak and trough levels should be measured.

Anti-convulsants

Carbamazepine Carbamazepine has fewer side effects, mainly neurotoxic, than phenytoin. Monitoring is of value in patients with poor control, since there is a variable relationship between dose and plasma concentration. The sample should be taken just before a dose.

Phenytoin Phenytoin has a low therapeutic ratio and is subject to variable rates of hepatic metabolism, leading to a non-linear relationship between dose and plasma concentration. Because of its undesirable side effects, which include neurotoxicity and increased frequency of fits, TDM is required in new patients, where there is an unexpected loss

in control, in pregnancy or when other drugs that interact with phenytoin are added or withdrawn.

Drugs that prevent graft rejection

A number of drugs are used to prevent graft rejection. TDM is recommended to ensure efficacy of each of these drugs since achieving the correct level of drug in the blood is essential to prevent rejection while minimising side effects such as nephrotoxicity. Some centres may use combinations of these drugs.

Ciclosporin is nephrotoxic, with signs that may mimic rejection in patients with transplants. The peak level (achieved 2 h after the dose, known as the C2 level) provides a better means of guiding dosage than the trough level.

Tacrolimus and *sirolimus* are relatively new immunosuppressive drugs that may have lower toxicity than ciclosporin. Therapeutic monitoring of blood levels of these drugs is still required.

Digoxin

Digoxin has little clinical effect at plasma concentrations below 1 nmol/L, whereas toxicity (often manifest as cardiac arrhythmia and vomiting) is common when plasma levels rise above 3.8 nmol/L. Digoxin results should always be interpreted together with a plasma potassium concentration, since hypokalaemia potentiates the effect of digoxin. Thus, toxic effects of the drug may occur in a hypokalaemic patient who has a plasma digoxin within the therapeutic range. A similar effect may be seen in hypercalcaemia, hypomagnesaemia and hypothyroidism. Equilibration of digoxin with cardiac tissue takes some time, and thus blood should not be taken for at least 6 h after the dose.

Lithium

Lithium is used for the treatment of depressive illness. It has a short half-life, and plasma levels should be determined 12 h after the last dose. TDM is essential because the drug is toxic, producing a range of symptoms including polyuria, hypothyroidism and, in severe cases, renal failure and coma. Patients with plasma [lithium] above 1.4 mmol/L are at risk of oliguria and acute renal

281

failure. TDM may also be necessary in order to monitor compliance.

Methotrexate

Methotrexate is a dihydrofolate reductase inhibitor, and therefore reduces intracellular folate, which in turn inhibits DNA synthesis. The drug is cytotoxic; high-dose regimens are used in the treatment of some cancers, and lower dose regimens are used for immunosuppression. TDM is of value in patients receiving high doses of methotrexate, to identify those at risk of toxic effects and to provide a guide to the dose and timing of leucovorin (a drug that restores the pool of reduced folate) rescue.

Theophylline

This drug is used to prevent or treat bronchoconstriction in some children or elderly patients who cannot use an inhaler easily. The drug commonly produces minor side effects such as nausea and headache, even at concentrations within the therapeutic range. Serious toxicity leading to cardiac arrhythmia can occur with plasma levels above 110 mmol/L. TDM is particularly valuable to optimise the dose, confirm toxicity or demonstrate poor compliance. Some believe that the metabolite caffeine should also be measured.

Pharmacogenomics

People have different responses to the same drug brought about by the presence of widespread polymorphisms in the expression of phase 1 and phase 2 drug-metabolising systems. For example, it was recognised over 40 years ago that succinylcholine (scoline) toxicity in some individuals was due to impaired metabolism of the drug by a genetic variant of pseudocholinesterase. There are now known to be marked variations in the ability of an individual to metabolise drugs catalysed by a wide range of phase I enzymes such as cytochrome P450 (CYP) 2D6 and the phase II enzyme TPMT. It has become clear that knowledge of the specific enzyme polymorphisms expressed by a patient allows the therapeutic action of a drug to be maximised with a low possibility of an adverse drug reaction.

Scoline apnoea and butylcholinesterase (BChE)

There are two principal choline esterases (ChEs): (1) plasma BChE (formerly known as pseudocholinesterase), is synthesised in the liver, and (2) acetylcholinesterase, which is present at nerve endings and in the erythrocytes, but not in plasma (formerly known as 'true' ChE). Assessment of plasma BChE is of particular value in the investigation of patients with Scoline apnoea and organophosphorus insecticide poisoning.

A few patients may exhibit prolonged apnoea, lasting several hours, after succinylcholine (Scoline, suxamethonium) administration. This drug is normally hydrolysed by plasma BChE but genetic variation means that in some individuals the phenotype has an impaired ability to metabolise Scoline. The common phenotype UU is present in more than 95% of the UK population. Phenotypes with impaired ability to metabolise scoline are AA, AS, AF, FF, FS, SS and to a variable degree UA. The action of suxamethonium can be increased from 30 min to several hours in these cases. The main four allelic genes are:

U codes for the *u*sual form of ChE, present in over 95% of the population in the U.

A codes for an *a*typical ChE that is resistant to inhibition by dibucaine.

F codes for an atypical ChE that is resistant to inhibition by *f*luoride.

S codes for a *s*ilent protein that has little or no ChE activity.

Most individuals with abnormal variants have low plasma ChE activity, but the only reliable way of demonstrating the variants is by means of inhibitor studies using dibucaine and fluoride or by carrying out genotyping. It is important to recognise these abnormalities of plasma ChE, since affected relatives can then be traced, and anaesthetists can be warned not to use Scoline.

Azathioprine and thiopurine methyltransferase (TPMT)

Azathioprine is widely used in the treatment of rheumatic disorders, hepatobiliary disease, skin disorders and following renal transplant. Azathioprine is metabolised by a number of pathways through 6-mercaptopurine (6-MP) eventually to form the therapeutically active 6-thioguanine nucleotides (TGNs). The TGNs are cytotoxic, being eventually incorporated into DNA as a false base, and cause cell death by a mismatch repair pathway. The 6-MP can also be methylated by TPMT and oxidised by xanthine oxidase (XO) to produce inactive metabolites. Variations in the extensive metabolism of 6-MP play a role in the toxicity and efficacy of azathioprine. TPMT has been extensively studied with respect to its variation in specific patient groups. The expression of TPMT in tissue is controlled by a genetic polymorphism inherited as an autosomal co-dominant trait. Patients with low expression of TPMT develop profound bone marrow toxicity, a consequence of the intracellular accumulation of grossly elevated cytotoxic TGN concentrations (Figure 20.2). A series of alleles have been identified that are associated with decreased levels of TPMT activity. The wild type is usually designated TPMT*1 and the

mutated genes assigned as TPMT*2–*8 (with TPMT*3 having three forms 3A, 3B, 3C). Thus, a total of 10 polymorphisms have so far been identified. The alleles TPMT*3A and TPMT*3C account for 80–95% of intermediate or low enzyme activity, with TPMT*3A being the most common allele in Caucasian populations and TPMT*3C being the most common in African and South East Asian populations. However, about 0.3% of the Caucasian population and as little as 0.04 of the Asian population express low levels of TPMT.

Patients who express intermediate or low activities of TPMT can accumulate high concentrations of toxic 6-thioguanine metabolites when given azathioprine, which puts them at increased risk of fatal bone marrow toxicity. Conversely, patients who express high activities of TPMT may not receive the maximum benefit from standard doses of the drug because of increased clearance. Genotyping or phenotyping for TPMT is thus advisable before initiating therapy with azathioprine.

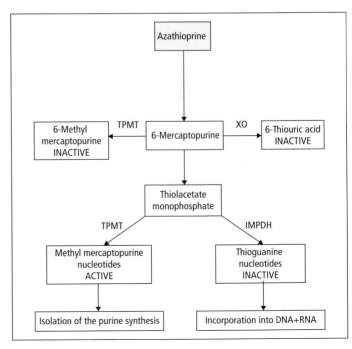

Figure 20.2 Azathioprine metabolism. TPMT = thiopurine *S*-methyltransferase; XO = xanthine oxidase; IMPDH = inosine monophosphate dehydrogenase. If TPMT activity is low, then more of the toxic thioguanine nucleotides will form.

Chemical toxicology

Although accidental poisoning does occur, intentional drug overdose is more common. If the patient is conscious and presents with specific signs and symptoms of toxicity, then a reliable history, with the clinical examination, will usually suggest which drug or drugs have been taken. This can be confirmed by laboratory investigations. Unfortunately, few of the drugs commonly taken in overdose have specific clinical signs. It is quite common for a combination of drugs to have been taken, sometimes with large amounts of alcohol.

Problems arise when the patient is unconscious and the history is unavailable or likely to be inaccurate. In such a situation, the laboratory may be asked to perform a drug screen to identify which drugs and poisons may have been taken.

Other important tests that should be performed on the patient with suspected poisoning include

- urea and electrolytes
- liver function tests
- blood glucose
- blood gases.

Treatment

A few drugs have a specific antidote (Table 20.2), but some antidotes may themselves have unpleasant side effects. For the majority of poisons, there is no antidote available, and the patient is treated conservatively until the drug has been eliminated from the body. If there is poor renal or liver function, it may be necessary to use haemodialysis or charcoal haemoperfusion to eliminate the drug and, in such a case, measurement of plasma levels is very important.

Online computer databases (e.g. TOXBASE) are now readily available to aid the doctor with advice regarding both the diagnosis and the treatment of the poisoned patient.

Table 20.2 The principal examples of substances that cause acute poisoning in the UK

Substance	Active treatment of overdose or toxin
Drugs commonly taken as overdose	
Benzodiazepines	Flumazenil
Ethanol	No specific treatment available
Paracetamol	*N*-Acetylcysteine
Salicylates	Sodium bicarbonate, haemodialysis, repeated oral activated charcoal
Tricyclic anti-depressants/SSRI	No specific treatment available
Drugs less commonly taken as overdose	
Carbamazepine	Repeated oral activated charcoal
Digoxin	Anti-digoxin antibody
Iron	Desferrioxamine
Lithium	Saline
Opiates	Naloxone
Phenobarbitone	Repeated oral activated charcoal
Phenytoin	Repeated oral activated charcoal
Quinine	Repeated oral activated charcoal
Toxic substances	
Carbon monoxide	Oxygen
Cyanide (non-fatal dose)	Cobalt edetate, hydroxocobalamin
Ethylene glycol	Ethanol, haemodialysis
Methanol	Ethanol, haemodialysis, fomepizole
Organophosphorus agents	Pralidoxime, atropine
Paraquat	No specific treatment available

Specific drugs and poisons

Paracetamol

Overdose with paracetamol is common. During the first few hours, there may be few symptoms, unless these arise from another drug that has been taken simultaneously. A very large overdose may produce symptoms of depressed consciousness and metabolic acidosis. In patients presenting after 20 h, biochemical evidence of liver dysfunction is often apparent.

Approximately 8% of ingested paracetamol is converted in the liver to a toxic metabolite, N-acetyl-p-benzoquinoneimine (NABQI), which is usually detoxified by conjugation with glutathione. If large amounts of paracetamol are taken, the hepatic stores of glutathione become depleted, and NABQI binds irreversibly to proteins within the hepatocyte, producing centrilobular necrosis. In some cases, renal damage is also produced by a similar mechanism. Increased production of NABQI occurs in patients with a chronic alcohol problem and in patients taking certain enzyme-inducing drugs such as phenytoin and phenobarbitone; these patients are at risk of hepatotoxicity at lower doses of paracetamol (Figure 20.3).

If paracetamol overdose is diagnosed quickly, a specific treatment is available (IV N-acetylcysteine or oral methionine). The decision to treat is based on the plasma paracetamol concentration related to the time from overdose (Figure 20.3), although 4 h should elapse from the time of ingestion to take into account drug absorption. These treatments show most benefit if instituted within 12 h of the overdose, and are unlikely to be effective if used after 24 h. When the time of the overdose is unknown, active intervention is advisable. The prothrombin time is usually the first liver function test to become abnormal (after ~12 h) and is of value in assessing prognosis. Other liver function tests do not show an abnormality until at least 24–36 h after the overdose.

Because effective treatment is available for paracetamol poisoning if diagnosed within 12 h of

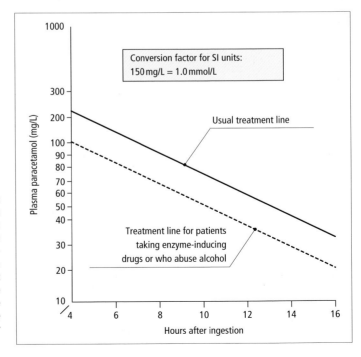

Figure 20.3 The decision to give antidote treatment depends on the time since the overdose and on the paracetamol concentration. The timing of specimen collection is important. Specimens need to be taken 4–16 h after suspected overdose. At less than 4 h, the drug may not have been fully absorbed; at over 16 h, the concentration is no longer a reliable indicator of whether to administer antidote.

ingestion, it is necessary to measure plasma paracetamol in

- patients who have taken paracetamol or combined formulations containing the drug
- patients who have taken unidentified tablets
- all unconscious patients.

Salicylates

Patients often present with nausea, vomiting and increased rate of respiration. Dehydration, due to vomiting, is often severe. Acid–base disturbances are common – usually a mixed respiratory alkalosis and metabolic acidosis, but if vomiting is severe a metabolic alkalosis can develop.

The diagnosis is confirmed by measuring plasma [salicylate]. Blood gas analysis may also be indicated. In patients with plasma [salicylate] above 3.6 mmol/L (500 mg/L) or, in children less than 5 years old, plasma [salicylate] above 2.5 mmol/L (350 mg/L), treatment with repeated oral administration of activated charcoal and IV infusion of sodium bicarbonate is often used to increase the excretion of the drug into urine. Haemodialysis may also be required in the severely poisoned patient [salicylate] above 5.1 mmol/L (700 mg/L), or if renal function is impaired.

Ethanol

The acute effects of overindulgence in ethanol sometimes lead to admission to hospitals. If the diagnosis is in doubt, plasma [ethanol] should be measured. Patients taking a deliberate drug overdose frequently take alcohol with the drug. Some patients may have drunk methylated spirits rather than ethanol, and rapid identification of both methanol and ethanol is then needed.

Methanol and ethylene glycol

Methanol is metabolised to formaldehyde and formic acid, while ethylene glycol is metabolised to a number of products including glycoaldehyde, glyoxylic and oxalic acids. Many of these are toxic, and also give rise to metabolic acidosis. Severe methanol poisoning frequently leads to perma-

nent visual impairment or complete blindness. Hypocalcaemia occurs with ethylene glycol poisoning. As little as 10 ml of methanol can cause blindness. Lethal doses can be as little as 30 ml for methanol and 100 ml for ethylene glycol. After ingestion, there are latent phases of 8–36 h for methanol and 4–12 h for ethylene glycol.

Urgent measurement of plasma concentrations of these substances is required if poisoning is suspected, but it may be difficult to get such measurements done out of normal laboratory hours. Measurement of the osmolar gap (i.e. the difference between the measured and calculated osmolality) is useful in all suspected cases of methanol/ ethylene glycol ingestion if the patient presents early after the overdose. An osmolar gap greater than 10 mos/kg is widely regarded as being indicative of an abnormality, but others have suggested that a value over 6 mos/kg should be regarded as abnormal. The osmolality must be measured using freezing point depression and not vapour pressure as the latter will produce falsely low results. A number of formulae have been published for the calculation of osmolality, for example $2 \times [Na^+ + K^+] + [urea] + [glucose]$. The osmolar gap may only be present early in the poisoning, while a high anion gap may only occur late in the presentation when the ingested poisons have been metabolised to the acidic products.

Treatment consists of giving ethanol or fomepizole to inhibit the metabolism of the methanol or ethylene glycol to their toxic metabolites. The metabolic acidosis and hypocalcaemia must also be corrected. Haemodialysis is also indicated.

Poisoning in children

Diagnosis is often more difficult than in the adult since the range of substances that may have been taken or administered is very large, symptoms may be atypical and often more severe, and the child may not be able to give useful information. The history obtained from parents may be vague or misleading, especially if one or both parents has been responsible for unauthorised drug administration. There are a number of urine drug-screening methods available which may, if necessary, be followed up by more accurate and specific methods such as gas chromatography–mass spectrometry (GC–MS).

Drug abuse

The marked growth in drug misuse has resulted in increasingly frequent requests for the screening of urine specimens from patients suspected of being drug abusers, for the possible presence of opiates, cocaine, lysergic acid diethylamide (LSD), benzodiazepines, methadone, buprenorphine, amphetamines and amphetamine derivatives such as ecstasy, etc.

It is important to screen for drugs of abuse
- to corroborate claims that drugs are being misused when patients request maintenance therapy
- to determine whether prescribed drugs (e.g. methadone) are being taken
- to determine whether drug abuse is continuing
- to monitor changing patterns of drug abuse
- for medicolegal reasons.

Drug-screening procedures used to be performed mainly on urine specimens, but salivary measurements are becoming more widely used. It is essential to ensure that the sample has not been tampered with by the patient, for example with the sample being diluted or exogenous drugs added. The preliminary drug screen uses immunoassays that are sensitive, but may lack specificity due to cross-reaction with related compounds. Confirmatory tests using specific chromatographic methods with mass spectrometry are required as a follow-up to positive results because of the possibly very serious implications for patients that can stem from being identified, correctly or incorrectly, as abusers of drugs.

Industrial and occupational hazards

Metal poisons

Mercury, cadmium and lead are all highly toxic to humans. Their effects depend partly on the type of compound involved, whether inorganic or organo-metallic, and partly on the route of absorption. In all cases, the kidney is liable to be severely damaged, and often the liver and the nervous system also. Whole blood and urine measurements of the metal are important to confirm diagnosis and assess the severity of the poisoning. Iron poisoning is particularly important in children who ingest iron tablets (p. 260). Hair or nail analysis can sometimes be used.

Patients with chronic renal failure maintained on haemodialysis regimes are particularly at risk from poisoning by dialysis fluid constituents. Aluminium toxicity leading to *dialysis dementia* and to *metabolic bone disease* has been described. Prevention of toxicity requires periodic checks of aluminium content in the water supply and in the effluent from deionisers used with dialysers.

Organic solvents

Many organic solvents used in industry are toxic (e.g. chlorinated hydrocarbons, ethylene glycol). Toxicity may be due to accidental exposure, or sometimes to solvent abuse. The toxic agent can usually be identified specifically (e.g. by gas chromatography). Other chemical investigations may be needed, to assess hepatic and renal function.

Pesticides and herbicides

Organophosphates (e.g. parathion, malathion) may cause poisoning among farm workers by inhibiting acetylcholinesterase; plasma BChE is also inhibited. Measurements of plasma BChE activity can help in the recognition of excessive exposure to organophosphates.

Paraquat and *diquat* are extremely dangerous herbicides, if ingested. Paraquat has severe effects, especially on the lungs and kidneys, and ingestion of more than 3 g is likely to be fatal. Clinical features usually suggest the diagnosis before the onset of complications, and the diagnosis can be confirmed by chemical examination of blood or urine for the presence of these herbicides or their metabolites. These measurements may help determine the prognosis.

Keypoints

- Therapeutic drug monitoring is required for drugs with a narrow therapeutic window, such as aminoglycoside antibiotics, phenytoin, carbamazepine, digoxin, lithium and ciclosporin. The time of the last dose of the drug should always be given.
- Paracetamol overdose is common, and may cause potentially fatal liver damage. Treatment with IV *N*-acetylcysteine is likely to be effective if started within 12 h of the overdose. Plasma [paracetamol] should be measured in patients who have taken paracetamol, either alone or in combined formulations, or unidentified tablets, and in all unconscious patients.
- Salicylate overdose often causes nausea, vomiting and increased respiration. Dehydration and acid–base disturbances are common. If plasma [salicylate] is >3.6 mmol/L, treatment with oral activated charcoal and IV sodium bicarbonate or haemodialysis may be required to increase the rate of elimination of the drug.
- In suspected poisoning with methanol or ethylene glycol, urgent measurement of these substances is required.
- Urinary tests for [drugs of abuse] are often required in order to monitor compliance in drug addicts on treatment and in employment screening.

Case 20.1

A 19-year-old student was admitted to an A&E department after calling his doctor to state that he had taken an overdose of aspirin 3 h previously. On admission, it was found that he had been vomiting and was now hyperventilating. The following results for blood tests were found:

Serum	Result	Reference range
Urea	7.3	2.5–6.6 mmol/L
Na	140	135–145 mmol/L
K^+	3.3	3.6–5.0 mmol/L
Total CO_2	10	22–32 mmol/L
Salicylate	3.8	mmol/L
Paracetamol	Not detected	

Comment on these results.

Comments: The results and presenting features are consistent with a salicylate overdose. There is an acidosis, and salicylate is present in plasma.

Paracetamol was measured, as some preparations of salicylate also contain paracetamol. The patient was treated conservatively, and made a full recovery.

Case 20.2

A 23-year-old woman was admitted to an A&E department after being found by a flatmate lying unconscious on her bed. Next to the patient was an empty bottle of vodka, and on the bedside table there was a bottle of paracetamol tablets that appeared about half-full. The patient had appeared normal when seen by the flatmate 6 h earlier. On admission, the patient's breath smelt strongly of alcohol, and the plasma paracetamol level was found to be 105 mg/L. Liver function tests were normal, as was the PT.

Comment on these results, and also on what treatment should be given.

Comments: The patient had taken a paracetamol overdose with vodka. The time of the paracetamol overdose was not known accurately, and the patient was therefore treated with IV *N*-acetylcysteine.

No abnormalities were found in liver function tests on admission. Plasma ALT activity showed a transient increase over the next few days, with levels peaking at 400 U/L and then gradually falling back to reference values. These results indicate that some mild degree of liver damage had occurred.

Case 20.3

A 65-year-old woman presented to her GP complaining of nausea. She had been treated with digoxin and diuretics for cardiac failure, and had tolerated the drugs well, with no previous evidence of poor compliance or poor therapeutic control. On examination, she was found to have bradycardia.

The following results were found (sampling at 14 h after last digoxin dose):

Serum	Result
Plasma digoxin	2.3 therapeutic range 1.0–2.6 nmol/L
Plasma K^+	3.1 reference range 3.6–5.0 nmol/L

What is the most likely cause of the patient's symptoms?

Comments: The patient is likely to be suffering from digoxin toxicity. Although the plasma level of digoxin is within the therapeutic range, it is at the upper limit. However, more importantly, the patient has hypokalaemia, which will potentiate the pharmacological effect of digoxin. Plasma digoxin concentrations are a poor guide to toxicity if there is hypokalaemia. A common cause of digoxin toxicity is concurrent administration of diuretics, which cause potassium depletion. The patient was treated successfully by giving potassium supplements to restore her plasma [potassium] to normal.

Case 20.4

A 43-year-old woman was admitted to the A&E department after she had complained of abdominal cramps, vomiting, dizziness and blurred vision. She had drunk about a quarter of a bottle of cheap vodka, which she had bought at the local market, approximately 8 h previously. The following were found:

Serum	Result	Reference range
Urea	7.0	2.5–6.6 mmol/L
Na^+	134	135–145 mmol/L
K^+	5.0	3.6–5.0 mmol/L
Total CO_2	15	22–32 mmol/L
Chloride	100	95–107 mmol/L
Osmolar gap	11	<10 mos/Kg

Calculate the anion gap and comment on the results. What treatment should be given?

Comments: The patient has a significant osmolar gap (>10 mos/kg) and an anion gap of 24 mmol/L. This together with the low [total CO_2] and presenting complaints suggests a marked metabolic acidosis caused by ingestion of methanol or ethylene glycol. A blood methanol concentration of 550 mg/L (17 mmol/L was detected with no ethylene glycol. She was treated with an ethanol infusion, IV bicarbonate and haemodialysis. She made a full recovery. The vodka she had bought was found to contain some methanol.

Chapter 21

Clinical biochemistry in paediatrics and geriatrics

Disorders of *children*, particularly the neonate, often differ from those in the adult. In the neonate, there may be problems associated with immaturity, problems in adapting to the new external environment and, rarely, inherited metabolic disorders. In childhood, disorders of growth, failure to thrive, etc., require investigation.

In *old age*, the differences from general adult medicine are fewer. However, multiple pathology is common, and diagnosis is often made difficult by the fact that symptoms may be minimal, atypical or confounded by drug treatment. For this reason, more reliance may have to be placed on laboratory tests.

Paediatrics

In this section, we discuss the following areas of diagnosis:

1 Causes and diagnosis of biochemical disturbances commonly found in the neonate and in early childhood.

2 Inherited metabolic disorders.

3 Biochemical abnormalities associated with failure to thrive, malnutrition and short stature.

Lecture Notes: Clinical Biochemistry, 8e. By G. Beckett, S. Walker, P. Rae & P. Ashby. Published 2010 by Blackwell Publishing.

Specimen collection from neonates and children

This should be done expertly, and the amount of blood taken minimised. Capillary blood is used in neonatal units and for newborn screening. Blood specimens from babies are obtained using an automated neonatal device by heel-prick from the fleshy (lateral) parts of the heel. In older children, finger-prick capillary sampling is used to monitor diabetes.

Pediatric reference ranges

Age-related reference ranges must always be used. In neonates, particularly when premature or small for gestational age, interpretation of results is especially difficult and requires considerable experience.

Causes and diagnosis of biochemical disturbances in the neonate and early childhood

Glucose

Neonates

The foetus utilises maternal glucose and any excess is stored as hepatic glycogen. Fat is also stored in

Table 21.1 Infants at risk of developing hypoglycaemia

Poor milk intake	*Hormone imbalance*
Establishment of breastfeeding	Hyperinsulinaemia
Decreased glycogen stores	Growth hormone
Prematurity	deficiency
Small for gestational age	Adrenal insufficiency
Some inborn errors	Hypopituitarism
Illness	
Increased demand	
Sepsis	
Hypoxia, hypothermia and	
pyrexia	
Inborn errors	

foetal adipose tissue during the last trimester. After birth the baby has to maintain its own blood glucose between feeds by fat and glycogen catabolism and gluconeogenesis. In some babies these mechanisms are insufficient to maintain blood [glucose], and hypoglycaemia occurs. In the neonate a blood [glucose] less than 2.5 mmol/L is widely regarded as being an intervention threshold. The principal causes of neonatal hypoglycaemia are as follows (see Table 21.1):

• Transient hypoglycaemia in healthy term infants is most commonly due to a low milk intake during establishment of breastfeeding. Premature infants, and infants that are small for gestational age, are particularly at risk from hypoglycaemia due to their lack of glycogen and fat stores.

• Hypoglycaemia may also become evident if there is an increased demand for glucose such as may occur in the septic, hypoxic, hypothermic or pyrexial infant.

• In rare cases the hypoglycaemia may be due to an inherited metabolic disorder or a deficiency or imbalance in a range of hormones including GH and glucocorticoids.

Hyperinsulinaemia is the most common cause of persistent or recurrent neonatal hypoglycaemia after the first 24 h of life. There are a number of causes including maternal hyperglycaemia due to poor diabetic control during pregnancy. Maternal hyperglycaemia induces hyperplasia of foetal islet cells, resulting in foetal hyperinsulinaemia that

cannot be suppressed in the neonate, and hypoglycaemia results. Rare genetic causes of persistent hyperinsulinism have been identified including deficiencies of glucokinase or glutamate dehydrogenase or recessive mutations of the genes for the sulphonylurea receptor (SUR 1) and the ATP-dependent potassium channel (KIR6.2) in the plasma membrane of the pancreatic β cells. The gene defects in SUR 1 and KIR 6.2 give rise to hyperplasia of insulin-producing cells in the pancreas, a condition known as 'nesidioblastosis'. Sporadic causes (e.g. Beckwith syndrome) have also been identified. Neonates at risk of hypoglycaemia should have their blood glucose monitored regularly by POCT, with low readings (<2.5 mmol/L) being confirmed by blood collection for laboratory measurement before treatment.

During childhood

Recurrent hypoglycaemia of infancy and childhood may be due to any of the causes listed in Table 6.5 (p. 100) as well as several other inherited metabolic disorders (e.g. fatty acid oxidation disorders and mitochondrial disorders). Although nesidioblastosis usually presents in the first few days of life, symptoms may be delayed for up to 6 months.

Calcium and magnesium

Plasma [calcium] falls, in normal full-term infants, by about 10–20% in the first 2–3 days of life. It then returns to normal (2.0–2.8 mmol/L) over the course of the next 3–4 days.

Neonatal hypocalcaemia within the first 48 h, sufficient to give rise to twitching, irritability and convulsions, occurs particularly in infants who are premature, those of diabetic mothers and those who have experienced birth asphyxia. Maternal vitamin D deficiency may be a factor (e.g. in Asian women). The mechanism is complex, but the hypocalcaemia tendency usually corrects spontaneously, although calcium gluconate may need to be given if convulsions occur, or if plasma [calcium] falls to less than 1.50 mmol/L. Rarely, hypocalcaemic convulsions in the neonate are associated with maternal hyperparathyroidism, which may produce temporary hypoparathyroidism in the neonate due to suppression of the foetal parathyroid glands by maternal hypercalcaemia.

Late neonatal hypocalcaemia, between the fourth and 10th days of life, may occur in full-term as well as in premature infants. Hyperexcitability of muscles is usually also present. This is liable to occur in infants whose mothers had a low intake of vitamin D during pregnancy; these infants may also have low plasma [magnesium]. Rarely, hypocalcaemia may be due to renal failure. Treatment with calcium, and often magnesium, may be required.

Neonatal rickets. Premature infants have increased requirements for calcium, phosphate and vitamin D for bone growth. The most sensitive indicator of inadequate intake is a rising plasma ALP, which precedes abnormalities in plasma calcium or phosphate.

Hypomagnesaemia is an occasional cause of neonatal convulsions. It can lead to hypocalcaemia by reducing PTH secretion. Plasma [magnesium] should be measured in all cases of hypocalcaemia.

Hypercalcaemia in the neonatal period is less common than hypocalcaemia. Inadequate phosphate supplements in rapidly growing pre-term infants can lead to hypophosphataemia, bone resorption and thus hypercalcaemia. Oversupplementation may also lead to hypercalcaemia. Much rarer causes include immobilisation, malignancy, hyperparathyroidism, familial hypocalciuric hypercalcaemia and William's syndrome.

Neonatal jaundice (Table 21.2)

Physiological unconjugated hyperbilirubinaemia

Approximately half of all infants develop hyperbilirubinaemia during the first week of life due to
- Increased production from breakdown of red cells, which have a shortened lifespan in the neonate.
- Decreased excretion, because of immaturity of hepatic bilirubin uptake, conjugation and biliary excretion.
- Reabsorption from the intestine. Bilirubin is deconjugated by the intestinal enzyme β-

Table 21.2 Causes of jaundice in the neonatal period

Early jaundice	Prolonged jaundice
Physiological	Breastfeeding
Haemolysis	Prematurity
Infection	Infection
Genetic defects of bilirubin metabolism	Biliary atresia
	Endocrine disorders
	Genetic disorders

glucuronidase. In adults it is further metabolised to urobilinogen by normal intestinal bacteria. The newborn's GI tract has not yet acquired these organisms, and some bilirubin is re-absorbed, a process which is stimulated by breast milk.

Pathological causes of unconjugated hyperbilirubinaemia

Babies may be at increased risk of severe hyperbilirubinaemia if they have one or more of the following, in addition to normal physiological factors.
- Dehydration, intercurrent infection, bruising, polycythaemia.
- Increased haemolysis
  - Lysis due to Rhesus incompatibility is now a rare occurrence; however, lysis may also result from ABO or other blood group incompatibility
  - Predisposition to lysis due to glucose-6-phosphate dehydrogenase deficiency, hereditary spherocytosis.
- Defective hepatic uptake or conjugation. This may occur in association with Gilbert's syndrome, mutations in anion transporters or rarely inherited disorders of bilirubin metabolism (Crigler–Najjar syndrome, p. 203).

In most infants, hyperbilirubinaemia is a self-limiting condition that requires no treatment. A tiny percentage of bilirubin exists free in the circulation, not bound to protein. Only free bilirubin can cross the blood–brain barrier, where high concentrations can cause bilirubin encephalopathy and kernicterus. The relationship between total plasma bilirubin and free brain bilirubin is complex because of:
- Variation in the concentration of circulating proteins (particularly albumin) that bind unconjugated bilirubin.

• Displacement of bilirubin from protein-binding sites by drugs (e.g. benzyl penicillin, phenobarbital, furosemide), free fatty acids (hypoglycaemic and ketotic infants) or hydrogen ions (acidotic infants).

• Impairment of the blood–brain barrier in premature and sick infants, allowing some albumin-bound bilirubin to penetrate the brain.

Total plasma bilirubin measurement is used routinely as a proxy for free bilirubin. First-line screen for healthy term babies is by visual assessment or transcutaneous bilirubin monitor. Confirmation requires laboratory measurement of total plasma bilirubin. Circulating unconjugated bilirubin is removed by phototherapy or, if concentrations are grossly elevated, by exchange transfusion. Action limits for treatment to prevent kernicterus are age related and are lower for preterm or sick infants.

Prolonged jaundice is defined as jaundice persisting beyond 14 days of age. It is most commonly breast milk jaundice, mainly due to increased enterohepatic circulation, and caused by unconjugated bilirubin alone. It does not usually require treatment. All prolonged jaundice requires measurement of total and conjugated (or direct) bilirubin.

Conjugated hyperbilirubinaemia

Any increase in conjugated (which may be measured as direct) bilirubin always indicates pathology and requires identification and further investigation of its aetiology by appropriate chemical and other tests.

Causes include infective, endocrine and genetic disorders (Table 21.3).

Biliary atresia. Extra-hepatic biliary atresia is a rapidly progressing condition where the bile ducts are rapidly obliterated. Diagnosis is confirmed by ultrasound scan to demonstrate absence of the gall bladder. Surgery before 60 days of age may be curative, otherwise the only treatment option is liver transplant. To identify potentially life-threatening but treatable causes, it is imperative to investigate all cases of prolonged jaundice without delay, by measurement of total and conjugated bilirubin, and liver function tests in the first instance. Further

Table 21.3 Causes of conjugated hyperbilirubinaemia in the neonate

Biliary atresia	Cystic fibrosis
Sepsis or neonatal hepatitis	Galactosaemia
Hypothyroidism	Tyrosinaemia
Hypopituitarism	α_1-Anti-trypsin deficiency
(± septo-optic dysplasia)	

tests such as thyroid function, urine reducing substances (for galactosaemia) and biliary tract imaging are carried out after clinical assessment of the infant.

Inherited metabolic disorders

Inborn errors of metabolism usually present in infancy or childhood. They result from alteration in a single gene, leading to a protein product that has suboptimal function. Most of these rare conditions show autonomic recessive inheritance: heterozygotes do not manifest the disorder. The affected protein may be an enzyme, a structural or transport protein or an enzyme cofactor affecting the activity of several enzymes (Table 21.4).

The consequences of an inherited defect affecting a metabolic pathway include:

• Accumulation of potentially toxic metabolites that occur in the pathway before the defect.

• Deficiency of essential metabolites produced by the pathway after the defect.

• Increased flux of potentially toxic metabolites through alternative metabolic pathways.

• Storage of macromolecules in organs such as liver and spleen if the defect is in their breakdown pathway.

• Negative feedback inhibition of the pathway activity may fail because production of the end-product is decreased.

Figures 21.1–21.3 illustrate these effects in PKU, defects in fatty acid oxidation and galactosaemia, respectively. The age at presentation depends on residual protein activity and is not constant for a given disorder.

In some cases addition or deletion of chromosomes or parts of chromosomes occur, leading to

Table 21.4 Examples of inherited metabolic disorders

General disorders	Examples
Amino acid metabolism	Phenylketonuria, tyrosinaemia
Organic acid metabolism	Methylmalonic aciduria
Fatty acid oxidation	Medium chain acyl-CoA dehydrogenase deficiency
Urea cycle defects	Ornithine transcarbamylase deficiency
Carbohydrate disorders	Galactosaemia
Defects of intermediary metabolism	Mitochondrial respiratory chain defects
Steroid synthesis defects	21-Hydroxylase, 11-hydroxylase deficiencies
Macromolecule breakdown defects	Lysosomal storage disorders
Transport protein defects	Cystic fibrosis
Cofactor defects	Biotinidase deficiency
Organelle assembly or uptake	Peroxisomal defects

clinically significant abnormalities (e.g. Down's syndrome, Turner's syndrome).

Diagnosis

The individual disorders are rare, but *collectively* they are not uncommon. The true incidence is unknown, except for those that are detected by screening programmes. In acute neonatal presentations, an infant assessed as normal at birth typically develops reluctance to feed, vomiting and abnormal breathing. Without treatment the affected infants rapidly progress to multiple organ failure, coma and death. A second group may have a more chronic and progressive course, with symptoms such as failure to thrive, progressive hepatomegaly or neurological deterioration developing over months or years. Several inherited metabolic disorders that present less acutely may nevertheless carry a very poor prognosis. Only a minority present with a clearly defined clinical syndrome.

For the index case in a family, the recognition that there is a metabolic disease present, and its identification, can present complex diagnostic problems.

The index case

In an acutely ill infant, or one presenting with chronic signs and symptoms, the results of routine laboratory tests may provide a clue to a potential inborn error of metabolism. These include positive urine reducing substances, metabolic acidosis identified by blood gas analyser or calculated anion gap, hypoglycaemia or haematological abnormalities such as neutropenia, haemolytic anaemia, megaloblastic anaemia and coagulation defects. Suggestive clinical features include dysmorphia, hepato- or splenomegaly, cardiomyopathy, neurological disorders, intractable feeding difficulties or onset of acute symptoms in response to fasting or weaning. Depending on the specific presentation, further blood testing by the local laboratory may include some of the following: liver function tests including coagulation screen, calcium, creatinine, urea, urate, glucose, lactate, urate, cholesterol, potassium, sodium, chloride and ammonia.

Samples may be referred to a regional paediatric laboratory for

- Urine, plasma or CSF amino acids
- Urine organic acids
- Galactosaemia screening test (red cell galactose-1-phosphate uridylyltransferase)
- Bloodspot acyl carnitine profile
- Mucopolysaccharide excretion
- Specific enzyme tests (to diagnose, for example, lysosomal storage disorders or mitochondrial respiratory chain defects).

For the correct interpretation of results it is essential to provide clinical details including fed/fasted status (fasting potentiates abnormalities in fatty acid oxidation and gluconeogenetic defects), transfusion history (any transfused red cells invalidate the galactosaemia screening test) and drug therapy (antibiotics mask amino acid abnormalities) at the time of specimen collection.

Confirmation of the diagnosis

Diagnostic confirmation may require tissue biopsy (skin, muscle, liver) to demonstrate deficient enzyme activity or a pathological DNA mutation. Specific therapy (e.g. enzyme replacement therapy for Gaucher's disease, biotin supplements in biotinidase deficiency) is available for some disorders. Even if no such therapy is available, precise diagnosis is essential to allow genetic counselling for the family, including investigation of siblings and other relatives, genetic advice on recurrence rates and potential pre-natal diagnosis during future pregnancies.

Fetal tissue can be obtained by the technique of chorionic villus biopsy for the purpose of pre-natal diagnosis. These techniques have been applied to a wide variety of diseases including the diagnosis of haemoglobinopathies, cystic fibrosis (p. 300) and Duchenne muscular dystrophy (p. 182). Heterozygote detection is not usually reliable by enzyme analysis, and is now done by mutation studies. It is particularly important for female relatives of boys diagnosed with an X-linked disorder (e.g. ornithine transcarbamylase deficiency, MPS II).

Examples of inherited metabolic disorders

Phenylketonuria (PKU)

This disease provides the best example of a treatable condition detected by neonatal screening. Screening for PKU has been performed for the past 40 years.

Phenylalanine is converted to tyrosine by hepatic phenylalanine hydroxylase (Fig. 21.1). In classical PKU, phenylalanine hydroxylase activity is undetectable or very much reduced. However, a minority (1–2%) of patients with inherited abnormalities of phenylalanine metabolism have defects in tetrahydrobiopterin (a cofactor for phenylalanine hydroxylase) metabolism. These rare forms of PKU must be differentiated from the classical form, as they require different treatment. Classical PKU illustrates many of the principles that underlie the diverse effects of inherited metabolic disorders.

1 *Accumulation of the substrate of the blocked reaction.* This occurs in the liver. Plasma [phenylalanine] is much increased, unless dietary phenylalanine is restricted.

2 *Reduced formation of product.* Tyrosine formation is severely affected in patients, but tyrosine deficiency is avoided by supplements.

3 *Alternative paths of metabolism of the precursor that accumulates.* There is increased formation and urinary excretion of phenyl-pyruvate, phenyl-lactate and phenyl-acetate, and of various *o*-hydroxyphenyl metabolites. Dietary phenylalanine restriction reduces the output of these metabolites.

4 *Effects on other reactions.* Accumulation of phenylalanine and its metabolites competes with transport of other amino acids into the brain, potentially causing cerebral deficiency of other essential amino acids.

Elevated brain phenylalanine and concomitant deficiencies of other amino acids lead to cerebral damage in early life. This is prevented by restricting natural dietary protein to supply only the tiny amount of phenylalanine required for growth. Other essential amino acids, vitamins and minerals are given as supplements. Dietary protein is adjusted in response to frequently measured capillary phenylalanine. Even patients with classical PKU may show some fall in circulating phenylalanine in response to treatment with high doses of the biopterin cofactor. A commercial preparation of this has recently been developed. Each patient with PKU will require detailed assessment of its potential use, along with, or instead of, dietary treatment.

Screening for phenylketonuria and other disorders

All infants in the UK are screened for PKU at 5–8 days old by use of dried blood spots on filter paper that are posted to screening centres for phenylalanine and other analyses. The screening test threshold of 240 µmol/L is set such as not to miss a single case (sensitivity of 100%) but without generating a large number of false-positive results.

Neonatal blood spots are also used to screen for other disorders, which vary from country to

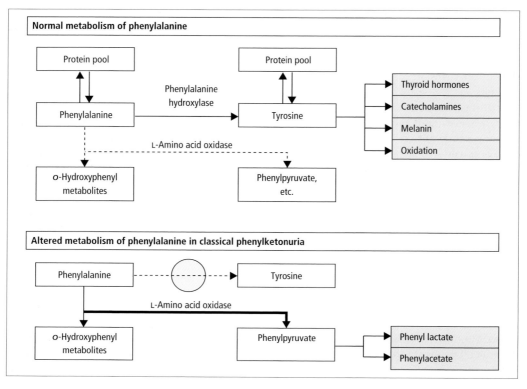

Figure 21.1 The metabolism of phenylalanine. In the classical form of PKU, the activity of phenylalanine hydroxylase is greatly reduced, and normally minor metabolites of phenylalanine are excreted in much increased amounts.

country. Screening programmes require considerable organisation. Before embarking on them, several questions need to be considered:

1 What is the incidence of the disease?
2 Is the disease life threatening or liable to be severe?
3 Is there an asymptomatic period before irreversible damage occurs.
4 Is acceptable treatment available?
5 Is a suitable screening test available?
6 Are the costs acceptable?

Screening programmes for PKU and neonatal hypothyroidism fulfil these criteria. Other conditions may be diagnosed if the same sample as that obtained for PKU can be used. These include tests for cystic fibrosis, sickle cell anaemia and galactosaemia. However, the screening arrangements may not be ideal for these other disorders. For

example many patients with galactosaemia will have life-threatening symptoms before the sixth day of life.

Medium chain acyl-CoA dehydrogenase (MCAD) deficiency

MCAD deficiency is the most common fatty acid oxidation defect in Europe, with an estimated incidence similar to PKU (1 in 10000). The primary defect affects β-oxidation of fatty acids (Figure 21.2). Patients characteristically present in the toddler age group, following a minor infection where vomiting with or without diarrhoea causes a longer than normal fast. At this age, glycogen stores are rapidly exhausted and energy production depends on the defective fatty acid oxidation. The patient becomes hypoglycaemic and encephalopathic, due to toxic fatty acid-related compounds. There is a relative lack of ketones; however, the presence of ketones does not rule out the diagnosis. The child responds rapidly to dextrose infusion, which restores glucose concentrations, increases insulin secretion and thus suppresses fatty acid oxidation and production of the toxic fatty acids. Prolonged hypoglycaemia and encephalopathy can result in irreversible neurological damage and death.

Diagnosis is readily made when the patient presents in hypoglycaemic crisis, by identification of the characteristic pattern of urinary dicarboxylic acids and acyl-glycines identified by GC–MS, or by the abnormal acyl-carnitine pattern on tandem mass spectrometry. These two sensitive techniques are also capable of detecting small amounts of diagnostic compounds when the patient is well (Fig. 21.2).

The clinical spectrum extends from fatal neonatal presentations to adults with no history of acute attack. The true incidence and natural history is unknown. Treatment consists of avoidance of prolonged fasting. If there is evidence of decompensation, dextrose infusion and carnitine replacement is urgently required.

Newborn screening programmes to include MCAD deficiency based on detection of elevated octanoyl-carnitine are in place in many countries and are currently being implemented across the UK.

Galactosaemia

Galactose is metabolised by the liver. Three rare defects have been described: deficiency of galactose-1-phosphate uridylyltransferase (Gal-1-PUT), galactokinase or UDP-galactose epimerase (Fig. 21.3). They all prevent normal metabolism of galactose, causing a rise in plasma and urine galactose. Galactose gives positive results if urinary tests for reducing substances are performed, and infants who have positive tests for reducing substances in urine should have the diagnosis ruled out by enzyme or metabolite tests.

Galactosaemia is rare (1–2 per 100000 live births). The most common and most severe enzymatic defect is due to Gal-1-PUT deficiency. This manifests itself in the neonatal period after feeding with galactose-containing milk, giving rise to vomiting, jaundice and abnormal liver function tests, and sometimes hypoglycaemia. Neonates in some countries are screened for defective galactose metabolism, but the response time is often too slow for this rapidly fatal condition, and the provisional diagnosis is nearly

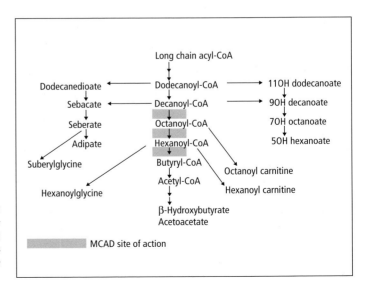

Figure 21.2 Pathways for fatty acid oxidation. In MCAD deficiency, fatty acid intermediates are metabolised by alternative β-oxidation pathways or excreted as glycine or carnitine conjugates.

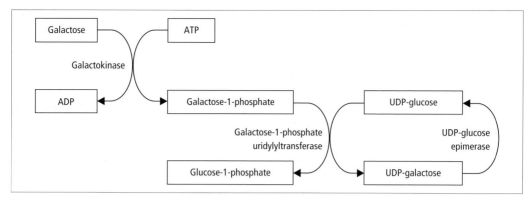

Figure 21.3 The enzymatic conversion of galactose to glucose. Galactosaemia may be caused by deficiency of any of these three enzymes, but the most common cause is deficiency of galactose-1-phosphate uridylyltransferase.

always made on clinical grounds, followed by withdrawal of galactose and lactose in foods until a final diagnosis is made. Definitive diagnosis requires enzyme measurements in erythrocytes. Treatment is by using a galactose-free diet. The disease has a poor outcome due to neurological impairment and primary ovarian failure in the majority of women.

In babies who exhibit a classic picture of galactosaemia, hereditary fructose intolerance and tyrosinaemia type 1 should also be considered as part of the differential diagnosis.

Tyrosinaemia type 1

This is due to a deficiency of fumarylacetoacetase hydrolase. It presents with hypoglycaemia, evidence of failure to thrive, irritability, jaundice, hepatomegaly, liver failure, cardiomyopathy and renal tubular defects. Radiologically, there are signs of vitamin D-resistant rickets and renal stones. As liver disease from any cause gives rise to increased plasma tyrosine, diagnosis of tyrosinaemia type 1 requires the measurement of urinary succinylacetone and fumarylacetoacetase hydrolase activity in cultured skin fibroblasts or leucocytes. It is treated by the drug NTBC, which inhibits an earlier step in the affected pathway and reduces the accumulation of toxic metabolites.

Congenital hypothyroidism

The incidence of congenital primary hypothyroidism is about 1 in 4000. Bloodspot [TSH] is used as the newborn screening test for this condition which is due to a defect in the development of the thyroid gland. The condition is amenable to treatment with thyroxine, particularly if started early, but it can be difficult to diagnose clinically.

Congenital adrenal hyperplasia (CAH)

Striking anatomical changes take place in the adrenal cortex immediately after birth; these are associated with marked alterations in the pattern of steroid output. There is a period of transition during the first 6 months of an infant's life during which the pattern of foetal steroid metabolism changes to the normal childhood pattern, which closely resembles the adult pattern. A number of enzyme deficiencies have been identified that are associated with abnormal steroid secretion or action. Figure 21.4 shows a simplified steroid biosynthetic pathway and some of the known sites of enzyme defect.

21-Hydroxylase deficiency (Fig. 21.4)

This is an autosomal recessive condition (about 1 in 10000 live births in Caucasians) that may impair synthesis of cortisol and aldosterone. It accounts

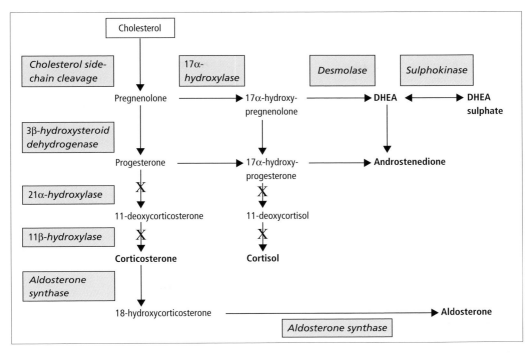

Figure 21.4 Defects in the steroid biosynthetic pathways leading to CAH. 21α-Hydroxylase deficiency leads to overproduction of androstenedione and 17α-hydroxyprogesterone. In 11β-hydroxylase deficiency, high concentrations of 11-deoxycortisol are found, The conversion of corticosterone to aldosterone is restricted to the zona glomerulosa. X indicates sites of enzyme defect.

for approximately 95% of all cases of CAH. The low cortisol promotes ACTH secretion, so that the adrenal gland becomes hyperplastic. Severe cases show evidence of mineralocorticoid deficiency, with salt and water loss and neonatal adrenal crisis. Steroids accumulate before the enzyme block, and are diverted to moderately strong androgens (e.g. androstenedione, which is metabolised to testosterone in peripheral tissues) causing virilisation of the female foetus and precocious sexual development in boys not diagnosed and treated in the neonatal period. Late presentation (adult life) is also possible in less severe cases (p. 147).

The diagnosis can be established by finding a raised concentration of 17-hydroxyprogesterone in a serum sample taken at least 2 days after birth. Earlier samples may contain maternally derived 17-hydroxyprogesterone, which complicates the interpretation of the results. Measurement of other steroids that accumulate before the block and by

gene probing for 21-hydroxylase can also be helpful. Treatment with glucocorticoids (e.g. cortisol) suppresses the excessive output of ACTH and limits the excessive androgen production. It may also be necessary to administer a mineralocorticoid. Monitoring of treatment requires measurement of serum 17-hydroxyprogesterone.

11β-Hydroxylase deficiency (Fig. 21.4)

Inherited deficiencies in the enzyme that converts cortisol to cortisone (11β-hydroxysteroid dehydrogenase) lead to the syndrome of apparent mineralocorticoid excess. Increased androgen production also gives rise to virilisation in the female. In this condition, high concentrations of 11-deoxycorticosterone are produced, a steroid that has mineralocorticoid properties. Diagnosis requires demonstration of high serum concentrations of 11-deoxycortisol or its urinary metabolites. Treatment involves giving cortisol alone, since the excess 11-deoxycorticosterone gives adequate mineralocorticoid effects even if aldosterone synthesis is impaired.

17-Hydroxylase, 18-hydroxylase and 3β-hydroxysteroid dehydrogenase deficiency are extremely rare causes of CAH.

Failure to thrive in childhood

Poor nutrition is by far the most common cause of this; however, it is important to exclude chronic disease, for example renal disease, coeliac disease and cystic fibrosis.

Malnutrition in children

PEM, in its severest forms, includes kwashiorkor and marasmus; there is a range of less severe clinical presentations. There may be other important factors, for example deficiency of essential fatty acids, or the consequences of immune defence mechanisms being impaired by malnutrition.

Plasma [albumin] is a widely used, though insensitive, test for malnutrition. Plasma [albumin] below 30 g/L should be regarded as abnormally low; values below 25 g/L are associated with increasing degrees of oedema. Parallel changes in plasma [pre-albumin] and [transferrin] also occur.

Malnutrition severe enough to cause hypoglycaemia is encountered in children with kwashiorkor and in starvation (e.g. due to gross parental neglect). If malnutrition is severe enough to cause liver failure to develop, many other chemical tests become abnormal.

Vitamin deficiency diseases make up a potentially important group of nutritional causes of failure to thrive, since the growing child has relatively greater requirements for vitamins than the mature adult. Rickets (p. 81) due to inadequate nutrition or lack of sunlight continues to occur, even in developed countries.

Cystic fibrosis

This autosomal recessive disorder is the most common inherited metabolic disease in Caucasians; occurring in about 1 in 2000 live births. Abnormalities of the cystic fibrosis transmem-

brane conductance protein, expressed in all epithelial cells, result in failure of cyclic adenosine monophosphate (cAMP)-regulated chloride transport across the cell membranes. The most common disease-causing mutation, ΔF_{508}, is found in about 70% of cystic fibrosis chromosomes in Northern Europe. Alterations in the ion concentrations in the secreted fluid lead to abnormally thick mucus in the lung, which predisposes to chronic infection and the development of obstructive airways disease. It also produces exocrine pancreatic insufficiency and high concentrations of chloride and sodium in secreted sweat. Chemical investigations used as part of the diagnostic process include sweat testing and measurement of stool elastase.

Newborn screening tests

Newborn screening for cystic fibrosis has been implemented in the UK, using first-line measurement of immunoreactive trypsin, which is greatly increased in specimens collected from infants with cystic fibrosis only in the first month of life. If elevated, cascade testing is by a panel of DNA mutations targeted to the population. In some cases, further tests, including a sweat test, may be required to establish the presence of atypical forms of cystic fibrosis.

Sweat test. This is used to confirm the diagnosis in atypical cases following newborn screening, and to investigate older children presenting with suggestive symptoms. Chloride or conductivity is measured in sweat obtained by iontophoresis from a small area of skin using standardised conditions; sweating is induced by applying pilocarpine to the skin under a low electric current. The test demands close attention to detail if reliable results are to be obtained, and should only be carried out by staff who are experienced in performing it.

In healthy children and adults, in pilocarpine-stimulated sweat, [chloride] is normally below 40 mmol/L. In patients with classical cystic fibrosis, the concentrations are nearly always above 60 mmol/L. Atypical forms of cystic fibrosis may give intermediate results between 40 and 60 mmol/L

Table 21.5 Disorders of growth

Growth abnormality and category	Examples
Short stature	
Genetic	Familial short stature, delayed development
Intrauterine	Small for gestational age infants
Nutritional	Inadequate food supply, malabsorption, coeliac disease[1], infections
Systemic disease	Chronic renal disease, congenital heart disease
Endocrine disease	GHD, hypothyroidism, corticosteroid excess
Tall stature	
Genetic	Familial tall stature, advanced development
Endocrine disease	Growth hormone excess, hyperthyroidism, precocious puberty
Miscellaneous	Klinefelter (XXY) syndrome, XYY anomaly

Short stature

Table 21.5 lists the principal categories of disordered growth, with examples. In this section, we shall only consider in detail the investigation of children for possible GH deficiency and for coeliac disease.

Growth hormone deficiency (GHD)

This may be an isolated defect, partial or complete, or it may be a component of panhypopituitarism. GH is released into the circulation in pulses, mainly at night. Random plasma [GH] in daytime specimens from normal children are often therefore undetectable. The investigation of suspected GHD requires provocation tests to test the function of the hypothalamic–pituitary–GH release axis. Hypothyroidism, chronic disease, Turner's syndrome and poor nutrition should be excluded before these tests are performed.

GH provocation tests

In suspected isolated GHD, two GH provocation tests (sequential or on separate days) are recommended. However, in those with defined CNS pathology, history of irradiation, multiple pituitary hormone deficiency or a genetic defect, one GH test may suffice. The second test is only required if there is an inadequate response in the first test. Other tests of pituitary function may also be required if indicated clinically, for example a GnRH test. Provocative agents used include clonidine, arginine, glucagon and insulin. The insulin hypoglycaemia test and glucagon tests are only safe in children if their performance can be properly supervised by staff who perform them on children regularly. If a second test is required it should employ a provocative agent other than that used in the first test.

In the *clonidine test*, clonidine is given orally to stimulate GH release; blood specimens are collected before giving clonidine (0.15 mg/m^2 body surface area) and at 30-min intervals for 2.5 h afterwards.

Arginine (0.5 g/kg body weight maximum 30 g) can be infused IV (10% arginine in 0.9% saline) at a constant rate over 30 min and samples taken before the infusion and at 30-min intervals for 2.5 h. Arginine provocation should not be used in patients with electrolyte disturbances, uraemia, diabetes or liver disease, and antihistamine and adrenaline should be available for treatment of anaphylaxis.

Glucagon normally stimulates the release of both GH and ACTH from the pituitary, therefore this test can be used to assess both the GH and cortisol responses to glucagon.

The *insulin hypoglycaemia test* uses a procedure modified slightly from the test as used in adults (p. 111), and the local laboratory should be consulted before performing the test. Specimens are taken before an IV injection of soluble insulin (0.075–0.10 U/kg) and at 20, 30, 45, 60 and 90 min after the injection. Plasma [GH] and [glucose] are measured in all the specimens, and serum [cortisol] in the 20-min and 45-min specimens if other panhypopituitarism is suspected. The test may be combined with a GnRH test if a combined pituitary function test is to be performed. For each of the above stimulation tests a post-stimulated GH of less than 5 μg/L supports the diagnosis.

Coeliac disease

This is a common cause of growth retardation. The first-line investigation is measurement of serum anti-tTG IgA antibodies, which are elevated in untreated coeliac disease. The definitive method of diagnosis is made by demonstrating abnormal villi in a duodenal biopsy collected by endoscopy. Other diagnostic features include the improvement that is brought about by a gluten-free diet, both physically and in the severity of diarrhoea and the relapse that follows dietary relaxation. Compliance with treatment with a gluten-free diet is monitored by measurement of anti-tTG IgA antibodies.

Neuroblastoma and ganglioneuroma

Neuroblastoma and related tumours, although rare, account for approximately one-third of childhood deaths from malignant disease. Most produce catecholamines. Marked pharmacological effects are uncommon, because the catecholamines are largely metabolised by the tumour tissue to form inactive metabolites. Only occasionally is there hypertension. Measurements of catecholamine metabolites are made in urine (4-hydroxy-3-methoxymandelic acid, homovanillic acid or 4-hydroxy-3-methoxyphenylacetic acid and dopamine) and are related to urinary [creatinine] because it is difficult to obtain complete 24-h urine collections in children. Age-related reference ranges are used. Elevated results may also occur in phaeochromocytoma which is uncommon in children.

Geriatrics

The additional diagnostic biochemical problems in the elderly arise mainly from the increased frequency of multiorgan disease, polypharmacy and the tendency for symptoms to be absent or atypical. There are a few aspects that merit emphasis.

Reference ranges in geriatrics

The concentrations of certain analytes show clear changes in the elderly, even when monitored in apparently healthy individuals. For the most part these changes merely represent the extension of changes that have been gradually occurring throughout adult life, and include a gradual increase in cholesterol, glucose, ALP, PSA and urate, with decreases in total protein and albumin. Whilst ideally laboratories should provide age-related reference ranges for the elderly, in practice few do.

Screening for disease in elderly patients

Because of the masking of clinical symptoms and signs, it is common practice to perform an admission biochemical screen on patients admitted to geriatric assessment units. Table 21.6 lists some of the tests that are commonly used.

Renal function, fluid and electrolyte balance

The GFR falls with age, as does the ability of the renal tubules to reabsorb and secrete various substances. There is also a progressive loss of nephrons that starts in middle age. The consequence of these changes is that creatinine clearance tends to fall and serum concentrations of creatinine and urea tend to rise slightly. The reduction in muscle mass and the smaller dietary intake of protein that tend to occur with older people may offset these effects to some extent in some patients. Some formulae (e.g. those derived from the Cockcroft–Gault equation) that are used to estimate the GFR from serum creatinine, age and body weight can be very misleading in the very elderly.

The regulatory mechanisms that control water and electrolyte balance become less efficient in the elderly. The renal response to vasopressin is reduced and, in addition, the sensation of thirst is impaired which makes water conservation less efficient. Renin and aldosterone levels decrease with

Table 21.6 Admission screening of elderly patients with chemical tests

Examination	Abnormalities commonly detected
Measurements on blood specimens	
Albumin, total protein	Evidence of poor nutrition
Creatinine, urea	Renal disease, post-renal uraemia
Glucose	Diabetes mellitus
Calcium	Hypocalcaemia (osteomalacia)
	Hypercalcaemia (hyperparathyroidism or malignancy)
ALPs	Increased in Paget's disease, malignancy and osteomalacia
Potassium	Hypokalaemia (often due to diuretic therapy)
	Hyperkalaemia (poor renal function and K^+-sparing diuretics)
Thyroid function tests	Hypothyroidism or hyperthyroidism
C-reactive protein (or ESR)	Non-specific indicator of the presence of organic disease
Point of care tests	
Urine	Glucosuria, proteinuria
Faeces	GI tract blood loss (e.g. haemorrhoids, carcinoma of the colon or of the rectum)

age, leading to problems with sodium conservation. The elderly also have an impaired ability to adapt to volume expansion since the secretion of ANP in response to hypervolaemia and the renal response to this hormone may both be diminished. In addition many elderly patients are on long-term diuretic treatment that in turn can produce hypovolaemia, postural hypotension, hyponatraemia, hypokalaemia and hyperuricaemia. Some patients taking diuretics may increase their water intake to an extent that it induces hyponatraemia. The maximum rate of secretion of hydrogen ions in response to an acid load is also impaired in the elderly.

These changes make the elderly patient particularly susceptible to disorders of fluid and electrolyte balance, and a full assessment of fluid and electrolyte balance is an essential component of the evaluation of an elderly patient who is ill

Bone disease

The incidence of bone disease rises markedly in old age.

• *Osteoporosis* is the most common cause, especially in women.

• *Paget's disease* is very common. It is one of the first diagnoses to be considered when increased serum ALP activity is found as an isolated abnormality in an elderly patient. It is occasionally necessary to determine whether the increased total enzymatic activity is due to the bone isoenzyme, as would be the case in Paget's disease, or to the liver isoenzyme (e.g. due to secondary deposits of carcinoma in the liver).

• *Osteomalacia* may contribute to fractures and falls in the elderly, and should be considered in a patient who has been housebound or who has a low dietary vitamin D intake. Often in such patients a lack of exposure to sunlight, combined with nutritional deficiency, is the cause. Serum [calcium] and [phosphate] may both be reduced and ALP activity increased in many cases. Serum [25-hydroxycholecalciferol] is often normal, but it may be reduced due to inadequate intake of vitamin D or lack of endogenous synthesis, or both (p. 81). It has been suggested that even minor vitamin D deficiency during the winter at higher latitudes can give rise to a PTH-driven negative bone balance and there are those that advocate the use of vitamin D supplements of 400–600 U/day during October to April.

The endocrine system

Although there is a small decline in the efficiency of a wide range of endocrine systems with ageing, there is no convincing evidence as yet to support the use of hormone supplements in the elderly. Despite this lack of evidence, there are still those that advocate that testosterone (in men), GH and DHEA replacement therapy may be of benefit to the elderly.

Some endocrine disorders are more common in the elderly than in other age groups.

Thyroid disease

Many geriatric assessment units have reported that screening for thyroid dysfunction is worthwhile, and hitherto unsuspected thyroid disorders are said to have been detected in 2–6% of patients. Classical features of hypothyroidism and hyperthyroidism are less common in the elderly. The elderly patient with hypothyroidism is more likely to present with a general decline in health, with depression being a common feature. The hyperthyroid patient may present with weight loss, GI or cardiovascular problems; in a small group of patients apathy and inactivity may dominate the clinical picture (apathetic hyperthyroidism).

Screening in the elderly frequently produces abnormal thyroid function test results in patients who subsequently are found not to have a thyroid disorder. For example, up to 3% of patients admitted to geriatric units may have an undetectable serum [TSH] without there necessarily being clinical or other biochemical evidence of thyroid serum. These abnormalities in thyroid function tests are often due to the effects of NTIs and drugs (see p. 125).

Thyroid function tests must be interpreted with extreme caution in the elderly.

Measurements of serum [TSH] provides the best screening test. The following conclusions can be drawn from its results:

1 A normal result excludes primary thyroid disease.

2 If, at the time the test is performed, the patient is not recovering from a recent NTI, a serum [TSH] greater than 10 mU/L indicates that the patient has hypothyroidism and may require treatment with thyroxine.

3 If the serum [TSH] is less than 0.1 mU/L, serum [FT4] or [total T4] and serum [total T3] or [FT3] should be measured. If the results for either the T4 or T3 measurements are raised, the patient should be referred for specialist advice, as treatment for hyperthyroidism may be required. If, however, the results for the T4 and T3 measurements are normal or low, this suggests that the cause of the low serum [TSH] is NTI, subclinical hyperthyroidism or, rarely, secondary hypothyroidism.

Diabetes mellitus

The diagnosis of diabetes in the elderly is often made as the result of routine testing during a concurrent illness or because of the development of peripheral vascular disease or cataracts. Few patients present with classical symptoms such as weight loss and polyuria. The presence of diabetes mellitus may not be detected by side-room testing of urine for glucose, as the renal threshold for glucose tends to rise with age and thus plasma glucose measurements may be needed (p. 93). Management of elderly diabetic patients may need to depend on the help of relatives.

Inadequate nutrition

Old people living alone are particularly at risk of having an inadequate diet, especially if they are poor, or are unable or unwilling to feed themselves properly. Although serum [albumin] may be low, its diagnostic value is limited.

Paediatrics

- In the neonatal period, particularly in premature babies, jaundice, hypoglycaemia and hypocalcaemia are common. These often differ in origin and treatment from the corresponding adult conditions.
- Some inherited metabolic disorders, notably PKU, are diagnosed by newborn screening; others require a staged biochemical investigation protocol.
- Family studies and genetic counselling absolutely depend on a definitive diagnostic test result, as does pre-natal diagnosis.
- Pre-natal diagnosis of some inherited metabolic diseases is possible by chorionic villus sampling and DNA or enzyme analysis.
- When an inherited abnormality is found, the whole family may need to be investigated to diagnose additional affected children.
- During early childhood, failure to thrive and short stature may be due to treatable biochemical abnormalities.

Geriatrics

- In old age, multiple pathology in one individual is common. Furthermore, some disorders tend to present in an atypical fashion or to be asymptomatic.
- There may be a case for more widespread use of screening programmes to detect inadequate nutrition, diabetes mellitus, and bone and thyroid disease.

Case 21.1

A female baby born at 38 weeks by normal vaginal delivery was discharged breastfeeding after 24 h. She was re-admitted to the hospital after 5 days with marked jaundice (total bilirubin 390 µmol/L; direct bilirubin 75 µmol/L). She was given light therapy but, despite this, after 6 weeks the jaundice persisted (total bilirubin was 190 µmol/L and direct bilirubin was 80 µmol/L). ALT was slightly raised at 60 U/L but GGT was markedly elevated at 600 U/L. What might be the differential diagnosis?

Comments: The baby has prolonged conjugated hyperbilirubinaemia. The differential diagnosis is between infection, inherited metabolic disorder and a biliary tree abnormality. Further investigations showed no evidence of infection. Urinary reducing substances were negative, as were urinary organic acids and amino acids. Thyroid function tests and serum cortisol were normal. Ultrasound of the liver demonstrated a small gallbladder. Further imaging, liver biopsy and laparotomy confirmed a diagnosis of extra-hepatic biliary atresia. The baby was treated surgically by Kasai hepatoportoenterostomy. Early diagnosis of this disease is very important. If surgery is performed before the baby is 2 months old, success is much more likely. For this reason, all infants who are jaundiced after the age of 4 weeks should be evaluated for biliary atresia if other causes cannot be found.

Case 21.2

A previously well 11-month-old boy was admitted to a hospital with a 1-day history of vomiting and diarrhoea, pyrexia and a red macular rash. On the ward he fed poorly, vomited three times overnight and the following morning suddenly became drowsy and floppy, with unrecordable glucose on BM sticks. At that time, selected biochemistry results were:

(continued on p. 306)

Case 21.2 *(continued)*

Plasma	Result	Age-corrected reference range
Glucose	<0.5	2.2–6.4 mmol/L
Urea	10.8	1.4–6.6 mmol/L
Cortisol	2137	100–610 (6 am to 10 am) nmol/L
Urine qualitative analysis		Ketones – moderate

What causes of hypoglycaemia can be ruled out from these results?
 What further tests should be requested?

Comments: It is important to confirm hypoglycaemia by laboratory measurement, and to collect sufficient sample for additional analyses to test the response to the provocation of falling plasma glucose. The cortisol response indicates an intact HPA axis and rules out adrenal failure and panhypopituitarism. The ketonuria rules out hyperinsulinism. The elevated urea reflects dehydration caused by vomiting and diarrhoea.

The remaining urine sample was analysed for organic acids. The pattern showed large peaks of fatty acid oxidation intermediates (adipate, suberate, sebacate, and their hydroxylated derivatives, with a relative lack of acetoacetate and β-hydroxybutyrate. Hexanoyl-, suberyl- and phenylprioninyl-glycine peaks were present. This pattern is diagnostic of MCAD deficiency presenting in crisis (see Figure 21.2).

The child responded rapidly to IV glucose and carnitine supplementation. He was discharged after the parents had been taught home glucose monitoring, and given advice on the importance of avoiding fasting and of bringing him to the hospital should he develop another vomiting illness. The diagnosis was subsequently confirmed by mutation studies. The identified mutations, along with organic acid analysis, were used to rule out the diagnosis in two siblings born subsequently. The patient had one further precautionary hospital admission at 15 months following a low home glucose measurement. Otherwise he has been well and developed normally. Once patients reach school age, their increased hepatic glycogen stores make them less vulnerable to decompensation following common childhood illnesses.

Case 21.3

A 73-year-old retired schoolteacher had been admitted to a hospital with exacerbation of her chronic asthma. She gave a history of having moderately severe hypertension, which her GP had been treating with a combined preparation of atenolol and chlorthalidone for the previous 2 years. She was treated with an increase in the dose of oral steroids that she was already taking and discharged home. Two weeks later, she was seen by her GP because her ankles had begun to swell, and he prescribed furosemide. However, her ankle swelling persisted, and she began to complain of feeling very weak. She was readmitted to the hospital, where examination of a blood specimen gave the following results:

Serum	Result	Reference range
Urea	5.0	2.5–6.6 mmol/L
Na$^+$	148	135–145 mmol/L
K$^+$	2.7	3.6–5.0 mmol/L
Total CO$_2$	30	22–30 mmol/L

Comment on the likely causes of this patient's hypokalaemia.

Comments: There are several drug-related reasons as to why this patient had developed marked hypokalaemia:
1 Chlorthalidone is a thiazide diuretic. It can cause modest K$^+$ depletion, although this is not usually sufficient by itself to require potassium supplements.
2 High doses of steroids cause potassium loss.
3 Furosemide causes K$^+$ loss. When using it for the treatment of oedema, it would be normal practice to use it in combination with a K$^+$-sparing diuretic.
The drug treatment of this patient was changed in the light of these analytical results.

Case 21.4

A 78-year-old retired civil servant was admitted to a geriatric assessment unit with a recent history of rapidly progressing dementia. Point-of-care tests and the results of admission screening investigations were all normal, apart from the results of thyroid function tests, which were as follows:

Serum	Result	Reference range
TSH	<0.1	0.2–4.5 mU/L
FT4	19	9–21 pmol/L
FT3	3.0	2.6–6.2 pmol/L

How would you interpret these results?

Comments: Undetectable serum [TSH] is reported in 1–3% of patients admitted to geriatric assessment units if thyroid function tests are performed as part of a routine admission screening of all patients. Although undetectable serum [TSH] is found in hyperthyroidism and in secondary hypothyroidism, in these elderly patients NTI and the effects of drug therapy are much more frequent reasons for this finding.

In this patient, the normal serum [FT4] and the low-normal serum [FT3] excluded overt hyperthyroidism and secondary hypothyroidism and suggest that the suppressed TSH was due to NTI. The final diagnosis was multiple cerebral infarctions caused by extensive atheromatous disease of the cerebral vessels, detected by CT scanning.

Self-assessment MCQs

Please answer True or False for each option. Each question may have more than one True option.

Chapter 1

1.1 Serum:
A Comprises the liquid component of clotted blood
B Is suitable for measurement of fibrinogen levels
C Can be used for analysis of most biochemical tests on blood
D Is obtained by taking blood into an anticoagulant and then comprises the liquid phase after centrifugation of the cellular elements
E Unlike plasma, is suitable for detection of a paraprotein on suspected multiple myeloma

1.2 Biochemical tests on serum may be affected by:
A Exercise
B Time of day
C Diet
D The menstrual cycle
E Patient's sex

1.3 In screening for phenylketonuria (PKU):
A A neonatal urine sample is required
B The best test would be one with high sensitivity but low specificity

C The best test should have low sensitivity but high specificity
D The best test is one with high sensitivity and high specificity
E A small number of false positives would be acceptable but false negatives would be unacceptable

1.4 Point of care testing:
A Eliminates the need for training staff who use these instruments
B Cannot be used to measure bilirubin
C Is best established independently from the central biochemistry lab
D Is less costly per unit test than analysis undertaken in the central laboratory
E Can be monitored for training and quality purposes through linkage to a central laboratory computer

Chapter 2

2.1 Vasopressin secretion
A Is controlled by ECF tonicity
B Is a cause of hypernatraemia
C Is suppressed by trauma
D Is increased by carbamazepine
E Causes excretion of dilute urine

2.2 In the control of total body sodium

A Renin is secreted in response to a rise in renal afferent arteriolar pressure

B Renin is secreted in a response to a reduction in supply of sodium to the distal tubule

C Angiotensin-converting enzyme (ACE) converts angiotensinogen to angiotensin I

D Sodium retention leads to expansion of the intracellular volume

E Aldosterone promotes sodium reabsorption at the proximal tubule

2.3 Hyperkalaemia

A Is a feature of digoxin poisoning

B Occurs in mineralocorticoid excess

C Can be treated with glucose and insulin infusion

D Is associated with alkaloses

E Is an early feature of chronic renal failure

2.4 Hyponatraemia

A Is usually due to excessive sodium losses

B Is commonly seen after surgery or trauma

C In the syndrome of inappropriate secretion of ADH is associated with low urine osmolality

D May be due to glucocorticoid deficiency

E May be a feature of hypothyroidism

Chapter 3

3.1 When investigating acid–base disturbances

A A normal [H$^+$] rules out any significant disturbance

B [HCO$_3^-$] is raised in a compensated respiratory alkalosis

C The anion gap is raised in an acidosis caused by gastrointestinal bicarbonate loss

D The 'total CO$_2$' is raised in a compensated respiratory acidosis

E In a patient with diabetic ketoacidosis a low P_{CO_2} suggests the presence of a respiratory alkalosis in addition to the metabolic acidosis

3.2 In a metabolic alkalosis

A ECF volume overload is a frequent finding

B Respiratory compensation results in a markedly raised P_{CO_2}

C Prolonged vomiting may be the cause

D Intravenous saline may be beneficial

E Potassium concentration is often high

3.3 A metabolic acidosis is an expected consequence of:

A Pyloric obstruction

B Common bile duct obstruction

C Ureteric implantation into an ileal conduit

D Unilateral ureteric obstruction

E Cushing's syndrome

3.4 Causes of respiratory acidosis include

A Severe asthma

B Opiate overdose

C Hepatic encephalopathy

D Pulmonary oedema

E Salicylate overdose

Chapter 4

4.1 When performing urinalysis with multitesting dipsticks, the test for proteinuria:

A Detects all proteins normally detectable in plasma with about equal sensitivity

B Often fails to detect Bence Jones protein when it is present

C Is not sensitive enough to detect the microalbuminuria of diabetic nephropathy

D Often gives false-positive results in patients with glycosuria

E Often gives false-positive results if the patient has recently had a pyelogram

4.2 Estimated GFR (eGFR)

A Is valid in all age groups

B Is a useful assessment of the progress of acute renal failure

C Can be used to assess renal function in pregnancy

D Is the basis for the classification of chronic kidney disease

E In the normal range rules out chronic kidney disease

4.3 In a patient with polyuria

A Lithium toxicity is a possible cause

B Hypocalcaemia is a possible cause

C Urine osmolality <800 mmol/kg in an early morning specimen indicates the need for further investigation

D Failure to concentrate urine in a fluid deprivation test is consistent with diabetes insipidus

E Failure to concentrate urine following DDAVP administration demonstrates a hypothalamic–pituitary cause of the diabetes insipidus

4.4 Plasma creatinine

A Is a useful screening test for the presence of renal tubular disease

B Is often reduced in patients with hepatic failure

C Is unaffected by changes in diet

D Tends to rise with age

E Assays may be subject to interference

Chapter 5

5.1 Hypomagnesaemia is associated with:

A Chronic alcohol abuse

B Vitamin D excess

C Hyperkalaemia

D Low circulating [PTH]

E Hypocalcaemia

5.2 In a hypercalcaemic patient which of the following are consistent with the diagnosis of primary hyperparathyroidism?

A An elevated plasma [HCO_3]

B Normal plasma alkaline phosphatase activity

C Serum [PTH] in the upper reference range

D Decreased plasma [phosphate]

E Increased plasma [chloride]

5.3 Circulating [PTH] is elevated in which of the following conditions?

A Magnesium deficiency

B Vitamin D deficiency

C Pseudohypoparathyroiism

D Milk alkali syndrome

E Osteoporosis

5.4 Which of the following statements relating to vitamin D metabolism is false?

A Elevated plasma [phosphate] inhibits renal 1α-hydroxylase

B PTH stimulates the synthesis of 24:25 dihydroxycholecalciferol

C Plasma [1:25 dihydroxycholecalciferol] may be elevated in sarcoidosis

D 1:25 dihydroxycholecalciferol promotes intestinal phosphate absorption

E PTH stimulates the synthesis of 1:25 dihydroxycholecalciferol

Chapter 6

6.1 In the diagnosis of diabetes

A An elevated HbA_{1c} is diagnostic

B Patients with results demonstrating impaired glucose tolerance are at increased cardiovascular risk

C A single elevated plasma glucose result is sufficient in itself

D The identification of monogenic diabetes enables family screening but makes little difference to the choice of treatment

E An oral glucose tolerance test is always required

6.2 With regard to the presence of micro-albuminuria:

A Significant urine albumin excretion is associated with an increased systemic vascular permeability

B Urine albumin excretion increases following strenuous exercise

C The presence of microalbuminuria in type 1 diabetes reflects irreversible renal disease

D Urine albumin excretion increases following trauma or surgery

E Microalbuminuria in non-diabetic populations carries an increased risk of coronary artery disease

6.3 Monitoring diabetes control

A Can be adequately achieved using urine tests for glucose

B By HbA$_{1c}$ measurement can be unreliable in patients with anaemia

C Using fructosamine reflects control over the previous 40–50 days

D Using home blood glucose measurement is essential in all patients

E By HbA$_{1c}$ measurement can give artefactually elevated results in patients with haemoglobinopathies

6.4 Hypoglycaemia

A May be caused by salicylate overdose in children

B May be caused by Cushing's syndrome

C Is continuously present in patients with insulinoma

D Is associated with undetectable C-peptide levels in patients with insulinoma

E In sulphonylurea overdose is associated with undetectable insulin levels

Chapter 7

7.1 The following tests are commonly used for the diagnosis of acromegaly

A Response of serum growth hormone to an oral glucose load

B Response of serum growth hormone to hypoglycaemia

C Serum IGF-1

D Serum gherelin

E Serum adiponectin

7.2 The following often lead to a raised serum prolactin

A Presence of macroprolactin

B Hypothyroidism

C Chronic renal failure

D Pregnancy

E Hypercalcaemia

7.3 The following pituitary hormones have a hypothalamic-stimulating factor

A TSH

B GH

C LH

D FSH

E Prolactin

7.4 The following are hormones released from the posterior pituitary

A Vasopressin (ADH)

B Oxytocin

C TSH

D Prolactin

E Growth hormone

Chapter 8

8.1 In subclinical hyperthyroidism

A TSH, FT4 and FT3 are all increased

B TSH, FT4 and FT3 are all decreased

C TSH is suppressed but FT4 and FT3 always fall within the reference range

D TSH is suppressed but FT4 or FT3 are always raised

E TSH receptor antibodies may be positive or negative

8.2 Patients who have subclinical hypothyroidsm

A Always have positive anti-thyroid peroxidase antibodies

B Should be given thyroxine replacement when TSH >10 mU/L

C Usually have positive TSH receptor antibodies

D Never have symptoms or features suggestive of hypothyroidism

E Always have a raised TSH for diagnosis

8.3 In the acute stage of a severe non-thyroidal illness

A TSH is often increased

B Reverse T3 is often increased

C Total T3 is often increased

D FT3 is often increased

E Peripheral conversion of T4 to T3 is decreased

8.4 TSH receptor antibody (TRAb) measurements are of value for

A Predicting neonatal hypothyroidism

B Distinguishing between postpartum thyroiditis and Graves' disease

C The investgation of suspected euthyroid Graves' ophthalmopathy

D The investigation of patients with hyperemesis gravidarum who have a low TSH

E Monitoring treatment of multinodular goitre

Chapter 9

9.1 The adrenal cortex synthesises the following hormones

A Aldosterone

B Catecholamines

C Cortisol

D DHEA

E Renin

9.2 In Cushing's syndrome

A The overnight dexamethasone suppression test is a good screening test

B The diurnal variation in serum cortisol is usually maintained

C The CRF test gives an exaggerated ACTH response in Cushing's disease

D Plasma ACTH is usually increased when an adrenal adenoma is the cause

E Hypokalaemic alkalosis is suggestive of ectopic ACTH production

9.3 In suspected Addison's disease

A A serum cortisol within the reference range at 8.00 am excludes the diagnosis

B A normal response to Synacthen effectively excludes the diagnosis

C Plasma ACTH is increased in primary adrenal failure

D Hypernatraemia is consistent with the diagnosis

E Hyperkalaemia is consitent with the diagnosis

9.4 In phaeochromocytoma

A The measurement of plasma metadrenalines is the best diagnostic test

B The plasma renin : aldosterone ratio is a useful test for diagnosis

C All tumours are always localised to the adrenal medulla

D The possibility of MEN I should be considered

E Tumours arise from chromaffin cells

Chapter 10

10.1 Causes of hypogonadism in males include:

A Klinefelter's syndrome

B Iron overload

C Hypopituitarsim

D Kallmans

E Hypercalcaemia

10.2 In the perimenopause

A FSH concentrations are usually low

B Oestradiol concetrations are always low

C A normal FSH concentration does not exclude the perimenopause

D Prolactin concentrations are elevated

E FSH is more sensitive than LH for assessing perimenopause

10.3 What measurement is made to assess if a patient has had an ovulatory cycle

A Day 14 progesterone

B Progesterone taken 7 days prior to next expected menses

C Day 21 oestradiol

D Day 21 testosterone

E Day 14 LH

10.4 Which of the following are androgens
A Testosterone
B Androstenedione
C Dehydroepiandrosterone
D 17-Hydroyprogesterone
E Corticosterone

Chapter 11

11.1 Which of the following statements relating to thyroid hormone metabolism in pregnancy is false?
A FT4 and FT3 decrease as the pregnancy progresses
B Total T4 and total T3 decrease as the pregnancy progresses
C TSH may be suppressed in hyperemesis gravidarum
D Patients on T4 replacement will need their daily dose increased
E High hCG has a mild stimulating action on T4 and T3 synthesis

11.2 Which of the following biochemical/physiological changes occur in pregnancy?
A Serum volume decreases
B Serum alkaline phosphatase activity increases
C GFR increases
D Serum [albumin] falls
E Serum [triglyceride] decreases

11.3 Which of the following maternal serum markers are used for first trimester screening for Down's syndrome?
A Inhibin A
B PAPP-A
C Oestriol
D Free β hCG
E AFP

11.4 Obstetric cholestasis is usually associated with
A Proteinuria >1 g/24h
B Generalised pruritus
C Elevated serum [bile acids]

D Elevated serum [urate]
E Normal liver function tests

Chapter 12

12.1 With regard to lipids and lipoproteins
A The main source of body cholesterol is the diet
B Apoprotein C-II activates lecithin cholesterol acyltransferase
C The principal apoprotein of HDL is apoA
D LDL particles are rich in cholesterol esters
E The LDL receptor binds apoB$_{48}$

12.2 Causes of secondary hyperlipidaemia include
A Hyperthyroidism
B Addison's disease
C Nephrotic syndrome
D Cholestasis
E Alcohol

12.3 Patients with familial hypercholesterolaemia
A Account for about 5% of patients with primary hypercholesterolaemia
B May develop tendon xanthomas
C Are homozygous for defects of the LDL receptor
D Are unlikely to benefit from treatment with cholesterol-lowering drugs
E Often have cholesterol levels in the range of 8–15 mmol/L

12.4 Regarding cardiac markers:
A Measurement of serum cardiac troponin I can be used to exclude rhabdomyolysis
B In the troponin–tropomyosin complex, troponin I binds calcium and regulates contraction
C Measurement of cardiac troponin T is of prognostic value in patients with unstable angina

D Successful reperfusion after thrombolytic treatment can be assessed by measuring cardiac markers

E The release of cardiac troponin T exhibits a biphasic response after myocardial infarction

Chapter 13

13.1 With regard to liver function tests:

A Raised GGT is specific for liver disease

B A low albumin always reflects pathological liver disease as a result of impaired synthesis

C A high ALT with minor changes in ALP and GGT is more consistent with hepatocellular injury

D Increases in both ALP and GGT with otherwise normal LFTs can be found in the case of a space-occupying lesion in the liver

E Normal GGT excludes alcohol excess

13.2 NAFLD:

A Is estimated to affect 2–3% of the adult population with obesity in developed countries

B Can be diagnosed with certainty from the typical liver function test profile changes

C Is characterised by fatty change in the liver without significant fibrosis on biopsy

D Is often accompanied by evidence of insulin sensitivity

E May progress to NASH

13.3 Wilson's disease:

A Shows autosomal recessive inheritance

B Is characterised by copper deposition in the liver

C Typically has raised serum levels of ceruloplasmin

D Is accompanied by decreased excretion of urine copper

E Requires liver biopsy for definitive diagnosis

13.4 Bilirubin:

A Is very high in Gilbert's syndrome

B Is present largely in the conjugated form in haemolytic anaemia

C Is present largely in the unconjugated form in the most common reason for neonatal jaundice

D May appear in the urine when unconjugated levels are increased

E Is usually normal in advanced primary biliary cirrhosis

Chapter 14

14.1 Malabsorption of fat may occur in patients with

A Hartnup disease

B Blind loop syndrome

C Chronic pancreatitis

D Biliary cirrhosis

E Crohn's disease affecting the terminal ileum

14.2 Bile salt insufficiency may occur in patients with

A Ileal disease

B Peptic ulcer

C Carcinoid syndrome

D Chronic pancreatitis

E Hepatic cirrhosis

14.3 Urinary 5-HIAA excretion is

A Increased by eating bananas

B Increased in patients with chronic diarrhoea

C Always increased in patients with carcinoid tumours

D Unaffected by dietary tomatoes

E Usually increased in patients with the carcinoid syndrome

14.4 Faecal calprotectin may be increased in patients with

A Coeliac disease

B Irritable bowel syndrome

C Colorectal cancer

D Inflammatory bowel disease

E Colonic polyps

Chapter 15

15.1 Parenteral nutrition:

A Is usually delivered via a central vein

B Can be used to maintain nutrition at home in some patients who require constant nutritional support

C Must provide adequate calories from carbohydrate, typically using 5% dextrose

D May lead to low levels of potassium, magnesium and phosphate as part of the re-feeding syndrome

E Requires a single, experienced individual to deal with all aspects of patient care

15.2 With regard to vitamins in the diet:

A Body stores of water-soluble vitamins are typically higher than those of fat-soluble vitamins

B Vitamin C is an anti-oxidant vitamin which helps maintain iron in the reduced (ferrous) form

C Thiamine deficiency can be found in chronic alcoholism when it may contribute to neurological and cardiac problems

D Folic acid in excess can lead to increased incidence of neural tube defects in pregnancy

E Retinol (vitamin A) can be partially derived from dietary hydrolysis of β-carotene

15.3 With regard to protein in the diet:

A It may contribute to the supply of energy

B About 40 g of protein of good biological value is the recommended minimum daily intake in an adult

C Supplies only seven of the eight essential amino acids

D Is a source of ammonia which is detoxified through urea production

E Must include an animal source to provide all essential amino acids in the diet

15.4 In the provision of dietary energy:

A Carbohydrates are preferred as they do not contribute to increasing body fat stores

B Fats are not required as all energy and essential nutrition requirements can be met from other sources

C The calorific value of fat exceeds that of carbohydrate

D Current recommendations are that no more than 40% total daily calorie intake should be from fat

E Stored carbohydrate in the liver (as glycogen) is depleted after 18–24 h starvation

Chapter 16

16.1 With regard to tumour markers

A CA-125 is used to monitor beast cancer

B hCG is used to monitor germ cell tumours

C Calcitonin is used to monitor medulary carcinoma of the thyroid

D Thyroglobulin is used to monitor papillary carcinoma of the thyroid

E Alpha-Fetoprotein is used to monitor colorectal cancer

16.2 Monoclonal gammopathy of unknown significance is characterised by

A The presence of a paraprotein on serum electrophoresis

B Monoclonal serum protein >30g/L

C Any myeloma-related organ impairment

D Clonal plasma cells <10% in bone marrow

E A requirement for long-tern follow-up

16.3 The following proteins increase in serum during the acute-phase response

A Albumin

B CRP

C Ceruloplasmin

D Anti-protease inhibitors

E Fibrinogen

16.4 Characteristic tumours in multiple endocrine neoplasia type I include

A Parathyroid adenoma

B Pituitary adenoma

C Phaeochromocytoma

D Medullary carcinoma of the thyroid

E Pancreatic adenoma

Chapter 17

17.1 The most useful laboratory tests for investigating suspected iron deficiency include

A Serum [iron]

B Serum [ferritin]

C Serum [transferrin]

D Faecal occult blood

E Serum transferrin receptor

17.2 Haemochromatosis is associated with

A A mutation of the *HFE* gene

B A reduced percentage saturation of TIBC

C Diabetes mellitus

D An increased plasma [ferritin]

E Testicular atrophy

17.3 In acute intermittent porphyria

A There is extensive allelic heterogeneity

B Faecal excretion of porphyrins is usually elevated

C The basic defect is a deficiency of hydroxylmethylbilane synthase

D Urinary excretion of PBG is always greatly increased during an acute attack

E Cutaneous manifestations may be the sole presenting feature

17.4 Lead poisoning is associated with

A Increased ferrochelatase activity

B Increased urinary ALA excretion

C Increased red cell zinc protoporphyrin

D Increased PBG synthase activity

E Increased coproporhyrin excretion

Chapter 18

18.1 Uric acid:

A Is highly soluble in urine, especially under acidic conditions

B Is reabsorbed in the proximal tubule

C Undergoes neither secretion nor reabsorbtion in the distal tubule

D Is the end-product of metabolism of both pyrimidine and purine bases of DNA

E Can be converted *in vivo* in man naturally to allantoin

18.2 Uric acid accumulation in plasma is found in the following situations:

A With impaired renal function

B When milk and dairy foods are consumed

C In association with fructose-containing beverages

D In lactate acidosis

E With coffee drinking

18.3 Gout:

A Is termed secondary when it arises in response to specific situations which lead to increased uric acid production or decreased renal excretion of urate

B May present as a monoarticular arthritis where the joint fluid contained crystals that show a positive birefringence

C May progress over many years and lead to joint damage and subcutaneous nodules containing uric acid (tophi)

D Always occurs when serum urate levels exceed 0.42 mmol/L, when the aqueous solution is supersaturated

E When primary, shows an association with hyperlipidaemia, metabolic syndrome and ischaemic heart disease

18.4 In the management of gout:

A Diets low in purine content with reduced alcohol intake may help

B Is best treated in the acute phase with allopurinol

C High fluid intake and alkalinisation of the urine may reduce urate stone formation

D Thiazide diuretic usage may improve the situation

E Rasburicase may be used to help prevent secondary gout in the tumour lysis syndrome

Chapter 19

19.1 The most useful test in the investigation of a suspected subarachnoid haemorrhage is

A CSF oligoclonal bands

B CSF total protein

C CSF glucose

D CSF asialotransferrin

E CSF bilirubin

Chapter 20

20.1 Paracetamol:

A Is metabolised to the toxic metabolite N-acetyl-p-benzoquinoneimine

B Depletes intracellular glutathione stores

C Causes both liver and renal damage

D Hepatotoxicity is less in heavy drinkers than in moderate drinkers

E Overdose is treated using intravenous glutathione

20.2 Methanol poisoning

A Gives a metabolic acidiosis by producing formic acid

B Can be treated by giving ethanol

C Can be treated by giving fomepizole

D Often causes hypocalcaemia

E Usually causes an increase in the osmolar gap soon after poisoning

20.3 Therapeutic drug monitoring is often required for

A Lithium

B Tacrolimus

C Paracetamol

D Digoxin

E Aminoglycoside antibiotics

20.4 Examples of enzymes that clinically have important polymorphisms are

A Choline esterase

B Alanine aminotransferase

C Thiopurine methyltransferase (TPMT)

D α_1-Protease inhibitor

E Alkaline phosphatase

Chapter 21

21.1 With regard to glucose metabolism in neonates:

A A glucose value <1.5 mmol/L is regarded as the threshold for intervention

B Transient hypoglycaemia in healthy term infants usually results from a low milk intake as breastfeeding is established

C After the first 24 h of life, hypoinsulinaemia is the most common cause of recurrent hypoglycaemia

D Deficiency of growth hormone may contribute to hypoglycaemia in infants

E Fatty acid oxidation disorders and mitochondrial disorders may present with hypoglycaemia

21.2 A raised bilirubin level in neonates:

A Is found in about half of all neonates in the first week of life

B Is most commonly due to an increase in unconjugated bilirubin

C Is defined as prolonged if it persists beyond 14 days of life

D Typically responds to phototherapy

E Should be regarded as pathological if the conjugated bilirubin is increased

21.3 With regard to plasma calcium in neonates:

A Levels commonly rise by 10–20% in the first 2–3 days of life

B Neonatal hypocalcaemia is well recognised in premature neonates

C Maternal primary hyperparathyroidism predisposes to neonatal hypercalcaemia

D Calcium gluconate may be required if calcium levels fall below 1.5 mmol/L

E Measurement of plasma magnesium is advised in the investigation of neonatal hypocalcaemia.

21.4 In the interpretation of biochemical tests in the elderly:

A Decreases in total protein and albumin with increases in glucose and cholesterol are often found

B Serum creatinine may progressively rise due to reduced muscle mass and deteriorating renal function with age

C Abnormalities in serum calcium arise due to the development of osteoporosis

D Thyroid screening is worthwhile, though interpretation can be affected by non-thyroidal illness

E The renal threshold for glucose may rise with age, improving the value of glucose dipstix measurement for the detection of diabetes

Answers to MCQs

The correct 'True' answers for each question are given below.

Chapter 1

1.1 A, C, E
1.2 A, B, C, D, E
1.3 D, E
1.4 E

Chapter 2

2.1 A, D
2.2 B
2.3 A, C
2.4 B, D, E

Chapter 3

3.1 D
3.2 C, D
3.3 C
3.4 A, B, D

Chapter 4

4.1 B, C
4.2 D
4.3 A, C, D
4.4 E

Chapter 5

5.1 A, D, E
5.2 C, D, E
5.3 B, C
5.4 A, C, D, E

Chapter 6

6.1 B
6.2 A, B, D, E
6.3 B
6.4 A

Chapter 7

7.1 A, C
7.2 A, B, C, D
7.3 A, B, C, D
7.4 A, B

Chapter 8

8.1 C, E
8.2 B, E
8.3 B, E
8.4 B, C, D

Chapter 9

9.1 A, C, D
9.2 A, C, E
9.3 B, C, E
9.4 A, E

Chapter 10

10.1 A, B, C, D
10.2 C, E
10.3 B
10.4 A, B, C

Chapter 11

11.1 A, C, D, E
11.2 B, C, D
11.3 B, D
11.4 B, C

Chapter 12

12.1 C, D
12.2 C, D, E
12.3 A, B, E
12.4 C, E

Chapter 13

13.1 C, D
13.2 C, E
13.3 A, B, E
13.4 C

Chapter 14

14.1 B, C, D, E
14.2 A, E
14.3 A, E
14.4 A, C, D, E

Chapter 15

15.1 A, B, D
15.2 B, C, E
15.3 A, B, D
15.4 C, E

Chapter 16

16.1 B, C, D
16.2 A, D, E
16.3 B, C, D, E
16.4 A, B, E

Chapter 17

17.1 B
17.2 A, C, E
17.3 A, C, D
17.4 B, C, E

Chapter 18

18.1 B
18.2 A, C, D
18.3 A, C, E
18.4 A, C, E

Chapter 19

19.1 E

Chapter 20

20.1 A, B, C
20.2 A, B, C, E
20.3 A, B, D, E
20.4 A, C, D

Chapter 21

21.1 B, D, E
21.2 A, B, C, D, E
21.3 B, D, E
21.4 A, D

Appendix

Reference ranges – SI units and 'conventional' units

Système International (SI) units express concentrations for substances of known atomic or molecular mass in molar units. In 1974, SI units were adopted in the United Kingdom for reporting the results of chemical investigations, and many other countries worldwide have also made the change from 'conventional' to SI units for these analyses. Mass units continue to be used for the results of analyses of mixtures and proteins, and some clinical pharmacologists in the United Kingdom retain a preference for mass units. The litre (L) is the systematic SI unit of volume in medicine.

In the United States and in parts of Europe, SI units have not been universally adopted, and 'conventional' mass units are still used. Thus, glucose concentrations are expressed as 'mg/dl' or 'mg/100 mL'. Some direct read-out chemical equipment used in side-rooms presents results in these units.

In this book, we have used SI units for nearly all values, and have not used conventional units. It is unsatisfactory, and potentially dangerous, to report results in two different sets of units, whether in SI units (with the corresponding result in 'conventional' units in brackets) or vice versa. However, in view of the continued use of both sets of units, conversion tables are presented in this appendix.

Table 1 lists the reference ranges for many of the routine analytes given in this book. Reference ranges for endocrine tests are not given as these are often very method dependent. The local laboratory handbook should be consulted for endocrine tests.

Table 1 Examples of reference ranges in SI and equivalent conventional units

Serum/Plasma constituent	SI units	Conventional units
Albumin	35–50 g/L	3.5–5.0 g/100 mL
Alkaline phosphatase	40–125 U/L	
Alanine aminotransferase	10–50 U/L	
Aspartate aminotransferase	10–45 U/L	
Bilirubin (total)	3–16 µmol/L	0.1–1.0 mg/100 mL
Calcium	2.1–2.6 mmol/L	8.5–10.5 mg/100 mL
Chloride	95–107 mmol/L	95–107 meq/L
Copper	13–24 µmol/L	76–165 µg/100 mL
Creatinine	60–120 µmol/L	0.6–1.3 mg/100 mL
Ferritin		
Male	20–300 µg/L	
Female	14–150 µg/L	
Gamma-GT		
Male	10–55 U/L	
Female	5–35 U/L	
Glucose (fasting)	3.6–5.8 mmol/L	65–105 mg/100 mL
Iron	10–32 µmol/L	80–180 µg/100 mL
Magnesium	0.7–1.0 mmol/L	1.6–2.4 mg/100 mL
Osmolality	280–296 mmol/Kg	
Phosphate (fasting, as P)	0.8–1.4 mmol/L	2.5–4.5 mg/100 mL
Potassium	3.6–5.0 mmol/L	3.6–5.1 meq/L
Protein (total)	63–80 g/L	6.3–8.3 g/100 mL
Sodium	135–145 mmol/L	135–145 meq/L
Transferrin	2.0–4.0 g/L	0.2–0.4 g/100
Transferrin saturation		
Male	20–50%	
Female	15–50%	
Urate		
Males	0.12–0.42 mmol/L	2.0–7.0 mg/100 mL
Females	0.12–0.36 mmol/L	2.0–6.0 mg/100 mL
Urea	2.5–6.6 mmol/L	15–40 mg/100 mL
Zinc	10–20 µmol/L	650–1300 µg/100 mL
Constituent (arterial blood)		*Other units*
Hydrogen ion	37–45 nmol/L	7.35–7.45 pH units
P_{CO_2}	4.5–6.0 kPa	34–46 mmHg
P_{O_2}	12–15 kPa	90–112 mmHg

Table 2 Examples of conversion factors between SI units and conventional units (as in Table 1).

Serum/Plasma constituent	Relative molecular mass (Da)	Multiplication factor to convert numerical values expressed in:	
		SI units to Conventional	Conventional to SI units
Albumin	66	0.1	10
Bilirubin	58	0.06	17
Calcium	40	4	0.25
Copper	63	6.4	0.16
Creatinine	113	0.011	88
Glucose	180	18	0.055
Iron	56	5.6	0.18
Magnesium	24	2.4	0.41
Phosphate	31	3.1	0.32
Protein (total)	A mixture	0.1	10
Transferrin	Approx 75,000	0.1	10
Urate	168	17	0.06
Urea	60	6	0.17
Zinc	65	6.5	0.15
Constituent (arterial blood)		SI units to mmHg	mmHg to SI units
P_{CO_2}		7.5	0.13
P_{O_2}		7.5	0.13

Index